Translational Studies on Inflammation

Edited by Ane C.F. Nunes

Published in London, United Kingdom

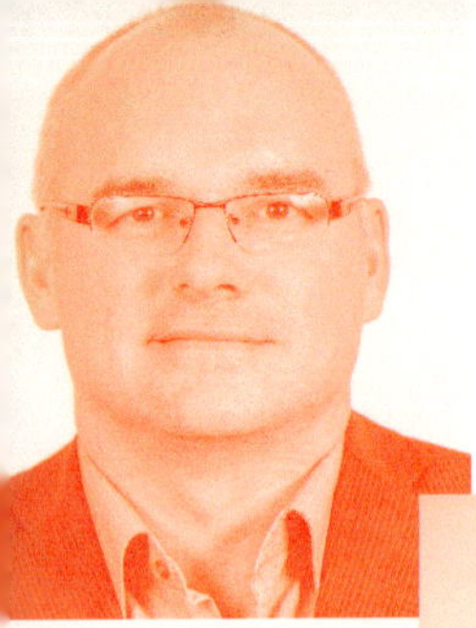
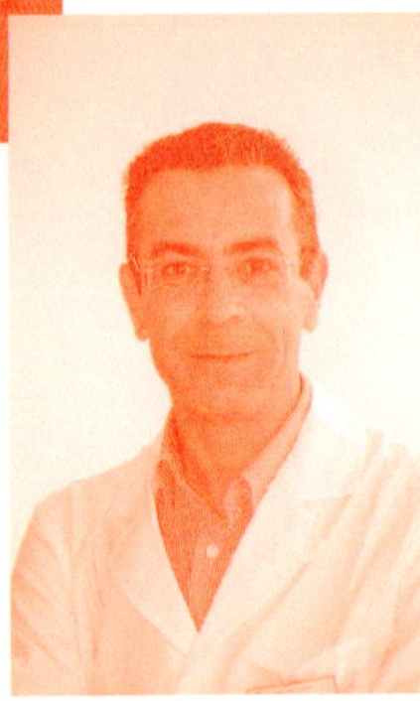
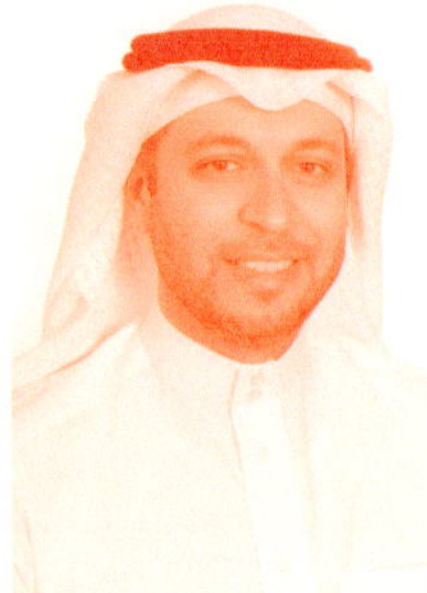
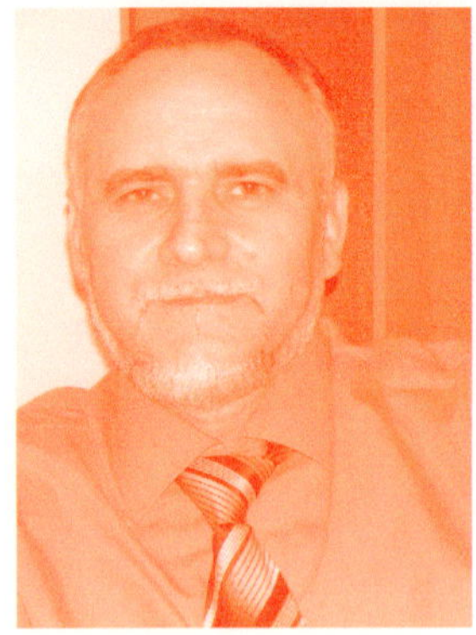
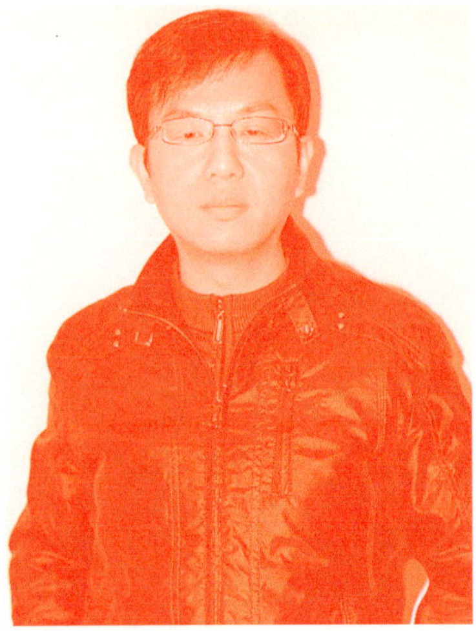
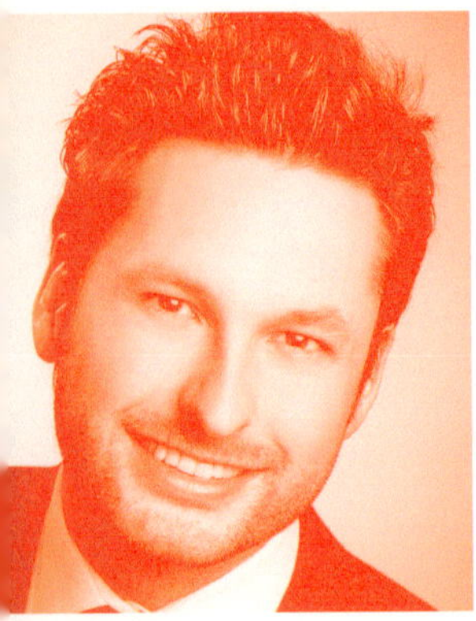
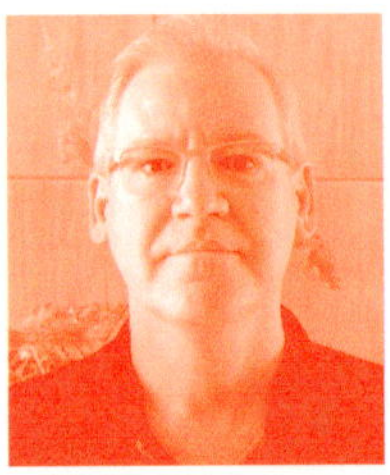

IntechOpen

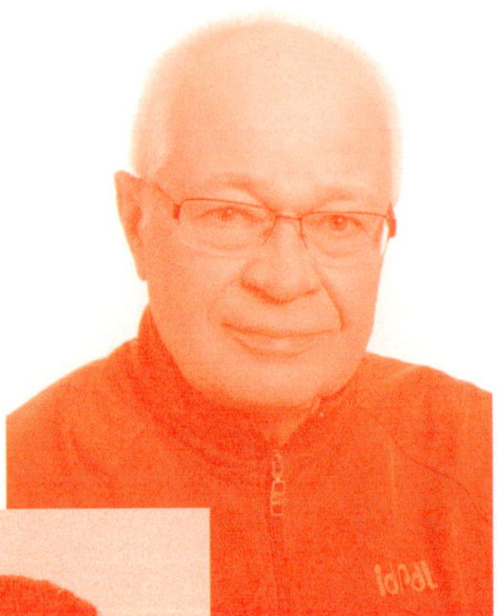
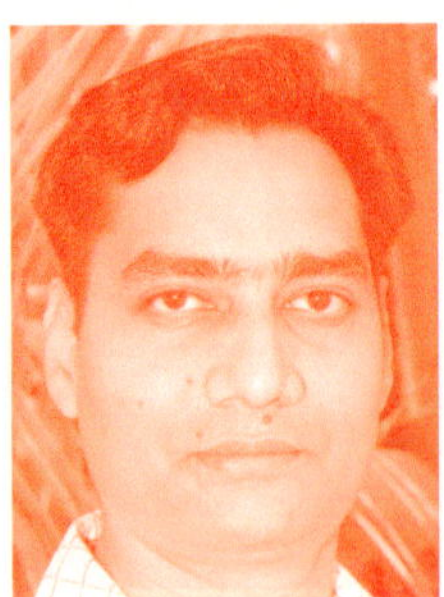
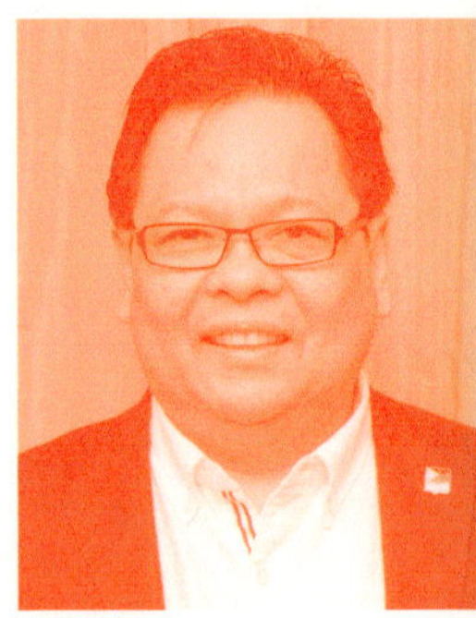
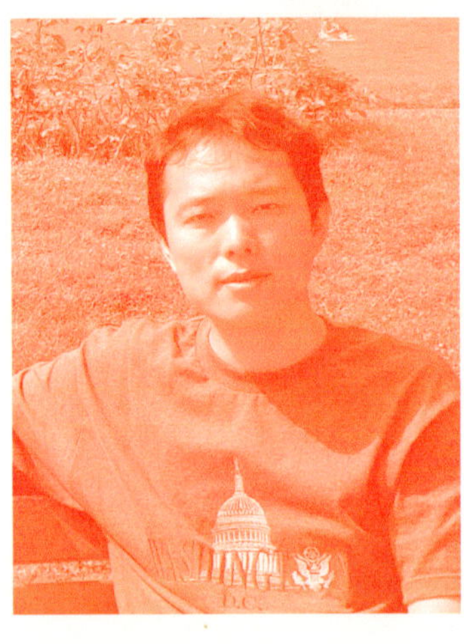
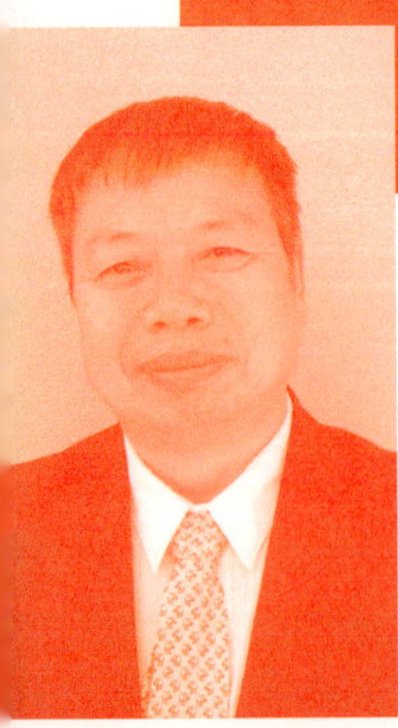
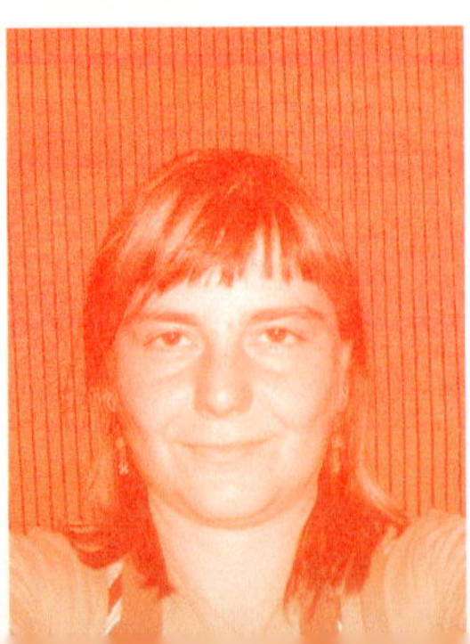

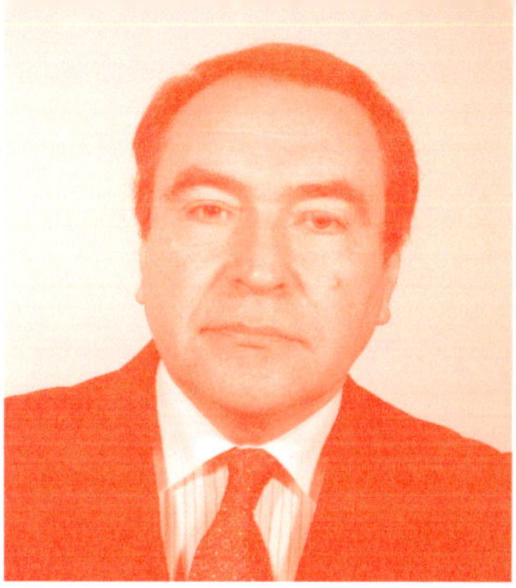
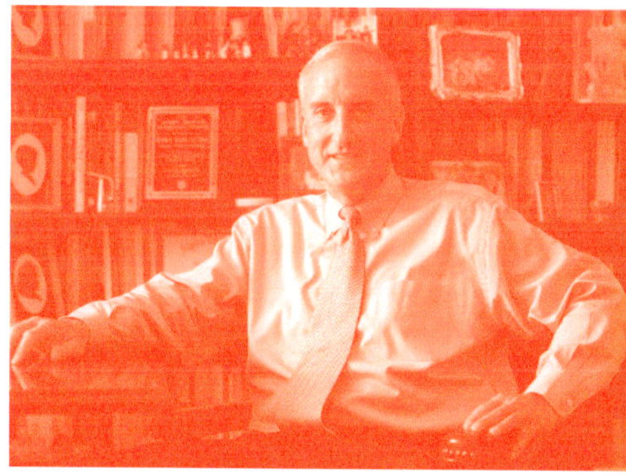
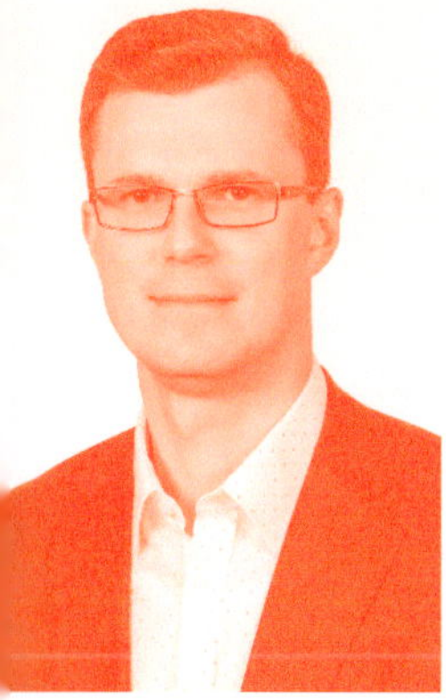
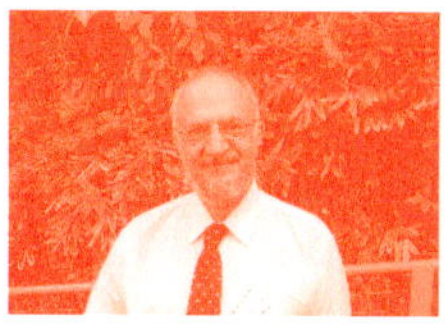
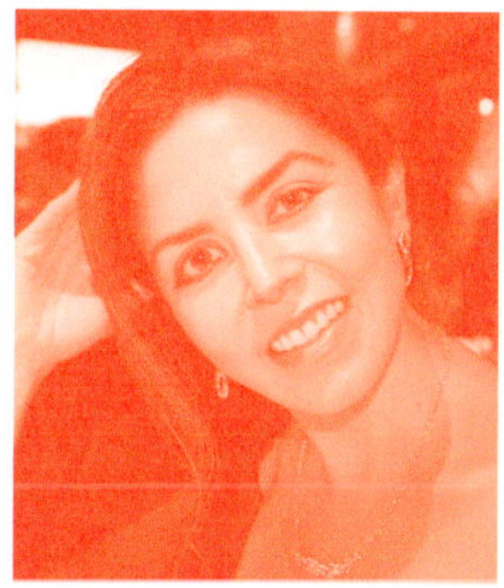

Supporting open minds since 2005

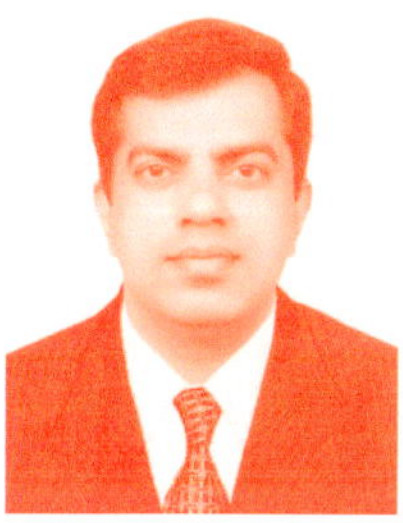
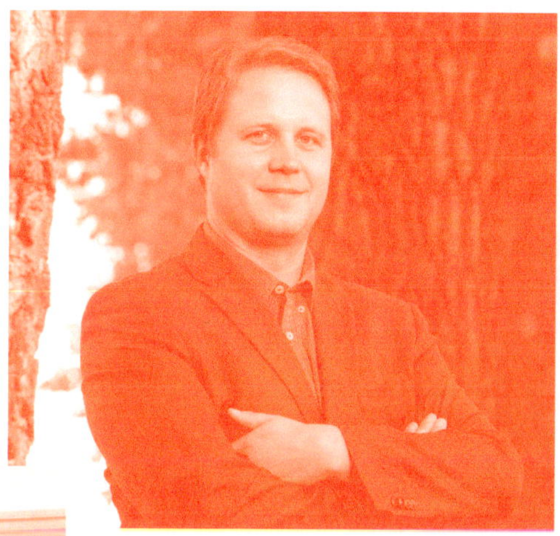
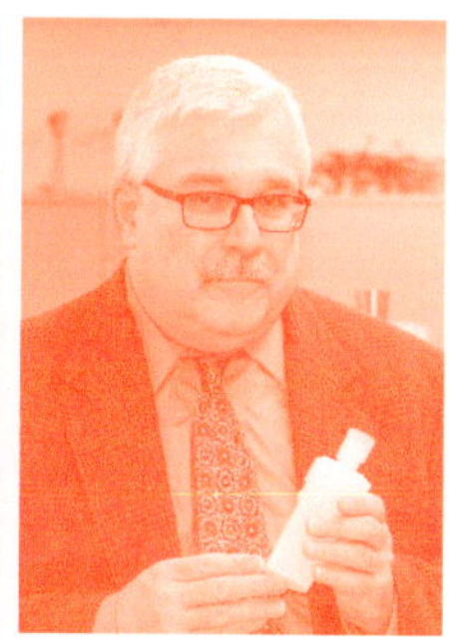
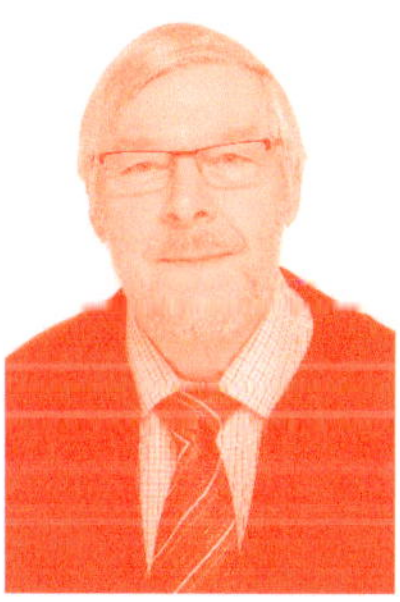
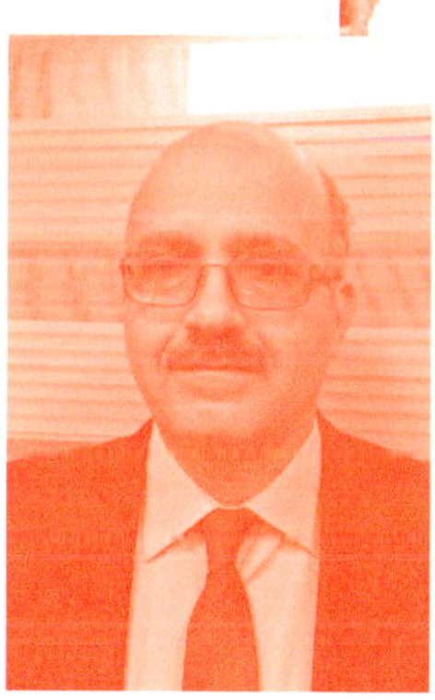
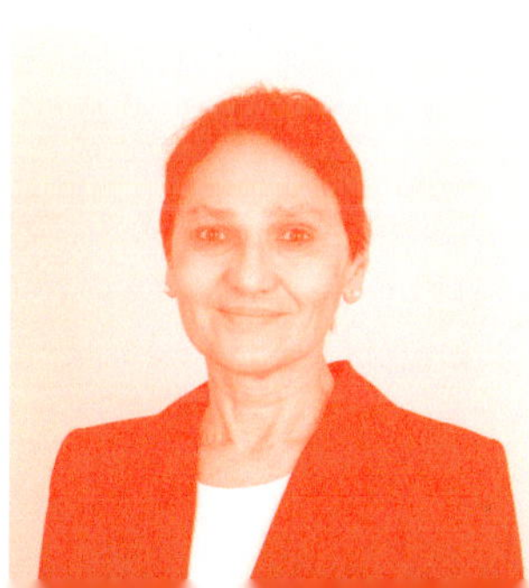
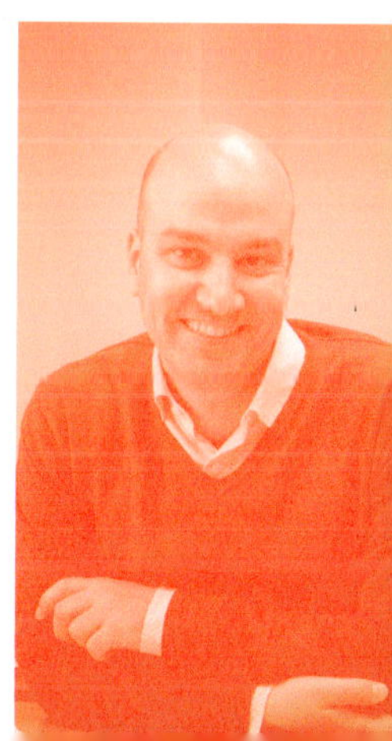

Translational Studies on Inflammation
http://dx.doi.org/10.5772/intechopen.78112
Edited by Ane C.F. Nunes

Contributors
Samantha Giordano-Mooga, Sari Terrazas, Lauren Brashear, Anna-Katherine Escoto, Shannon Lynch, Dylan Slaughter, Neena Xavier, Norman Robert Estes II, Alireza Ziaei, Forough Kheiry, Mario Rosemblatt, Cristian Doñas, Alejandra Loyola, Mona A. Elsayed, Ayman Noreddin, Martijn Bastiaan Adriaan Van Doorn, Robert Rissmann, Salma Assil, Jaime Arias, Ana Arias, Maria Angeles Aller, Javier Blanco-Rivero, Sophia Ran, Nihit Bhattarai, Radhika Patel, Lisa Volk-Draper, I.N. Bolshakov, Anatoly V. Svetlakov, A.V. Eremeev, Yu.I. Sheina, Márcia Guimarães Da Silva, Natália Prearo Moço, Mariana De Castro Silva, Ramkumar Menon, Bruna Ribeiro de Andrade Ramos, Jossimara Polettini, Ane C.F. Nunes, Uma Ranjan Lal, Inder Pal Singh

First published in London, United Kingdom, 2020 by IntechOpen
IntechOpen is the global imprint of INTECHOPEN LIMITED, registered in England and Wales, registration number: 11086078, 7th floor, 10 Lower Thames Street, London, EC3R 6AF, United Kingdom
Printed in Croatia

British Library Cataloguing-in-Publication Data
A catalogue record for this book is available from the British Library

Additional hard and PDF copies can be obtained from orders@intechopen.com

Translational Studies on Inflammation
Edited by Ane C.F. Nunes
p. cm.
Print ISBN 978-1-78984-357-6
Online ISBN 978-1-78984-358-3
eBook (PDF) ISBN 978-1-83968-001-4

For EU product safety concerns:
IN TECH d.o.o., Prolaz Marije Krucifikse Kozulić 3, 51000 Rijeka, Croatia, info@intechopen.com or visit our website at intechopen.com.

Meet the editor

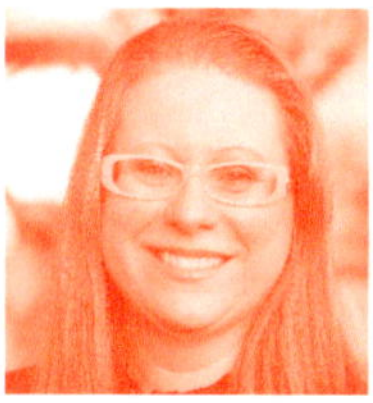

Dr. Ane C.F. Nunes is a geneticist, with her Masters and PhD. in Medical Sciences and Nephrology from the UFRGS/Brazil, and with postdoctoral experience in renal physiology from the UFRJ/Brazil, clinical medicine and nephrology from the USP/Brazil, and nephrology and hypertension from the UCI/USA. She is a Professor of medical genetics, human genetics and molecular biology. Her research fields are human genetic diseases, cellular and molecular biology applied to nephrology, biochemistry, and microbiology with projects mainly in the following subjects: inflammatory markers, molecular diagnosis, DNA polymorphisms, chronic kidney disease (CKD), polycystic kidney disease, Fabry disease, rare diseases, cellular and murine models for CKD, RNA processing, fluorescent image analysis, nanoparticles development, and nanomedicine.

Contents

Preface

Inflammatory processes, their causes, and parameters are, by themselves, elements of considerable debate in the medical-scientific community. Faced with a wide range of questions and lines of action, it is pertinent to address studies on inflammation using a translational approach. Based on this aspect, the idea of this book grew.

Although this was an arduous task considering the many equally appropriate titles that were submitted, the chapters that follow fulfill this interdisciplinary goal and we selected them based on quality and variety.

Readers will find in these four sections different translational studies about inflammation from different points of view:

(1) General Aspects of Inflammatory Process and Immune System Network: This is the introductory unit and the first chapter presented by me as the Academic Editor summarizes the basis of inflammation and its interactions. An extension of this approach is presented in the second chapter produced by Dr. Guimarães da Silva group, which brings to this book an interest aspect of the ontogenetic effect of the molecular panel related to innate immune system and oxidative stress.

(2) Clinical and Pharmacological Approaches: Four chapters that link experimental models and clinical information make up this unit. In the first one, Dr. Van Doorn and collaborators report the pharmacological properties of some models used for drug development. The second chapter, which was prepared by the Dr. Giordano-Mooga group, is a comprehensive review on the impact of sex differences over obesity, cardiovascular disease, diabetes, kidney disease, and its links with the inflammatory process. The third chapter by the Dr. Arias group brings to this book a well-detailed review on wound-healing response, with special emphasis on the immunological and ontogenetic features of portal hypertensive inflammation. Closing this section, the fourth chapter is an in-depth presentation produced by Dr. Lal, which features the implications of the traditional Indian System of Medicine for management of the inflammatory bowel disease.

(3) Role of Chronic Inflammation in Cancer: Because of its complex network of interactions, cancer itself deserved an entire section to cover its specific inflammatory characteristic. In this book, two comprehensive chapters compose this subject. In the first chapter, Dr. Ziaei describes the process by which chemotherapy compounds act under an inflammatory condition. In the second chapter of this section, Dr. Ran and colleagues reviewed the role of the TLR4 pathway and its intricate performance in inflammation and tumor spread.

(4) Therapeutic Perspectives for Inflammation: The final section of this book presents three chapters that cover some innovative proposals for inflammation management. Opening this section is the chapter by Dr. Elsayed and Dr. Noreddin. They present an overview of inflammation and nanomedicine. In the second chapter of this section, Dr. Rosemblatt and colleagues review the role of epigenetic processes

and the impact of these events in the development and management of the immune system and its inflammatory consequences. Closing this section and the book is an original study conducted by Dr. Bolshakov and group, which presents an innovative strategy based in cellular therapy to revert the damage in an experimental vertebral-spine trauma, controlling potential clinical endpoints beyond inflammation.

As an Academic Editor, this project was a challenge that brought me tremendous pleasure to be in charge of reviewing such high-level proposals as those received.

We are grateful to all authors, contributors, and experts who took considerable effort to ensure that each chapter provided updated and innovative data for this special issue.

Thanks to the IntechOpen team for their support, especially to Ms. Sandra Maljavac for her constant assistance.

I wish all readers could reach same satisfaction as I have attained by editing this book.

Ane C. F. Nunes, Ph.D.
University of California,
Irvine, USA

Section 1

General Aspects of Inflammatory Process and Immune System Network

Chapter 1

Introductory Chapter: Overview of the Cellular and Molecular Basis of Inflammatory Process

Ane C.F. Nunes

1. Introduction

Tissue or cell injuries and assorted infections are targets to major studies on inflammation. These conditions play a central role for the understanding of the inflammatory mechanism as a pathophysiological process. In addition, tissue-resident macrophages can create an adaptive response against stressed or unwell environments, which may lead to various pro-inflammatory pathways. Together, these conditions may be associated with a broad spectrum of acute and chronic inflammation in some of contemporary human disorders [1].

In general, inflammation is a natural response to avoid the progress from fester to deadly in any kind of injury. Its very well-balanced network of anti- and pro-factors should be constantly checked by the immune system to make sure the healing process does not miss your goal and becomes unreliable to the point of creating an incorrigible damage [1, 2].

Regardless of its etiology, patients suffering from inflammatory episodes or disorders have higher risk of facing other clinical complications. Acute and chronic inflammations have their particular dynamics and prognostics but, even if it is unclear in several aspects, it has been pertinent in addressing any analysis on inflammation under a translational approach.

In face of that, the following review is a summary report on essential aspects related to inflammation as a biological event, considering the potentially wide range of questions and action lines, from its molecular basis to some potential clinical outcomes.

2. Causes and early stages of inflammation

Different agents can promote inflammatory events, such as (a) necrosis, due to the decrease in blood flow and lack of nutrients and oxygen in the target tissue, which results in tissue death; (b) chemical or physical traumas, like radiation, burn, frostbite, corrosion by oxidizing, alkalis, or acid; (c) displaced or delayed immunological response due to genetic conditions or unstable metabolism; and (d) infections or coexistent microbiome unbalanced status, mainly from very common performers as bacteria, through endotoxins release, and virus, which encroach cells for its proliferation until the host wrecking [2–6].

Basic signs of inflammation are (1) edema or swelling caused by gradual deposit of fluid outside of blood vessels; (2) pain, caused by mechanical action of edema and/or direct response to prostaglandin, serotonin, and bradykinin

IntechOpen

reactions; (3) redness, as a consequence of vasodilation at damage site; and (4) fever caused by pro-inflammatory mediators that contribute to the rise of local and/or systemic temperature [1, 2].

Vasoconstriction, the constriction of blood vessels, which increases blood pressure, is one of the first and brief reactions to inflammatory process. In the beginning of inflammatory process, it is followed by a counterreaction, the vasodilation. During vasodilation the blood flow increases into the target area, and it can take from few minutes to long-time periods to be released. These contractile events on the vessel affect the blood flow and, for consequence, the blood vessel wall permeability. When the vessel wall becomes more permeable, the transit of fluids also is raised, beyond usual salt- and water-based liquids [7].

A protein-rich fluid, the exudate, increases its transposition through the wall, which affects the distribution of anti-inflammatory elements, as coagulation factors and antibodies, in the sense to refrain the spreading of infectious agents.

3. Cellular setup and molecular mediators

The inflammatory environment with fluid leaking out the blood vessels creates the conditions for white cell adhesion to the blood vessel wall since the blood flow starts to slowdown. This is the initial step of a serial process moving out the white cells from the vessel lumen to the interstitium of the damaged tissue.

Two major aspects related to the body's reaction to inflammation are the speed and the amount of white cells taken to the target tissue. Phagocytes are the predominant form of leukocytes designated to clean up the site of injury, eating bacteria and strange elements, removing the cellular remains produced during the injury progress [2].

Neutrophils are a class of white cells involved in acute inflammation. This particular type of phagocyte holds granules of enzymes capable of destroying toxic substances, such as reactive oxygen species, proteins, and cells, making these cells the major components in the injury processing. For local and weak damages, the amount of circulating neutrophils is enough for inflammatory response. However, for wide damages, sources of neutrophils from the bone marrow are constantly requested for acting on the injured site as the early agents. Even if in its immature form, neutrophils can reach the local spot quickly after the inflammatory process starts [2].

Monocytes are the second group of blood cells requested for acting on the inflamed area, usually several hours after the beginning of this process. These white blood cells when matured are called macrophages, and they are responsible for the ultimate step of engulfing and disposing the invasive cells and foreign elements. Macrophages are also the predominant agents in the chronic inflammation healing [1–2].

The cells required to act at the site of inflammation actually move from blood vessels to injured tissue. Both neutrophils and macrophages use chemical recognition properties, called chemotaxis, to guide themselves through the pathway. While the lesion itself has an important role in the inflammation healing initiation, chemotaxis is responsible for determining how far fast and effective will be its processing. It is a complex network working from the chemical signals given out by the injured tissue. Structural compounds, such as endothelial cells, operate together with blood plasma elements, platelets, and mast cells, creating a chemical communications to address the differentiated white blood cells to the right site, according to each role and time frame [8, 9].

The blood plasma is an important source of inflammatory mediators. Some complex proteins are connected through its elaborate cascade pathways, such as the complement, coagulation factors, the fibrinolytic system, and the kinins.

Activated complement proteins, for example, are able to increase vascular permeability, make mast cells release histamine, and work for neutrophils as chemotactic elements.

On the other hand, the vascular permeability is directly influenced by a serial process among the coagulation, fibrinolytic, and kinin systems. Coagulation, in a cascade of activations, contributes to fluid exudate formation, polymerizing fibrinogen to fibrin, which is part of the exudate. Fibrin, in its turn, is quickly broken by the plasmin produced from fibrinolytic system, resulting in chemical compounds that interfere with the permeability of blood vessels. Overlapping these events, the kinin system also generates mediators responsible to increase vascular permeability. Moreover, an essential kinin named bradykinin is in charge of two of the main uncomfortable effects of inflammation, itching and pain.

Prostaglandins are considered major inflammatory mediators. This type of fatty acids plays an essential role on the platelet cluster formation, also interfering on clotting process. Some prostaglandins can promote vascular permeability too. This group of molecules is targeted for many anti-inflammatory drugs, since they are related to fever and pain caused by inflammation [10, 11].

Another group of inflammatory mediators, including histamine, cytokines, and lysosomal compounds, has a significant role on the capacity to exchange the permeability of vessels, even with its distinct characteristics. Histamines, for example, are the first line of agents released to increases vascular permeability, since they are easily accessed from mast cells and basophils. The activation of histamine H1 receptors promptly changes some pro-inflammatory pathways. Moreover, the histamine regulates the synthesis of cytokine in some inflammation process, such as allergies. In turn, cytokines released by different cells exhibit features that affect vessel dilatation and the ability to chemically transport white blood cells through the blood vessel into the interstitium of injured parenchyma [7].

Closing this overview, it is important to highlight that the time of inflammation processing is the key to distinguish an acute response, which usually takes a couple of days, from a chronic inflammation, which trends to request long time for healing and its outcomes may persist. From autoimmune diseases to long-term inflammatory sequels, many different targets may be addressed in classic inflammatory pathway, alternative networks, and its upshots. From microbiome interactions, richly reported in recent studies [3–6], to chronic side effects of traditional or innovative treatments, many therapeutics targets have being studied to develop new inflammation mediators that could be helpful, either in scientific or clinical decisions.

Author details

Ane C.F. Nunes
University of California, Irvine, California, USA

*Address all correspondence to: nunes.acf@gmail.com

References

[1] Medzhitov R. Inflammation 2010: New adventures of an old flame. Cell. 2010;**140**(6):771-776. DOI: 10.1016/j.cell.2010.03.006

[2] Nathan C, Ding A. Nonresolving inflammation. Cell. 2010;**140**(6):871-882. DOI: 10.1016/j.cell.2010.02.029

[3] Lau WL, Vaziri ND. The leaky gut and altered microbiome in chronic kidney disease. Journal of Renal Nutrition. 2017;**27**(6):458-461. DOI: 10.1053/j.jrn.2017.02.010

[4] Lau WL, Savoj J, Nakata MB, Vaziri ND. Altered microbiome in chronic kidney disease: Systemic effects of gut-derived uremic toxins. Clinical Science (London). 2018;**132**(5):509-522. DOI: 10.1042/CS20171107

[5] Lau WL, Vaziri ND. Gut microbial short-chain fatty acids and the risk of diabetes. Nature Reviews. Nephrology. 2019;**15**(7):389-390. DOI: 10.1038_s41581-019-0142-7

[6] Jazani N, Savoj J, Lustgarten M, Lau WL, Vaziri ND. Impact of gut dysbiosis on neurohormonal pathways in chronic kidney disease. Diseases. 2019;**7**(1):pii:E21. DOI: 10.3390/diseases7010021

[7] Marone G, Granata F, Spadaro G, Genovese A, Triggiani M. The histamine-cytokine network in allergic inflammation. Journal of Allergy and Clinical Immunology. 2003;**12**(4):S83-S88. DOI: 10.1016/S0091-6749(03)01881-5

[8] Strassheim D, Gerasimovskaya E, Irwin D, Dempsey E, Stenmark K, Karoor V. RhoGTPase in vascular disease. Cell. 2019;**8**(6):551. DOI: 10.3390/cells8060551

[9] Erlinger TP, Platz EA, Rifai N, Helzlsouer KJ. C-reactive protein and the risk of incident colorectal cancer. JAMA. 2004;**291**(5):585-590. DOI: 10.1001/jama.291.5.585

[10] Rodríguez-Hernández, Heriberto et al. Obesity and inflammation: Epidemiology, risk factors, and markers of inflammation. International Journal of Endocrinology. 2013:**2013**:678159. DOI: 10.1155/2013/678159

[11] Serhan CN, Chiang N, Dalli J, Levy BD. Lipid mediators in the resolution of inflammation. Cold Spring Harbor Perspectives in Biology. 2015;**7**(2):a016311. DOI: 10.1101/cshperspect.a016311

Chapter 2

Spontaneous Prematurity, Innate Immune System, and Oxidative Stress at the Maternal-Fetal Interface: An Overview

Natália Prearo Moço, Bruna Ribeiro de Andrade Ramos, Mariana de Castro Silva, Jossimara Polettini, Ramkumar Menon and Márcia Guimarães da Silva

Abstract

Despite the multifactorial etiology of prematurity, intra-amniotic infection is present in 25–40% of preterm pregnancies. Bacteria in amniotic cavity synthesize phospholipases associated with the production of prostaglandins that leads to rupture of fetal membranes and uterine contractions. Bacterial pathogen-associated molecular patterns (PAMPs) activate pattern recognition receptors (PRRs) such as Toll-like (TLRs) and NOD-like receptors (NLRs), triggering pathways that culminate in the production of cytokines that further increase prostaglandin release. Importantly, endogenous molecules called damage-associated molecular patterns (DAMPs) released under stressful conditions can also activate PRRs. Risk factors for both preterm labor (PTL) and preterm premature rupture of membranes (PPROM), including infection-induced inflammation, may cause an increase of ROS release and depletion of antioxidant defenses. In spite of the similarity between the pathophysiology of PTL and PPROM, there are significant differences regarding molecular mediators, degree of tissue damage, and oxidative stress present in these two conditions. PPROM seems to be a consequence of notable tissue damage resulting from chronic oxidative stress, while PTL is associated with minimal tissue degradation resulting from acute exposure and greater antioxidant status. A better understanding of prematurity pathophysiology and the differences between PTL and PPROM can benefit therapeutic approaches to prevent these important inflammatory syndromes.

Keywords: prematurity, innate immune system, oxidative stress

1. Introduction

Innate immune responses play a critical role at different stages of gestation, and a successful pregnancy depends on the balance between anti- and pro-inflammatory molecules. In addition, normal pregnancy is marked by increased oxidative stress, due to increased fetal metabolism, decreased maternal antioxidant reserves,

 IntechOpen

or maternal supply of substrate. Disruption of these two major mechanisms, inflammation and oxidative stress, is closely linked to spontaneous prematurity.

2. Innate immunity and pattern recognition receptors (PRRs)

Innate immunity is a primordial defense system implicated in the identification and eradication of infectious agents that also recognizes products from damaged cells and works to eliminate them. The innate immune system acts through the recognition of molecular structures common to microorganisms, called pathogen-associated molecular patterns (PAMPs) and endogenous molecules called damage-associated molecular patterns (DAMPs) [1], which are passively released from damaged and dying cells, or actively secreted by immune cells or severely stressed cells [2].

PAMPs and DAMPs are recognized by pattern recognition receptors (PRRs) expressed by several cell types [1, 3]. Their ubiquitous localization in cells enables PRRs to recognize microorganisms present in distinct compartments. Membrane-bound PRRs are located in the plasma membrane, endosomal and lysosomal membranes, while cytosolic PRRs are located in the cytoplasm of cells [1, 3].

Toll-like receptors (TLR) are PRRs coupled to the cell membrane [4], composed of type I integral membrane glycoproteins, comprised of an ectodomain with a leucine-rich repeat domain (LRR), an endodomain with Toll/IL-1 receptor (TIR), that shares a 200-amino acid conserved region with interleukin-1 (IL-1) and IL-18 receptors, and a short transmembrane domain [1, 5]. The ectodomain recognizes specific PAMPs, while the endodomain recruits adaptor molecules, enabling the intracellular cascade [5].

The first group of TLRs is responsible for the recognition of structural components of microorganisms and comprises receptors expressed on the cell surface, including TLR-1, TLR-2, TLR-4, TLR-5, TLR-6, and TLR-11 [4]. The second group includes receptors exclusively expressed in intracellular vesicles, TLR-3, TLR-7, and TLR-9, which recognize nucleic acids from microorganisms [4, 6].

PAMPs' recognition by TLRs activates intracellular pathways that lead to the activation of transcription factors responsible for the expression of genes involved in inflammatory and antiviral responses [1, 5, 6]. Among the transcription factors activated by TLR signaling, the most common factors are nuclear factor kappa-B (NF-κB), activating protein 1 (AP-1), interferon regulatory factor 3 (IRF3), and IRF7 [1]. Activation of NF-κB and AP-1 results in the transcription of several genes of pro-inflammatory effector molecules, such as cytokines and chemokines, while the activation of IRF3 and IRF7 leads to the production of type I interferons that are involved in antiviral immunity [1, 3].

Intracellular signaling through NF-κB and AP-1 is very well characterized [4, 7], and TLR-4 and TLR-9 are shown as examples of TLRs on the cell surface and in endosomes, respectively, in **Figure 1**. The activation of TLRs by PAMPs and DAMPs triggers the formation of a signaling complex, a myddosome, composed of protein MyD88 and interleukin-1 receptor-associated kinase 1 (IRAK1) and IRAK4, leading to activation of pro-inflammatory transcription factors, NF-kB and AP-1.

Although infection is the main stimulus for inflammation, it can also be induced in sterile conditions [8]. Therefore, DAMPs are as important to sterile inflammation as PAMPs are to innate response to microorganisms. DAMPs are endogenous factors that in physiologic conditions are protected from cellular receptors. During

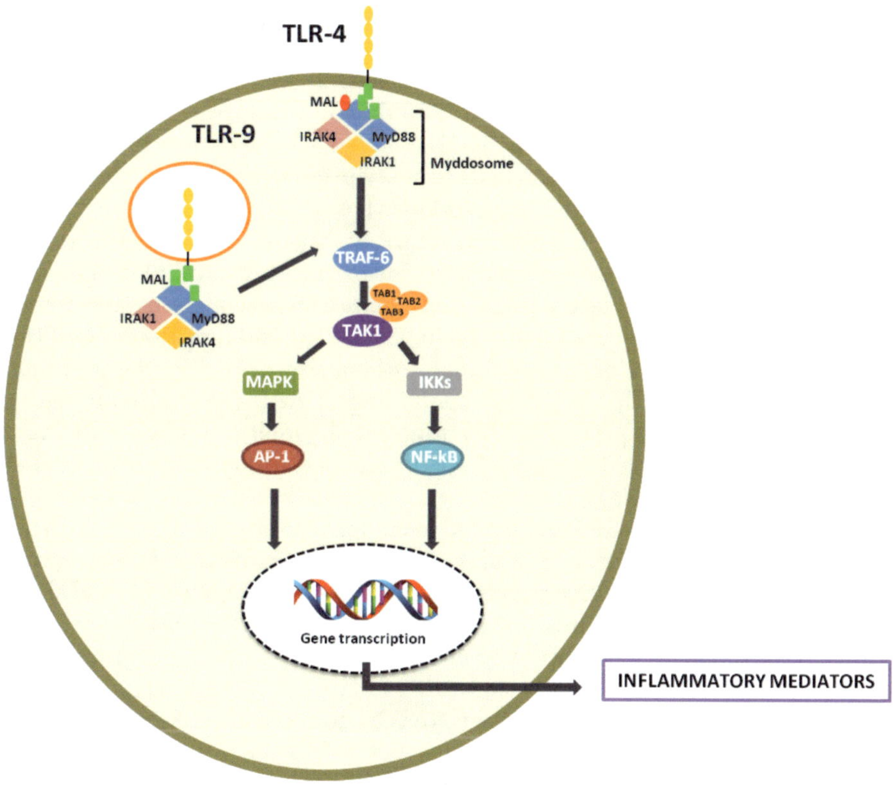

Figure 1.
Overview of TLR signaling pathways. Activation of TLRs on the cell surface or endosomal membranes and formation of myddosome complex, leading to activation of pro-inflammatory transcription factors NF-kB and AP-1. Communication between TLR and the myddosome occurs through interaction of the TIR domain of the Toll-like receptor with the TIR domain of MyD88 and depends on the adapter molecule called MAL, allowing the myddosome to form a helical structure. IRAK-4 activates IRAK-1, which undergoes autophosphorylation. Phosphorylated IRAK-1 then binds to TRAF-6, resulting in the activation of the TAK-1, which results in activation of the cascade of KKs that phosphorylate the inhibitory protein of NF-kB, leading to activation of NF-kB. Additionally, the activation of TAK-1 protein also results in activation of MAPKs, leading to activation of the transcription factor AP-1. AP-1, activator protein 1; IKK, IκB kinase; IRAK, interleukin-1 receptor-associated kinase; MAL, MyD88-adapter-like protein; MAPK, mitogen-activated protein kinase; MYD88, myeloid differentiation primary response protein 88; TAB, TAK1-binding protein; TAK1, transforming growth factor β (TGF-β)-activated kinase 1; TRAF6, tumor necrosis factor receptor-associated factor 6. Adapted from Kawasaki and Kawai [4].

tissue damage, DAMPs are liberated from cells and are recognized by immune cells [9]. DAMPs can also be actively secreted by immune and severely stressed cells [2]. Evidence shows that PAMPs and DAMPs act in different ways to stimulate innate immunity. Antigen-presenting cells that are unresponsive to lipopolysaccharide (LPS) can be activated by necrotic cells, indicating that TLR-4 activation, regardless of LPS, occurs in response to endogenous ligands [10]. Similarly, TLR-3 recognizes cells that undergo necrosis during acute inflammatory events, independently of the presence of viral PAMPs [11].

Among the cytosolic PRRs, nucleotide-binding oligomerization domain (NOD)-like receptors (NLRs) are of great importance [1]. The NLR family is a class of intracellular receptors that lead to intracellular signaling associated to inflammation, after recognition of PAMPs and DAMPs [1]. Members of the NLR family are characterized by at least three domains: the first one is an LRR domain, responsible for the recognition of the ligand; the second is a NACHT domain that allows the formation of oligomers of NLRs; and the third is the effector domain, usually a caspase recruitment domain (CARD), responsible for the recruitment of accessory proteins [12].

The first NLRs described were NOD-1 and NOD-2 [13], which recognize peptides from degradation of peptidoglycan (PG) that occurs during bacterial growth or destruction. Recognition of PGs by NOD-1 and NOD-2 leads to activation of intracellular pathways, which activate the transcription factor NF-κB, and results in the synthesis of several inflammatory cytokines [14, 15].

Members of the NLR family known as NLRP are capable of responding to cytoplasmic PAMPs and DAMPs through the formation of intracellular signaling complexes, termed inflammasomes [1]. Inflammasomes activate proteases from the caspase family during immune regulation in physiologic and pathologic conditions [16]. The typical structure of the inflammasome consists of NLRP, adaptor protein apoptosis-associated speck-like protein containing a CARD (ASC; also known as PYCARD), and pro-caspase [17]. This transient oligomer starts a cascade that culminates with activation of caspase-1 and production of the active form of IL-1β [18] and IL-18 [19].

The inflammasome NLRP3 is activated in response to several PAMPs, such as flagellin, muramyl dipeptide, LPS, and pore-formation toxins [1]. Moreover, it can be activated by DAMPs, reactive oxygen species (ROS), and environmental signals [16, 20]. Three models describing mechanisms of NRLP3 inflammasome activation have been suggested, which may not be mutually exclusive [21–23] (**Figure 2**). In the absence of activation mechanisms, NLRP3 inflammasome complex is autorepressed, owing to an interaction between NATCH domains and LRRs. When one or

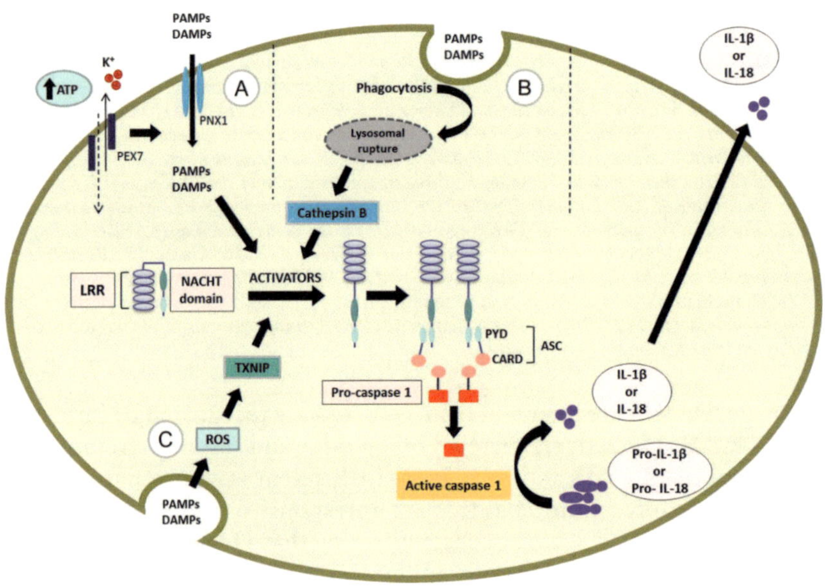

Figure 2.
Mechanisms of NLRP3 inflammasome activation. PAMPs and DAMPs are able to induce the activation of the NLRP3 inflammasome by three principal mechanisms: (A) high concentrations of extracellular ATP lead to opening of PANX1 channels by binding to the P2X7 receptor, which results in K+ efflux and influx of PAMPs and DAMPs; (B) phagocytosis of PAMPs and DAMPs leads to disruption of the lysosomal membrane and consequent release of a putative NLRP3-activating molecule, such as cathepsin B; and (C) PAMPs and DAMPs can induce the production of ROS, which may active TXNIP to trigger NLRP3 activation. Activation of the NLRP3 inflammasome results in maturation of caspase-1 and release of mature forms of IL-1 and IL-18. ATP, adenosine triphosphate; DAMPS, damage-associated molecular patterns; LRR, leucine-rich repeat domain; PAMPs, pathogen-associated molecular patterns; PANX1, pannexin-1; ROS, reactive oxygen species; TXNIP, thioredoxin-interacting protein. Adapted from Tschopp and Schroder [23].

more activation mechanism is present, this autorepression is removed, resulting in NATCH domain exposure. After this exposure, NLRP3 oligomerizes and recruits ASC and pro-caspase 1, leading to activation of caspase 1 and, consequently, maturation and secretion of IL-1β and IL-18 [21, 22]. The immune response initiated by inflammasome activation shows a close relationship with both physiologic and pathologic processes, as immunological defense and development of inflammatory diseases [20].

3. Pregnancy, maternal immunity, and oxidative stress

During pregnancy, a tightly regulated immune system allows for fetal survival and its adequate development. Among the several modifications made by the maternal immune system to raise tolerance to the allograft fetus, changes in cytokine profiles at the maternal-fetal interface are of great importance [24].

Recent data have shown that a successful pregnancy depends on a complex balance between anti- and pro-inflammatory molecules that changes throughout pregnancy [25, 26]. First trimester is characterized by prevalence of the T helper cell type 1 (Th1) profile. During this stage, an inflammatory microenvironment is necessary for repair and remodeling of the uterine epithelium damaged during implantation and for removal of cellular debris [27]. In the second trimester, there is a prevalence of a Th2 profile [28–30]. The increased anti-inflammatory activity is important for maintenance of gestation. During the third trimester and labor, the Th1 profile is again predominant systemically [31] in the placental tissue and amniotic fluid, supporting the theory that proinflammatory overload in the intrauterine environment is required for initiation and progression of labor [32, 33]. The final trimester is characterized by an influx of immune cells at the maternal-fetal interface and increased production of pro-inflammatory cytokines [34, 35]. This scenario is essential for the development of the physiologic processes of cervical remodeling, weakening and rupture of fetal membranes, and initiation of uterine contractility, which together culminate in labor [36, 37].

Recent studies have also demonstrated that normal pregnancy is marked by increased oxidative stress, due to increased fetal metabolism, decreased fetal antioxidant reserves, or maternal supply of substrate [38, 39]. Oxidative stress results from exacerbated production of ROS and/or decreased production of antioxidants. Increased oxidative stress has been described in the third trimester of normal pregnancies and labor [38]. During the process of labor, the intensity of uterine contractions increases uterus pressure and can cause interruption or reduction in the uteroplacental blood flow, causing cycles of cellular hypoxia and reoxygenation. These events of parturition are responsible for inducing increased oxidative stress in pregnant women, which must be controlled by their antioxidant system [40, 41].

3.1 Prematurity, inflammatory response, and oxidative stress

Prematurity is the leading cause of neonatal mortality and is also responsible for several short- and long-term morbidities. The risk for these complications is inversely proportional to gestational age at birth [42–44]. Preterm delivery (PTD) is defined as birth before 37 weeks of gestation, and the incidence of PTD among singleton pregnancies is 9.6% worldwide [45]. Spontaneous PTD can be divided into PTD, which is preceded by preterm labor (PTL) with intact membranes, or by preterm premature rupture of membranes (PPROM) [43, 46]. The incidence of PTL is approximately 60 and 30–40% for PPROM [27, 35, 47].

The etiology of prematurity is multifactorial and includes maternal, paternal, and genetic risks [48–52], as summarized in **Table 1**. Despite this multifactorial etiology, studies show that intra-amniotic infections (IAI) are present in 25–40% of preterm pregnancies; however, these frequencies are believed to be underestimated [43, 53].

The main infection route into the amniotic cavity (AC) is the ascending of bacteria present in the lower genital tract through the endocervical canal. Ascending bacteria can then cross the membranes and invade the AC, with subsequent proliferation in the amniotic fluid. Once microorganisms reach this site, they may travel to the amnion, connective tissue, and even chorion and decidua [54]. The establishment of inflammation in the chorioamniotic membranes in response to bacteria is called chorioamnionitis. Clinical chorioamnionitis (cCAM) occurs in 1–2% of term labors and in 5–10% of PTLs, and this prevalence increases in case of PPROM due to

Maternal		
	Sociodemographic characteristics	African-American ethnicity
		Extreme maternal ages
		Low socioeconomic index
		Smoking
		Drugs and alcohol abuse
	Clinical and gynecological history	Previous prematurity
		Diabetes
		Hypertension
		Cervical cone biopsy
	Gestational characteristics	Multiple gestation pregnancies
		Placenta previa
		Placenta abruption
		Preeclampsia
		Polyhydramnios or oligohydramnios
		Uterine and cervical anomalies
		Assisted conception
		Infections
		Bacterial vaginosis
		Periodontal infection
		Chlamydial infection
		Intrauterine infection
Paternal	**High paternal age**	
Genetics	**Polymorphisms**	IL-1R,IL-1β, IL-6, IL-10, MMP-1, MMP-9, TLR-4, TNF-α, HPS47

IL-1R, interleukin 1 receptor; IL-1β, interleukin 1 beta; IL-6, interleukin 6; IL-10, interleukin 10; MMP-1, matrix metalloproteinase 1; MMP-9, matrix metalloproteinase 9; TLR-4, Toll-like receptor 4; TNF-α, tumor necrosis factor alpha; HPS47, heat shock protein 47.

Table 1.
Risk factors for spontaneous prematurity.

the compromised immune status of the fetal membranes [55]. Histological chorioamnionitis (hCAM) is defined by the presence of polymorphonuclear cells (PMN) in the chorioamniotic membranes. Most cases of hCAM are not followed by clinical signals and symptoms of infection; however, the diagnosis is made in approximately 20% of term pregnancies and over 50% of PTLs [56–58].

The main microorganisms found in the AC of pregnant women with IAI are *Ureaplasma urealitycum*, *Mycoplasma hominis*, and *Fusobacterium* sp. Gram-negative bacilli such as *Bacteroides* sp. and *Prevotella* sp. are also occasionally found, along with *Escherichia coli*, *Gardnerella vaginalis*, and group B *Streptococcus* [59–61].

The main mechanism by which IAI leads to prematurity is through the production of prostaglandins. Bacteria present in amniotic fluid synthesize phospholipases that, in turn, activate the liberation of arachidonic acid that is metabolized via cyclooxygenase, culminating in the production of prostaglandins. Concomitantly, activation of TLRs and NLRs by PAMPs present in these bacteria initiates production and release of inflammatory cytokines, which increase the release of prostaglandins by macrophage, decidual, and amniotic cells [62, 63].

PTL and PPROM pathways are similar in etiology; however, according to Menon et al. [64], the major difference is the presence of molecular factors associated with infection, such as metalloproteinases and pro-apoptotic factors that are responsible for structural modifications and weakening of fetal membranes in patients undergoing PPROM. These same factors are absent or minimally expressed in PTL. Other differences between PTL and PPROM include the distinct response to microorganisms present in the AC [65–67] and the intensity of the inflammatory response [68].

Recently, new data have demonstrated the participation of oxidative stress in the physiopathology of PPROM [69, 70], suggesting that this pathology is similar to term pregnancies with regard to degradation, apoptotic signals, oxidative stress, and premature aging of fetal membranes [71, 72]. Increased levels of oxidative stress markers have been not only associated with the third trimester of normal pregnancy and labor [73] but also observed during second trimester pregnancy disorders, such as preeclampsia and low birth weight [74]. Hence, early senescence, a mechanism leading to fetal membrane aging and immunological dysfunction, is a feature of PPROM [72, 75, 76]. Risk factors for both PTL and PPROM, including infection-induced inflammation, may cause an increase of ROS release and depletion of antioxidant defenses [76, 77]. In this way, Menon suggests that PPROM is characterized by pronounced tissue damage resulting from oxidative stress and proteolysis, while PTL has minimal tissue damage [76]. The greater tissue damage present in PPROM may be a consequence of chronic exposure to oxidative stress risk factors. PTL, in turn, may result from acute oxidative stress associated with a better antioxidant status, a scenario in which the capacity of cell resistance is maintained, while the inflammatory response required for initiation of labor pathway is preserved. PPROM also differs from PTL in its molecular signature linked to senescence of fetal membranes, where premature aging and tissue injury cause DAMPs' release from fetal membranes, which can also contribute to rupture and secondary invasion of microbes due to an immunocompromised environment. Therefore, sterile inflammation by senescent fetal tissues is also a major contributor to PPROM pathology. We have reported differences in antioxidants, telomere length (marker of aging), F2-isoprostanes (markers of oxidative lipid peroxidation), and senescence-associated β-galactosidase (senescence) in fetal membranes and amniotic fluid between PPROM and spontaneous preterm births without PPROM, illustrating the molecular differences between the two phenotypes [75, 78, 79].

3.2 TLRs and NLRs at the maternal-fetal interface and pregnancy complicated by chorioamnionitis and prematurity

Regarding the maternal-fetal interface, expression of TLRs has mainly been investigated in chorioamniotic membranes and the placenta. TLR-2 and TLR-4 are able to recognize most PAMPs present in pathogens involved in AC infections, which are associated with precocious activation of inflammatory response in amniochorionic membranes. Due to this, they are evaluated in most studies concerning TLR expression at maternal-fetal interface.

TLR-2 recognizes microbial lipoproteins, peptidoglycans, and lipoteichoic acid from Gram-positive bacteria, lipoarabinomannan from mycobacteria, zymosan from fungi, and hemagglutinin from smallpox virus [80]. The large capacity of recognition shown by TLR-2 can be explained by its ability to form heterodimers with TLR-1 and TLR-6. The heterodimer TLR-1/TLR-2 recognizes tri-acetylated lipopeptides, while TLR-2/TLR-6 recognizes zymozan and diacetylated lipopeptides [80, 81]. TLR-4 recognizes LPS from Gram-negative bacteria, an important macrophage activator and initiator of septic shock [82].

Kim et al. [83] showed increased expression of TLR-2 in chorioamniotic membranes with hCAM. Our group provided the first report of increase in TLR-1 and TLR-2 mRNAs in fetal membranes of preterm pregnancies with hCAM, when compared to preterm membranes without hCAM [84]. Kumazaki et al. [32] showed that placental macrophages from preterm pregnancies complicated by CAM had increased immunoreactivity to TLR-4, when compared to those without inflammatory infiltrate or term placentas. Using immunohistochemistry techniques, Rindsjö et al. [85] demonstrated an important reduction in TLR-2 expression in placentas in the setting of hCAM and reasoned that the expression of this receptor is probably affected by inflammatory processes in the membranes. Moreover, Kacerovsky et al. [86, 87] showed that pregnant women with PPROM and microbial invasion of the AC had higher levels of soluble TLR-1, TLR-2, TLR-4, and TLR-6 in amniotic fluid.

The expression of TLR-2 and TLR-4 by amniotic epithelium suggests that the epithelium not only works as a mechanical barrier against microorganisms but also plays an important part in the activation of innate immunity [83]. According to Kim et al. [83], the increased expression of these receptors in term membranes reinforces the association between labor and inflammation, as described by Keelan et al. [88]. This upregulation of TLRs may enhance maternal and fetal protection against microbial invasion of the AC. However, Holmlund et al. [89] did not observe differences in TLR-2 and TLR-4 expression between trophoblastic cells, stimulated with zymozan and LPS, and nonstimulated trophoblasts. A possible explanation is that both receptors may be overexpressed in uterine tissue as a defense mechanism, which can protect the fetus against infection during pregnancy and labor. Gonzalez et al. [90] showed that pregnant and nonpregnant mice present different TLR expression in their uterine tissue and that the expression of TLR-2, -3, -4, and -9 increases throughout pregnancy. This finding is in agreement with those of Beijar et al. [91], who reported lower expression of TLR-4 in first trimester villi, when compared to term villi. The apparent disagreement among studies may reflect differences in response to infection in distinct sites of the placenta and gestational tissues.

While several studies showed that gestational tissues express TLRs and are capable of responding to pathogens who present TLR-specific ligands, few studies have discussed the expression of NLRs at the maternal-fetal interface during normal and complicated pregnancies [92–97]. Gene expression of NOD1 was observed in the placenta of pregnant women at term [92, 93], while first trimester placenta villi expressed NOD1 and NOD2 mRNA, both by syncytiotrophoblast and cytotrophoblast cells [94]. This differential expression is also observed functionally; the first trimester trophoblast cells trigger an inflammatory response following exposure to the NOD1 and NOD2 protein ligands, while trophoblast cells from term pregnancies only respond to the NOD1 ligand [94]. Interestingly, Wang et al. demonstrated that expression of NOD1 and NOD 2 in placental villi and decidua was higher in epithelium than in tissue stroma, reinforcing the idea that epithelial tissues are strongly involved in the host defense response at the maternal-fetal interface [96].

Regarding chorioamnionitis, Romero et al. [95] observed that the expression of NOD2 and NLRP3 in chorioamniotic membranes was higher during labor at term in the presence of histologic chorioamnionitis (hCAM), than in membranes without hCAM; however, only the NLPR3 protein concentration was increased in chorioamniotic membranes in the presence of hCAM. Additionally, Pontillo et al. [97] observed that LPS from Gram-negative bacteria increases expression of the NLRP3 inflammasome in trophoblast and decidual stromal cells, suggesting that this multiprotein complex could be important in placental immune defense against invading pathogens.

4. Conclusion

Inflammation and oxidative stress are important to the success of normal pregnancy, and their disruption is closely related with pregnancy complications. Regarding inflammatory responses, special receptors of the maternal innate immune system are capable of responding to microbial ligands present in amniotic fluid during intra-amniotic infection, resulting in an exacerbation of inflammatory mediator production, which is associated with the precocious activation of the parturition pathway. Additionally, studies have demonstrated the participation of oxidative stress in the physiopathology of PPROM, highlighting the similarity between PPROM and term pregnancies in relation to degradation and aging of fetal membranes. In this way, PPROM would be a consequence of notable tissue damage resulting from chronic oxidative stress, while PTL would be associated with minimal tissue degradation, resulting from acute exposure associated with a better antioxidant status. This indicates that exacerbation of the maternal inflammatory response and oxidative stress operates in an interdependent way in the pathophysiology of spontaneous preterm birth, including PTL and PPROM.

Acknowledgements

This work was supported by Unesp (PROPG/PROPE Edital 12/2019).

Conflict of interest

The authors declare that this research was conducted in the absence of any commercial or financial relationship that could be construed as a potential conflict of interest.

Author details

Natália Prearo Moço[1], Bruna Ribeiro de Andrade Ramos[1], Mariana de Castro Silva[1], Jossimara Polettini[1], Ramkumar Menon[2] and Márcia Guimarães da Silva[1*]

1 Department of Pathology, Botucatu Medical School, Botucatu, São Paulo, Brazil

2 Division of Maternal-Fetal Medicine and Perinatal Research, Department of Obstetrics and Gynecology, The University of Texas Medical Branch at Galveston, Galveston, Texas, United States of America

*Address all correspondence to: marcia.guimaraes@unesp.br

References

[1] Abbas AK, Lichtman AH, Pillai S. Imunologia Celular e Molecular. Vol. 7a. Rio de Janeiro: Elsevier; 2011. pp. 125-130

[2] Tang D, Kang R, Coyne CB, Zeh HJ, Lotze MT. PAMPs and DAMPs: Signal 0s that spur autophagy and immunity. Immunological Reviews. 2012;**249**(1):158-175

[3] Murphy KM, Travers P, Walport M. Janeway Immunologie. Vol. 7. Aufl., Wiesbaden, Deutschland: Spektrum Akademischer Verlag GmbH; 2009. 1119 p

[4] Kawasaki T, Kawai T. Toll-like receptor signaling pathways. Frontiers in Immunology. 2014;**5**(September):461

[5] Anwar MA, Basith S, Choi S. Negative regulatory approaches to the attenuation of toll-like receptor signaling. Experimental and Molecular Medicine. 2013;**45**(2):e11

[6] Akira S, Uematsu S, Takeuchi O. Pathogen recognition and innate immunity. Cell. 2006;**124**(4):783-801

[7] De Nardo D. Toll-like receptors: Activation, signalling and transcriptional modulation. Cytokine. 2015;**74**(2):181-189

[8] Rock KL, Latz E, Ontiveros F, Kono H. The sterile inflammatory response. Annual Review of Immunology. 2010;**28**:321-342

[9] Chen GY, Nuñez G. Sterile inflammation: Sensing and reacting to damage. Nature Reviews. Immunology. 2010;**10**(12):826-837

[10] Lee KM, Seong SY. Partial role of TLR4 as a receptor responding to damage-associated molecular pattern. Immunology Letters. 2009;**125**(1):31-39

[11] Cavassani KA, Ishii M, Wen H, Schaller MA, Lincoln PM, Lukacs NW, et al. TLR3 is an endogenous sensor of tissue necrosis during acute inflammatory events. The Journal of Experimental Medicine. 2008;**205**(11):2609-2621

[12] Mathews RJ, Sprakes MB, McDermott MF. NOD-like receptors and inflammation. Arthritis Research and Therapy. 2008;**10**:228

[13] Girardin SE, Boneca IG, Viala J, Chamaillard M, Labigne A, Thomas G, et al. Nod2 is a general sensor of peptidoglycan through muramyl dipeptide (MDP) detection. The Journal of Biological Chemistry. 2003;**278**(11):8869-8872

[14] Chamaillard M, Hashimoto M, Horie Y, Masumoto J, Qiu S, Saab L, et al. An essential role for NOD1 in host recognition of bacterial peptidoglycan containing diaminopimelic acid. Nature Immunology. 2003;**4**(7):702-707

[15] Uehara A, Fujimoto Y, Kawasaki A, Kusumoto S, Fukase K, Takada H. Meso-diaminopimelic acid and meso-lanthionine, amino acids specific to bacterial peptidoglycans, activate human epithelial cells through NOD1. Journal of Immunology. 2006;**177**(3):1796-1804

[16] Paiva-Oliveira EL, Silva AC, de Melo HA, Lagrota-Candido J, Quirico-Santos T. Inflamassoma e sua repercussão clínica: revisão da literatura. Rev Ciências Médicas e Biológicas. 2012;**11**(1):96-102

[17] Srinivasula SM, Poyet JL, Razmara M, Datta P, Zhang Z, Alnemri ES. The PYRIN-CARD protein ASC is an activating adaptor for caspase-1. The Journal of Biological Chemistry. 2002;**277**(24):21119-21122

[18] Hazuda DJ, Lee JC, Young PR. The kinetics of interleukin 1 secretion from activated monocytes. Differences between interleukin 1α and interleukin 1β. The Journal of Biological Chemistry. 1988;**263**(17):8473-8479

[19] Ghayur T, Banerjee S, Hugunin M, Butler D, Herzog L, Carter A, et al. Caspase-1 processes IFN-gamma-inducing factor and regulates LPS-induced IFN-gamma production. Nature. 1997;**386**:619-623

[20] Tsuchiya K, Hara H. The inflammasome and its regulation. Critical Reviews in Immunology. 2014;**34**(1):41-80

[21] Chen I-Y, Ichinohe T. Response of host inflammasomes to viral infection. Trends in Microbiology. 2015;**23**(1):55-63

[22] Saxena M, Yeretssian G. NOD-like receptors: Master regulators of inflammation and cancer. Frontiers in Immunology. 2014;**5**:1-16

[23] Tschopp J, Schroder K. NLRP3 inflammasome activation: The convergence of multiple signalling pathways on ROS production? Nature Reviews Immunology. 2010;**10**(3):210-215

[24] Clark GF, Schust DJ. Manifestations of immune tolerance in the human female reproductive tract. Frontiers in Immunology. 2013;**4**:e1-e14

[25] Chaouat G. The Th1/Th2 paradigm: Still important in pregnancy? Seminars in Immunopathology. 2007;**29**:95-113

[26] Wilczyński JR. Th1/Th2 cytokines balance—Yin and yang of reproductive immunology. European Journal of Obstetrics, Gynecology, and Reproductive Biology. 2005;**122**(2):136-143

[27] Mor G. Inflammation and pregnancy. Annals of the New York Academy of Sciences. 2008;**1127**(1):121-128

[28] Raghupathy R. Maternal anti-placental cell-mediated reactivity and spontaneous abortions. American Journal of Reproductive Immunology. 1997;**37**(6):478-484

[29] Makhseed M, Raghupathy R, El-Shazly S, Azizieh F, Al-Harmi JA, Al-Azemi MMK. Pro-inflammatory maternal cytokine profile in preterm delivery. American Journal of Reproductive Immunology. 2003;**49**(5):308-318

[30] El-Shazly S, Makhseed M, Azizieh F, Raghupathy R. Increased expression of pro-inflammatory cytokines in placentas of women undergoing spontaneous preterm delivery or premature rupture of membranes. American Journal of Reproductive Immunology. 2004;**52**(1):45-52

[31] Arntzen KJ, Lien E, Austgulen R. Maternal serum levels of interleukin-6 and clinical characteristics of normal delivery at term. Acta Obstetricia et Gynecologica Scandinavica. 1997;**76**(1):55-60

[32] Kumazaki K, Nakayama M, Yanagihara I, Suehara N, Wada Y. Immunohistochemical distribution of toll-like receptor 4 in term and preterm human placentas from normal and complicated pregnancy including chorioamnionitis. Human Pathology. 2004;**35**(1):47-54

[33] Patni S, Flynn P, Wynen LP, Seager a L, Morgan G, White JO, et al. An introduction to toll-like receptors and their possible role in the initiation of labour. BJOG. 2007;**114**(11):1326-1334

[34] Osman I, Young A, Ledingham MA, Thomson AJ, Jordan F, Greer IA, et al. Leukocyte density and pro-inflammatory cytokine expression in human fetal membranes, decidua,

cervix and myometrium before and during labour at term. Molecular Human Reproduction. 2003;**9**:41-45

[35] Romero R, Espinoza J, Gonçalves LF, Kusanovic JP, Friel LA, Nien JK. Inflammation in preterm and term labour and delivery. Seminars in Fetal and Neonatal Medicine. 2006;**11**(5):317-326

[36] Mor G, Cardenas I, Abrahams V, Guller S. Inflammation and pregnancy: the role of the immune system at the implantation site. The Annals of the New York Academy of Science. 2011;**1221**:80-87

[37] King AE, Kelly RW, Sallenave J-M, Bocking a D, Challis JRG. Innate immune defences in the human uterus during pregnancy. Placenta. 2007;**28**(11-12):1099-1106

[38] Hung T-H, Lo L-M, Chiu T-H, Li M-J, Yeh Y-L, Chen S-F, et al. A longitudinal study of oxidative stress and antioxidant status in women with uncomplicated pregnancies throughout gestation. Reproductive Sciences. 2010;**17**(4):401-409

[39] Little RE, Gladen BC. Levels of lipid peroxides in uncomplicated pregnancy: A review of the literature. Reproductive Toxicology. 1999;**13**:347-352

[40] Salas-Pacheco JM, Lourenco-Jaramillo DL, Mendez-Hernandez EM, Sandoval-Carrillo AA, Hernandez Rayon YI, Llave-Leon O, et al. Oxidative stress equilibrium during obstetric event in normal pregnancy. The Journal of Maternal-Fetal and Neonatal Medicine. 2016;**7058**:1-5

[41] Li C, Jackson RM. Reactive species mechanisms of cellular hypoxia-reoxygenation injury. American Journal of Physiology. Cell Physiology. 2002;**282**:C227-C241

[42] Moura E, Daher S, Souza E, Mattar R. Aspectos imunogenéticos do parto pré-termo espontâneo. Femina. 2009;**1**:499-503

[43] Goldenberg RL, Culhane JF, Iams JD, Romero R. Epidemiology and causes of preterm birth. Lancet. 2008;**371**(9606):75-84

[44] Birth P, Survival L. Preterm Birth, Long-term Survival, and Fertility. 2016;**300**(2)

[45] Beck S, Wojdyla D, Say L, Betran AP, Merialdi M, Requejo JH, et al. The worldwide incidence of preterm birth: a systematic review of maternal mortality and morbidity. The Bulletin of the World Health Organization. 2010;**88**(1):31-38

[46] Goldenberg RL, Gravett MG, Iams J, Papageorghiou AT, Waller SA, Kramer M, et al. The preterm birth syndrome: Issues to consider in creating a classification system. American Journal of Obstetrics and Gynecology. 2012;**206**:113-118

[47] Menon R. Spontaneous preterm birth, a clinical dilemma: Etiologic, pathophysiologic and genetic heterogeneities and racial disparity. Acta Obstetricia et Gynecologica Scandinavica. 2008;**87**(6):590-600

[48] Sayres WG. Preterm labor. American Family Physician. 2010;**81**(4):477-484

[49] Murphy DJ. Epidemiology and environmental factors in preterm labour. Best Practice and Research. Clinical Obstetrics and Gynaecology. 2007;**21**(5):773-789

[50] Anum EA, Springel EH, Shriver MD, Strauss JF. Genetic contributions to disparities in preterm birth. Pediatric Research. 2009;**65**:1-9

[51] Holst D, Garnier Y. Preterm birth and inflammation—The role of genetic polymorphisms. The European Journal

of Obstetrics and Gynecology and Reproductive Biology. 2008;**141**(1):3-9

[52] Ribeiro de Andrade Ramos B, da Silva MG. The burden of genetic and epigenetic traits in prematurity. Reproductive Sciences. 2017;**25**(4):471-479

[53] Goldenberg RL, Hauth JC, Andrews WW. Intrauterine infection and preterm delivery. The New England Journal of Medicine. 2000;**342**(20):1500-1507

[54] Kim MJ, Romero R, Gervasi MT, Kim J-S, Yoo W, Lee D-C, et al. Widespread microbial invasion of the chorioamniotic membranes is a consequence and not a cause of intra-amniotic infection. Laboratory Investigation. 2009;**89**(8):924-936

[55] Gibbs RS, Duff P. Progress in pathogenesis and management of clinical intraamniotic infection. American Journal of Obstetrics and Gynecology. 1991;**164**(5 PART 1):1317-1326

[56] Edwards RK. Chorioamnionitis and labor. Obstetrics and Gynecology Clinics of North America. 2005;**32**(2):287-296

[57] Conti N, Torricelli M, Voltolini C, Vannuccini S, Clifton VL, Bloise E, et al. Term histologic chorioamnionitis: A heterogeneous condition. European Journal of Obstetrics, Gynecology, and Reproductive Biology. 2015;**188**:34-38

[58] Newton ER. Preterm labor, preterm premature rupture of membranes, and chorioamnionitis. Clinics in Perinatology. 2005;**32**(3):571-600

[59] Sperling RS, Newton E, Gibbs RS. Intraamniotic infection in low-birth-weight infants. The Journal of Infectious Diseases. 1988;**157**(1):113-117

[60] Romero R, Miranda J, Chaiworapongsa T, Korzeniewski SJ, Chaemsaithong P, Gotsch F, et al. Prevalence and clinical significance of sterile intra-amniotic inflammation in patients with preterm labor and intact membranes. American Journal of Reproductive Immunology. 2014;**72**(5):458-474

[61] Gibbs RS, Blanco JD, St Clair PJ, Castaneda YS. Quantitative bacteriology of amniotic fluid from women with clinical intraamniotic infection at term. The Journal of Infectious Diseases. 1982;**145**(1):1-8

[62] Abrahams VM. The role of the nod-like receptor family in trophoblast innate immune responses. Journal of Reproductive Immunology. 2011;**88**(2):112-117

[63] Challis JRG, Sloboda DM, Alfaidy N, Lye SJ, Gibb W, Patel FA, et al. Prostaglandins and mechanisms of preterm birth. Reproduction. 2002;**124**:1-17

[64] Menon R, Fortunato SJ. Infection and the role of inflammation in preterm premature rupture of the membranes. Best Practice and Research. Clinical Obstetrics and Gynaecology. 2007;**21**(3):467-478

[65] DiGiulio DB. Diversity of microbes in amniotic fluid. Seminars in Fetal and Neonatal Medicine. 2012;**17**(1):2-11

[66] Zaga-Clavellina V, Garcia-Lopez G, Flores-Herrera H, Espejel-Nuñez A, Flores-Pliego A, Soriano-Becerril D, et al. In vitro secretion profiles of interleukin (IL)-1beta, IL-6, IL-8, IL-10, and TNF alpha after selective infection with *Escherichia coli* in human fetal membranes. Reproductive Biology and Endocrinology. 2007;**5**:46

[67] Menon R, Peltier MR, Eckardt J, Fortunato SJ. Diversity in cytokine response to bacteria associated with preterm birth by fetal membranes.

American Journal of Obstetrics and Gynecology. 2009;**201**(3):306.e1-306.e6

[68] Park CW, Yoon BH, Park JS, Jun JK. A fetal and an intra-amniotic inflammatory response is more severe in Preterm labor than in Preterm PROM in the context of funisitis: Unexpected observation in human gestations. PLoS One. 2013;**8**(5)

[69] Menon R, Yu J, Basanta-Henry P, Brou L, Berga SL, Fortunato SJ, et al. Short fetal leukocyte telomere length and preterm prelabor rupture of the membranes. PLoS One. 2012;**7**(2):e31136

[70] Chai M, Barker G, Menon R, Lappas M. Increased oxidative stress in human fetal membranes overlying the cervix from term non-labouring and post labour deliveries. Placenta. 2012;**33**(8):604-610

[71] Menon R, Fortunato SJ. The role of matrix degrading enzymes and apoptosis in rupture of membranes. Journal of the Society for Gynecologic Investigation. 2004;**11**(7):427-437

[72] Menon R, Boldogh I, Hawkins HK, Woodson M, Polettini J, Syed TA, et al. Histological evidence of oxidative stress and premature senescence in preterm premature rupture of the human fetal membranes recapitulated in vitro. The American Journal of Pathology. 2014;**184**(6):1740-1751

[73] Stoll BJ, Hansen NI, Adams-Chapman I, Fanaroff AA, Hintz SR, Vohr B, et al. Neurodevelopmental and growth impairment among extremely low-birth-weight infants with neonatal infection. Journal of the American Medical Association. 2004;**292**(19):2357-2365

[74] Hsieh T-T, Chen S-F, Lo L-M, Li M-J, Ych Y-L, Hung T H. The association between maternal oxidative stress at mid-gestation and subsequent pregnancy complications. Reproductive Sciences. 2012;**19**(5):505-512

[75] Dutta EH, Behnia F, Boldogh I, Saade GR, Taylor BD, Kacerovský M, et al. Oxidative stress damage-associated molecular signaling pathways differentiate spontaneous preterm birth and preterm premature rupture of the membranes. Molecular Human Reproduction. 2015;**22**(2):143-157

[76] Menon R. Oxidative stress damage as a detrimental factor in preterm birth pathology. Frontiers in Immunology. 2014;**5**:e1-e14

[77] de Andrade Ramos BR, Witkin SS. The influence of oxidative stress and autophagy cross regulation on pregnancy outcome. Cell Stress and Chaperones. 2016;**21**(5):755-762

[78] Menon R, Bonney EA, Condon J, Mesiano S, Taylor RN. Novel concepts on pregnancy clocks and alarms: Redundancy and synergy in human parturition. Human Reproduction Update. 2016;**22**(5):535-560

[79] Menon R, Behnia F, Polettini J, Saade GR, Campisi J, Velarde M. Placental membrane aging and HMGB1 signaling associated with human parturition. Aging (Albany NY). 2016;**8**(2):216-230

[80] Kawai T, Akira S. The role of pattern-recognition receptors in innate immunity: Update on toll-like receptors. Nature Immunology. 2010;**11**(5):373-384

[81] Takeuchi O, Sato S, Horiuchi T, Hoshino K, Takeda K, Dong Z, et al. Cutting edge: Role of toll-like receptor 1 in mediating immune response to microbial lipoproteins. Journal of Immunology. 2002;**169**(1):10-14

[82] Akira S. Mammalian toll-like receptors. Current Opinion in Immunology. 2003;**15**(1):5-11

[83] Kim YM, Romero R, Chaiworapongsa T, Kim GJ, Kim MR, Kuivaniemi H, et al. Toll-like receptor-2 and -4 in the chorioamniotic membranes in spontaneous labor at term and in preterm parturition that are associated with chorioamnionitis. American Journal of Obstetrics and Gynecology. 2004;**191**(4):1346-1355

[84] Moço NP, Martin LF, Pereira AC, Polettini J, Peraçoli JC, Coelho KIR, et al. Gene expression and protein localization of TLR-1, −2, −4 and −6 in amniochorion membranes of pregnancies complicated by histologic chorioamnionitis. European Journal of Obstetrics, Gynecology, and Reproductive Biology. 2013;**171**(1):12-17

[85] Rindsjö E, Holmlund U, Sverremark-Ekström E, Papadogiannakis N, Scheynius A. Toll-like receptor-2 expression in normal and pathologic human placenta. Human Pathology. 2007;**38**(3):468-473

[86] Kacerovsky M, Andrys C, Hornychova H, Pliskova L, Lancz K, Musilova I, et al. Amniotic fluid soluble toll-like receptor 4 in pregnancies complicated by preterm prelabor rupture of the membranes. The Journal of Maternal-Fetal and Neonatal Medicine. 2012;**25**(7):1148-1155

[87] Kacerovsky M, Andrys C, Drahosova M, Musilova I, Hornychova H, Lesko D, et al. Soluble toll-like receptor 1 family members in the amniotic fluid of women with preterm prelabor rupture of the membranes. The Journal of Maternal-Fetal and Neonatal Medicine. 2012;**25**(9):1699-1704

[88] Keelan JA, Marvin KW, Sato TA, Coleman M, McCowan LM, Mitchell MD. Cytokine abundance in placental tissues: Evidence of inflammatory activation in gestational membranes with term and preterm parturition. American Journal of Obstetrics and Gynecology. 1999;**181**(6):1530-1536

[89] Holmlund U, Cebers G, Dahlfors AR, Sandstedt B, Bremme K, Ekström ES, et al. Expression and regulation of the pattern recognition receptors Toll-like receptor-2 and Toll-like receptor-4 in the human placenta. Immunology. 2002;**107**(1):145-151

[90] Gonzalez JM, Xu H, Ofori E, Elovitz MA. Toll-like receptors in the uterus, cervix, and placenta: Is pregnancy an immunosuppressed state? American Journal of Obstetrics and Gynecology. 2007;**197**(3):e1-e6

[91] Beijar ECE, Mallard C, Powell TL. Expression and subcellular localization of TLR-4 in term and first trimester human placenta. Placenta. 2006;**27**(2-3):322-326

[92] Bertin J, Nir WJ, Fischer CM, Tayber OV, Errada PR, Grant JR, et al. Human CARD4 protein is a novel CED-4/Apaf-1 cell death family member that activates NF-??B. The Journal of Biological Chemistry. 1999;**274**(19):12955-12958

[93] Inohara N, Koseki T, Peso L, Hu Y, Yee C, Chen S, et al. Nod1, an Apaf-1-like activator of caspase-9 and nuclear factor-kappaB. 1999;**274**(21):14560-14567

[94] Costello MJ, Joyce SK, Abrahams VM. NOD protein expression and function in first trimester trophoblast cells. American Journal of Reproductive Immunology. 2007;**57**(1):67-80

[95] Romero R, Xu Y, Plazyo O, Chaemsaithong P, Chaiworapongsa T, Unkel R, et al. A role for the Inflammasome in spontaneous labor at term. American Journal of Reproductive Immunology. 2016;**79**(6):e12440

[96] Wang Z, Liu M, Nie X, Zhang Y, Chen Y, Zhu L, et al. NOD1 and NOD2 control the invasiveness of trophoblast cells via the MAPK/p38 signaling pathway in human first-trimester pregnancy. Placenta. 2015;**36**(6):652-660

[97] Pontillo A, Girardelli M, Agostinis C, Masat E, Bulla R, Crovella S. Bacterial LPS differently modulates inflammasome gene expression and IL-1β secretion in trophoblast cells, decidual stromal cells, and decidual endothelial cells. Reproductive Sciences. 2013;**20**(5):563-566

Section 2

Clinical and Pharmacological Approaches

Chapter 3

Pharmacological Challenge Models in Clinical Drug Developmental Programs

Salma Assil, Robert Rissmann and Martijn Bastiaan Adriaan van Doorn

Abstract

Early phase clinical research for drug development requires the investigation of safety, tolerability and efficacy of novel compounds. The latter is hampered by the absence of the disorder in healthy volunteers, which is why challenge models are often applied in order to demonstrate 'proof of pharmacology.' These challenge models can often be translatable from animal work and can inform the drug developer which dose, dosing regimen or application frequency should be selected prior to phase II studies in the target population. Furthermore, these challenge models represent well-controlled settings to perform activity screening of the compound. The following skin challenge models will be reviewed in this chapter: inflammation induced by Toll-like receptor agonists such as imiquimod, KLH challenge, UV-B irradiation and histamine.

Keywords: skin inflammation, immune system, imiquimod, translational model, pruritus, drug development

1. Introduction

Drug development programs are well-established and long-lasting processes, taking between 10 and 15 years, from discovery to market availability. Clinical trials with drug candidates are the final stage in drug development programs [1, 2]. These clinical trials are often classified into four stages of experimentation, phase I—IV, which are used as a general guideline in clinical trial research for development of a new treatment in specific diseases, i.e., skin diseases [3]. In general, safety, tolerability and pharmacokinetic properties are assessed in healthy volunteers during phase I. The candidate drug will move on to phase II when the initial safety and tolerability has been determined. The main aim of phase II is to establish the safety and efficacy of the drug in the target population. Phase III studies involve large-scaling testing to provide more and extended information on the effectiveness of the drug and on the benefits and possible adverse events. The last phase, IV, also known as the post marketing surveillance trials, is executed after the drug enters the market. The main purpose of this monitoring phase is to determine the long-term effectiveness and patient's quality of life and cost-effectiveness [4, 5].

Translational research focuses on the transcription of the animal model into humans, also known as first-in-human-dose. In general, efficacy, safety and tolerability are examined in the early phases of clinical research. However, the absence of the disorder in healthy volunteers may hamper investigation of the above-mentioned hallmarks of drug development. Inflammation, for example, plays an important role in diseases and is often an indication for a certain skin disease. Difficulties occur when testing drugs against inflammation in volunteers who do not have this condition. Therefore, pharmacological challenge models have been established to mimic physiological and pathophysiological conditions of several skin diseases. These models distort the physiological condition and lead to temporary effects that mimic the pathophysiology of the disease.

Table 1 gives an overview of established skin challenge models.

This approach includes translating basic scientific discoveries into clinical applications. Several recent developments in plaque psoriasis are noteworthy, which serve as an example of research with many translational aspects [42, 43]. Psoriasis is a chronic, inflammatory skin disease that is characterized by erythematous, itchy plaques covered by course scales on the extensor surface of the elbows and knees, as well as the scalp, dorsal hands and lumbar area. Also, the nails and joints (psoriatic arthritis) can be affected [44, 45]. Psoriasis is a multifactorial disease but the

Challenge	Application	Mode of action	Condition induced	Immune response	Reference
Inflammation					
BCG	Intradermal	TLR 4, 9 agonist	Local inflammation, systemic immune response	Adaptive	[6–8]
Imiquimod	Local under occlusion	TLR7 agonist	Local inflammation	Innate + adaptive	[9–13]
LPS challenge + $Al(OH)_3$	Intra dermal	TLR 4 agonist	Inflammatory response	Innate + adaptive	[14, 15]
Cantharidin	Paper disc with cantharidin	Neutrophils	Local inflammation	Innate	[14, 16]
Injected UV killed E. coli	Intradermal	Neutrophils	Erythema, heat, swelling and pain	Innate	[14, 17]
KLH	Intradermal, Intramuscular	Neo-antigen	Local inflammation, systemic immune response	Adaptive	[18–22]
ITCH					
Capsaicin	Intradermal, intra muscular, topical	TRPV 1 receptor	Itch	Innate	[23–25]
Histamine	Intradermal, intramuscular	H1, 2, 3, 4 receptor C_{MIA} fibers	Itch	Innate	[26–33]
Cowhage	Cutaneous	CMH-fibers	Itch Burning	Unknown	[34, 35]
UV-exposure					
UV-B irradiation	Local thermode	PI3K/AKT/mTOR-upregulation	Pain, pigmentation, erythema, inflammation	Innate Adaptive	[23, 36–41]

BCG: Bacillus Calmette-Guérin; LPS challenge: lipopolysaccharide; injected UV killed E. coli: Injected ultraviolet killed Escherichia coli; KLH: keyhole limpet hemocyanin; UV-B: Ultraviolet B.

Table 1.
Overview of human skin challenge models.

hallmarks of pathophysiological pathways (Th1/Th17) with interleukin-12/23 and IL-17 have been clearly established as most important players. Over the last decade many new compounds have been in development for psoriasis yielding a total of 11 registered, targeted monoclonal antibodies today. In these drug development programs *in vivo* models in mice are of great importance for the setup of clinical programs. These mouse models needed to be made suitable to display certain features of psoriasis, since mice are unable to develop psoriasis themselves [10]. This research resulted in development of diverse mouse models i.e., spontaneous mutation model, genetically engineered model, cytokine injection model and transplantation model. All of the mentioned animal approaches represent more or less psoriasis-like cutaneous characteristics. Despite expression of psoriasis like features, the models also have some limitations including the need for special experimental facilities and lack of effectiveness of anti-psoriatic drugs [46–49]. In general, animal models are far from perfect especially in terms of pharmaco- and toxicokinetics.

Animals are not able to predict health effects in humans better than humans themselves. Monkeys reflects the human being the best, however, even they can differ as became clear in 2016. An anti-CD28 antibody caused multiple organ failures in six healthy volunteers within hours, despite multiple normal tests in monkeys. This shows that animal models may have limited predictability for safety in humans. Ethical concerns with regard to need for animal testing may also be a factor underlining the need for pharmacological challenge models in humans [50].

This chapter will provide a detailed overview of four different, local inflammation models: inflammation by Toll-like receptor agonists such as imiquimod (inflammation), UV-B irradiation (inflammation and pain), histamine provocation (itch) and KLH challenge (delayed type hypersensitivity).

2. Imiquimod skin inflammation model

Skin inflammation is a common response of our immune system to penetrating pathogens, skin trauma, exposure of xenobiotics, microbes and parasites [51–53]. Inflammation is clinically recognizable by erythema, pain, heat and swelling [54]. Generally, in inflamed skin, various immune cells, of both the innate and adaptive system are involved to combat the pathogens. However, imbalance of these immune cells may lead to chronic skin diseases such as psoriasis vulgaris, atopic dermatitis and acne vulgaris. Currently, many investigations are addressing the biomolecular mechanisms of inflammation; however, the pathophysiology of the skin remains complex and needs further investigation [55, 56].

Hence, various models in healthy volunteers were developed that mimic inflamed skin conditions [57]. One of the examples is the challenge model with topical application of imiquimod, the active ingredient of Aldara cream. Imiquimod is a small molecule with a low molecular weight and high lipophilicity which is preferable for absorption in the skin after topical administration. This small molecule is also a ligand for toll-like receptor seven and eight (TLR), which belongs to the class of immunomodulatory agents and is able to induce the production of several cytokines (interferon-1 response) with antiviral and tumoricidal properties. The mechanism of action of imiquimod is complex and three main pathways are required including TLR signaling, inflammasome activation and inhibition of the adenosine receptor. However, limited information is available on the mechanism of imiquimod on the adenosine receptor. The first pathway is TLR dependent and activates nuclear factor kappa B (NF-κB) signaling *via* My-D88, which is important in an early immune response. Herewith, activation of c-Junk and IRAK pathways occur which are involved in the production of several pro-inflammatory cytokines. The second pathway is TLR independent. Imiquimod is able to activate the inflammasome *via* the NALP3 pathway, which also triggers an immune response and leads to production of interleukin-1β (IL-1β, a pro-inflammatory cytokine) [10, 11, 13, 58–60].

Aldara 5% cream is registered as a topical product that is indicated for the treatment of superficial basal cell carcinoma, actinic keratosis and genital and peri-anal warts (condyloma acuminata). Topical administration of imiquimod appears to be safe and reasonably tolerated according to the mouse model. This murine imiquimod challenge model has been widely used to examine the mechanisms involved in psoriasis vulgaris, since it is simple, inexpensive and develops an acute inflammatory response with psoriasiform features. However, in general, the main limitation of murine models is that no single mouse model is able to reflect human disease precisely, as the physiology and the pathophysiology of the skin differs in both species [61]. Therefore, recently, human studies been conducted that study skin inflammation after topical application of imiquimod.

Vinter et al. successfully developed an imiquimod-induced psoriasis- like skin inflammation model in humans by applying imiquimod topically under occlusion on non-lesional psoriatic skin of the lower back. A group of patients (n = 7) received the treatment and vehicle for 2 days, while the other group (n = 3) received the same treatment for 7 days. All the treatments were applied on tape stripped skin resulting in perturbation of the skin barrier. After 2 days of treatment with imiquimod, a significant upregulation in mRNA expression was observed for the pro- inflammatory cytokines tumor necrosis factor a (TNF-a), IL-1β and IL-6, whereas TNF-a and IL-6 are keratinocyte driven cytokines. Additionally, a high level of IFN-γ and IL-10 was found, the latter has an important role in suppression of the inflammatory response in the skin, as it influences the regulatory T-cells. In this model, inflammation and psoriasis-like characteristics were induced; however, typical psoriasis lesions were not observed and therefore appear to be the main limitation of the study.

A different approach to study skin inflammation was established by Van der Kolk et al. by applying imiquimod topically to healthy volunteers under occlusion. A distinction between the two groups was made. The first cohort received a topical treatment for 24, 48 and 72 hours on the intact skin barrier, while the second cohort received exactly the same treatment on a compromised skin barrier, through tape stripping (**Figure 1**). In this open label, dose-ranging study, erythema and blood perfusion were monitored by means of erythema index photo analysis, erythema colorimetry, erythema visual grading and laser speckle contrast imaging (LSCI). A dose-dependent increase in erythema was observed for all measurements, with a more rapid and pronounced effect in the tape stripped group. This model showed no clear differences in erythema intensity between the treatments after 48 and 72 hours, which is in concordance with observations in the murine model [9, 13]. Additionally, an increased skin perfusion was found after treatment with imiquimod, however this was only observed in the tape stripped cohort. A similar effect was found for the biomarkers in skin biopsies. Tape-stripping combined with imiquimod treatment resulted in an upregulation of gene expression of CXCL10, MX-A, ICAM-1 and hBD-2 after 48 and 72 hours. The same results were observed after treatment with imiquimod only compared to vehicle, however to a lesser extent. Imiquimod has a three-step mechanism, which entails an initial (24 hour), intermediate (24–72 hour) and late phase (>72 hour). In the intermediate phase of imiquimod, activation of both the innate and adaptive immune response takes place, which is characterized by infiltration of neutrophils, lymphocytes, and macrophages, based on the findings reported in the review of translational imiquimod skin inflammation

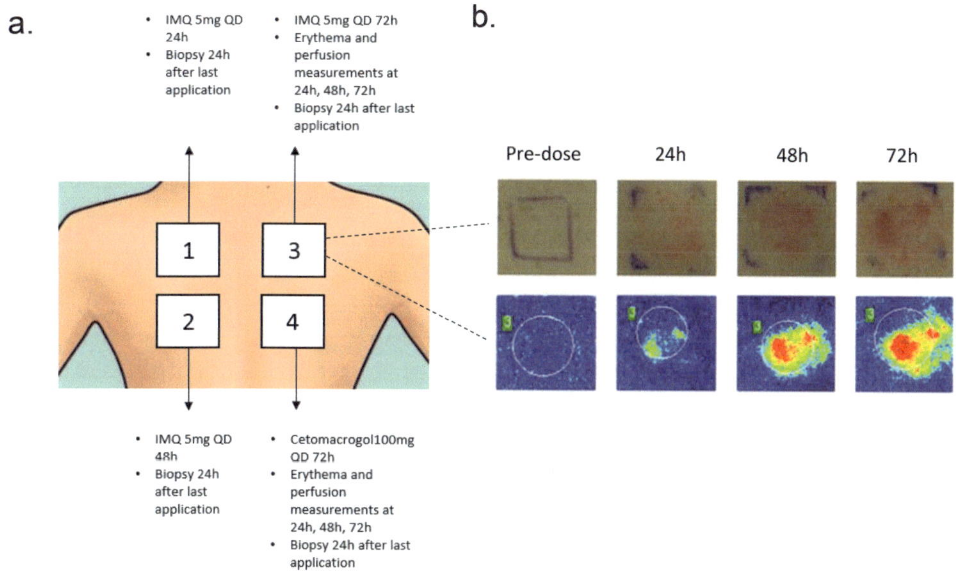

Figure 1.
Overview of the treatment schedule. (a) Treatment areas 1, 2 and 3 were treated with 5 mg imiquimod respectively for 24, 48 and 72 hours. All treatments were applied under occlusion by a 12 mm Finn chamber. (b) Clinical impression of site 3 of the tape stripped cohort after 72 hours of imiquimod treatment [9]. Permitted for non-profit use.

models [59]. In addition, histologically, infiltration of CD11+, HLA-DR, CD4+ and CD8+ into the dermis was observed. Increased infiltration was more pronounced in the tape stripped cohort, however, no differences were observed between 48 and 72 hours of treatment [9].

This chapter focuses mainly on translating skin inflammation into a model that can be used in healthy human volunteers. In the past decades, a lot of research has been performed in this field; however, murine models remained the gold standard. Since skin inflammation plays a crucial role in skin diseases such as psoriasis and atopic dermatitis, Vinter et al. established a human counterpart to the mouse model of imiquimod- induced psoriasis like skin inflammation [13]. Despite the expression of different pro-inflammatory cytokines and the presence of psoriasis-like features, typical psoriasis lesions were not observed. However, this study formed the base to the inflammation model developed by Van der Kolk et al. where imiquimod has been applied under occlusion to challenge the skin. This model resulted in expression of certain cytokines and chemokines that are involved in activation of innate as well as adaptive immune system. Chemokines such as CXCL10 are expressed through activation of keratinocytes in inflamed skin. Expression of MX-A, a downstream interferon, which corresponds with the activation of plasmacytoid dendritic cells (pDCs), was also upregulated in the tape stripped cohort. The presence of interferons reflects the antiviral response, which is in concordance with the antiviral characteristics of imiquimod, used for HPV-induced diseases [62, 63]. Based on these findings, the murine imiquimod skin inflammation model was translated to a safe, human model in healthy volunteers. Skin erythema, skin perfusion and expression of cytokines had high intensity in the tape stripped cohort due to the enhanced transepidermal drug delivery. This model is suitable as a challenge model and can be used in drug developmental programs where TLR 7 is involved. Currently, several drugs are under development targeting TLR7/8 that have anti-tumor characteristics with more than 30 leads to be explored within the next years [64, 65].

3. Models for itch: histamine and cowhage provocation

Itch, interchangeably used as pruritus, is a common skin sensation and together with pain are crucial symptoms in many chronic and allergic skin diseases. Itch can be induced by mechanical, thermal and chemical stimuli. Additionally, itch can lead to impairment of the skin and thereby affect a person's quality of life. Yosipovitch et al. defined different types of pruritus that are involved in chronic itch including pruriceptive, neuropathic, neurogenic and psychogenic itch. Skin inflammation, dryness, or other skin damage are the main factors causing pruriceptive itch and are found in diseases such as scabies, urticaria and insect bite reactions [66, 67]. Neuropathic itch, is usually caused by nerve injury and can arise at any point along the afferent pathway of the neurons. This itch is observed for example after a varicella zoster infection or nerve trauma. Itch that is originated from activation of the central nervous system is called neurogenic itch. The underlying mechanism is complex since it involves pruriceptive itch as well. This itch is often observed in visceral disease states such as end state renal disease or kidney failure. The last subtype of itch is termed psychogenic itch. This type of itch arises with somatization and the delusional state of parasitophobia [66–68]. In this chapter, we will focus on pruriceptive itch and the translational model for it.

Generally, theories have been proposed that explained the relation between itch and pain. Itch is mediated through weak activation of nociceptors and stronger activation would result in weak pain. This is also called, the intensity theory. However, further research has elucidated new aspects that explain pruriceptive sensory mechanism in the nervous system. This resulted in two main pathways including specificity and pattern theories. The specificity theory, explains that there are different sets of neuron fibers transferring information to the central nervous system which send responsive signals including itch and pain [25, 35]. The pattern theory stipulates that many sensory receptors and spinal cord neurons are involved in sensation of itch [69]. Although, the neural mechanism of pruritus has been investigated extensively, there remains much to be learned. Therefore, studies that use chemical agents to induce itch have been designed to study the sensory patterns of itch and pain in humans.

One of the most frequently and widely used pruritic agent, that evokes itch, is histamine [70]. Originally, histamine is a neurotransmitter that is associated with pathological processes such as inflammation, pruritus and vascular leak. Histamine is stored in several immune cells, basophils and mast cells and is quickly released after stimulation. Stimulation with histamine, triggers the unmyelinated nerve fibers, also known as C-fibers. A subset of C-fibers (CMi or CMh) is stimulated according the intensity of the stimulus. In case of histamine stimulation, sustained response of CMi occurs [71]. Histidine decarboxylase (HDC), an enzyme that is responsible for histamine production, increases through stimulation with certain mediators that are found in skin lesions of patients with atopic dermatitis. Hence, this enhancement is associated with upregulated histamine release and thus with increased itch sensitivity [28, 70].

Histamine has been used in literature as an important inflammatory mediator that is responsible for vascular and inflammatory effects [33]. In the early 1900s the first studies were conducted regarding the potential vascular role of histamine *in vivo*, however, only a couple of years ago a clinical study was conducted that investigated the cutaneous inflammatory response in human skin. Falcone et al. has developed an easy-to-use model to study the early stages of skin inflammation. Eighteen (18) subjects with Fitzpatrick skin type II and III received topically applied histamine after performing histamine iontophoresis. The subject had to rate their perceived itch on visual analog scale (VAS) with 3 being the threshold for willingness to scratch the skin. Additionally, different skin assessments were performed including trans-epidermal water loss, skin redness and punch biopsy to process immunohistochemistry. Itch was observed up to 30 minutes after stimulation with histamine iontophoresis and was above the itch threshold (VAS > 3). Immunohistochemistry showed an increase of the epidermal thickness, after 72 hours of histamine iontophoresis challenge. In summary, this model can be used as an *in vivo* model to provoke local and acute skin inflammation, without having an impact on the barrier function. However, no data are available on cell level or cytokine expression profiles [29].

As was earlier described, increased production of histamine has been related to several skin diseases including atopic dermatitis. In addition, histamine has been the main prototypical pruritogen that has been used for experimental purposes. The working mechanism of histamine is going *via* G- protein coupled receptors: H1 up and till H4. It appears that the H1 and H4 receptors play a role in the histamine involved itch response in mice. In humans, the involvement of other receptor subtypes (H2 and H3) in itch is not well-examined in literature [31, 32]. Generally, the classical anti-histamines bind to H1 receptor and are prescribed in patients suffering from atopic dermatitis. However, recent research clarifies that histamine pathway is not playing a major role in atopic dermatitis. Also, the clinical use of anti-histamines in atopic dermatitis population has been ineffective and questionable which corroborates these findings [27, 32, 72].

Therefore, there was a need to establish an alternative itch model, relating to another pathway. The pruritus pathway has physiological functions such as skin barrier homeostasis, inflammation, itch and pain and is the protease-activated receptor (PAR) pathway. PARs are classified as G-protein-coupled receptors and consist of four members, PAR-1, PAR-2, PAR-3 and PAR-4, whereas PAR-2 pathway is mainly associated with skin diseases such as atopic dermatitis [26]. Papoiu et al. established a simple human model based on exogenously stimulation of the PAR-2 pathway in order to provoke itch by applying Cowhage spicules. Additionally, the Cowhage model was compared to the traditional histamine iontophoresis model and the effect of the combined model (histamine iontophoresis and Cowhage) was observed. VAS rating was increased in both atopic dermatitis patients and healthy volunteers, the Cowhage and combination model compared to the histamine model, resulting in no synergy between the Cowhage and the combined model. This finding suggests that Cowhage was the major contributor of itch after stimulation of both pathways simultaneously [34]. The Cowhage model is simple and easy to use and could serve to study itch related skin diseases such as atopic dermatitis. On the other hand, less is known about this pathway and more research is required to examine the mechanism behind this model.

In conclusion, two main skin challenge models were described to provoke itch: histamine iontophoresis and Cowhage. Both models are suitable to use, however, both have a different underlying mechanism to elicit the itch sensation. Evidence-based, induction of the PAR-2 pathway plays a major role in atopic dermatitis, causing pruritus, compared to the histamine model. Therefore, from a therapeutic point of view, drugs that inhibit PAR-2 itch pathway, could be promising, leading to development of a new treatment for chronic pruritus. Since less is known about the underlying cellular mechanism of Cowhage, it would we useful to examine biomarker expression, conduct different skin photography assessments and look at the skin vascularity flow. Furthermore, an advanced challenge study is required in healthy volunteers and patients with atopic dermatitis to examine and monitor the inflammation of both models. In addition, the efficacy of anti-histamine agents and PAR-2 antagonists could be evaluated as well.

4. Model for inflammation and pain: UV-B skin irradiation

Ultraviolet (UV) radiation is classified as a carcinogenic compound since it has the ability to initiate and promote malignant skin tumors. Additionally, increased exposure to UV radiation can lead to other skin problems such as inflammation and degenerative aging. UV energy is subdivided into three main classes based on physical properties: UV-A, UV-B and UV-C. UV-B can cause physiological skin alterations leading to a cascade of cytokine activation and resulting in an inflammatory response, so called "sunburn". Furthermore, exposure to UV-B is related to the accumulation of epidermal keratinocytes and thereby increases the epidermal thickness. UV-B radiation has an additional effect on the skin, it is able to up-regulate the production and the accumulation of melanin in the skin and is also linked to cancer susceptibility.

In well-controlled clinical settings, exposure to UV-B is widely used as a human and animal challenge model to induce local cutaneous hyperalgesia (pain) and inflammation. Primary hyperalgesia is induced after 24 hours and remains for more than 48 hours which makes the model suitable for studies where multiple dosing is required. The amount of UV-B radiation applied to the skin needs to be adjusted to a subject's skin type, according the classification of Fitzpatrick Skin Type [73, 74]. Hereafter, prior the start of the challenge, the Minimal Erythema Dose (MED) is determined and subsequently a one-, two- or threefold multiple of this dose is applied to the skin. After 24 hours, skin inflammation occurs.

This UV model is one of the pain models that can be used as a screening tool for early stage clinical drug development. However, in research, the UV model is used to examine the effects of anti-analgesic or local anesthetics [75, 76]. Recently, an article was published where the UV-B model was one of the models that was applied to compare the effects of several analgesic to placebo. The following analgesic compounds were investigated in the first part: fentanyl, phenytoin, (S)-ketamine and placebo. For the second part of the study imipramine, pregabalin, ibuprofen and placebo were examined. Different pharmacodynamic (PD) assessments were performed which are part of the pain cart including thermal grill, thermode testing and UV-B, electrical stimulation test, pressure stimulation and cold pressure test [41]. Whilst, this study was performed to examine systemic effects of analgesic compounds, the topical effect of UV-B radiation was not determined. One article published the effects of single doses of UV-A, UV-B and UV-C on skin blood flow and barrier function by laser-Doppler flowmeter and evaporimetry. Radiation with various UV light resulted in skin inflammation characterized by erythema, however, assessed visually. Visual perception of erythema correlated with the increase in blood flow assessed by laser-Doppler flowmeter. However, UV radiation has not damaged the skin barrier function, since the trans- epidermal water loss was not increased. An exception formed the three MED, an increase in blood flow was observed after 2 weeks [38]. This study has examined the effects of analgesics on UV-B radiation and other models evoking pain, while skin inflammation occurs as well. Only a few *in vivo* studies attempted to examine the effect of UV-B radiation on skin inflammation. In general, UV-B radiation triggers the production of inflammatory cytokines in the human keratinocyte cell line HaCaT, including IL-1, IL-6, IL-8, IL-10 and TNF-a, which are leading to alterations of immune cells of the skin [39]. However, involvement of immune cells in skin inflammation after UV-B radiation has not yet been examined and monitored in healthy volunteers.

For future perspectives, the UV-B challenge model could be applied to induce temporarily skin inflammation that could be monitored with additional dermatological tests, such as multispectral imaging, thermography and laser speckle contrast imaging.

5. KLH challenge

Challenge models that are described in this chapter, were mostly initiating an innate response, except the imiquimod challenge model. However, in auto-immune skin diseases, activation of the adaptive immune system is crucial as well as the involvement of T-cells [77]. It is quite challenging to evaluate the efficacy of novel drugs in healthy volunteers that target T-lymphocytes, since these are in the resting phase. Hence, challenge models could provide the desirable solution by activating autoreactive T-cell pathways in healthy volunteers. Earlier research investigated keyhole limpet hemocyanin (KLH) as a potential immunization candidate for studying the cell- mediated immune response [78]. KLH is a large molecule (~8000 kDa) consisting of several subtypes and has been widely used in animal and human research for more than 40 years to outline cellular and humoral responses [79–81]. Additionally, KLH can be used as a carrier protein for cancer vaccines and for bladder cancer immunotherapy [20, 82]. Because of the xenogeneic properties to the human immune system, KLH is able to promote a reliable primary immune response. The following administration routes are known and have been used in earlier research—intradermal, subcutaneous, intramuscular and inhalational [21, 22, 83–87]. Furthermore, KLH is considered to be clinically safe, since no reports are available on significant adverse events as reported in the comprehensive review by Harris & Markl. Only mild adverse events were reported including itch, rash and mild injection site reactions (soreness) [19, 88]. In summary, single dose immunization with KLH evokes a predictable primary T-cell dependent immune response. An additional intradermal dose of KLH will result in an additional immune response and thereby induces a delayed type IV hypersensitivity reaction around the site of injection [78].

Presence of erythema and induration are features of a cell-mediated immune response and are generally scored by visual inspection, which is a subjective method and may lead to significant interrater variability. Saghari et al. established a challenge model to activate T-cells in healthy volunteers after immunization with KLH, whereas both the cellular response and the delayed type hypersensitivity are objectively quantified. Adaptive immunity was measured by anti-KLH IgM and IgG blood serum level titers. Additionally, cutaneous blood perfusion, erythema and swelling were objectively measured by respectively laser speckle contrast imaging (LSCI), multispectral imaging and colorimetry. An increase in anti-KLH IgM and IgG was observed after intramuscular KLH administration compared to placebo. This was the case for the cutaneous blood perfusion quantified by LSCI and for the erythema and swelling quantified by multispectral imaging and colorimetry. So far, none of the studies have quantified induration and erythema response by using non-invasive instruments. This model is developed as proof-of-concept to determine the feasibility and to quantify the features of cell-mediated response [89]. Therefore, the delayed type hypersensitivity model can serve as a candidate to study the pharmacological and pharmacodynamic effects of immunomodulators in healthy volunteers.

6. Conclusion

Generally, *in vivo* mice models are a crucial part in pre-clinical drug developmental programs, assessing safety. However, often animal models lack the disease or differ in morphological and physiological properties. Ethical concerns with regard to animal studies are an additional issue which prompts to search for new solutions. Currently, safety is assessed in healthy volunteers who hamper the disease.

Therefore, challenge models that mimic the disease temporarily, could provide a possible solution and act as translational models. This chapter has provided an overview (**Table 1**) of various challenge models that are known to initiate skin inflammation by triggering the human immune system. First, the human imiquimod challenge model was introduced as a safe and well-tolerated model to study temporarily induced skin inflammation by targeting the TLR7/8 receptor. The effect on erythema, cutaneous perfusion and biomarker expression was more pronounced in the group with the perturbed skin barrier due tape stripping. Nowadays, this imiquimod model can be applied to test agents that target TLR7/8 receptor with anti-tumor characteristics.

Furthermore, two models for pruritus were described focusing on two different mechanisms. The first model used histamine as pruritogen to evoke itch *via* a subset of C-fibers. An upregulation of HDC is associated with an increase in histamine release and is found in the lesions of patients suffering from atopic dermatitis. Anti-histamines are often prescribed against itch in patients with atopic dermatitis even though they are ineffective. Therefore, an alternative model was developed targeting the PAR-2 pathway. In this model, itch was initiated by applying Cowhage spicules to the forearm of healthy volunteers and patients with atopic dermatitis. The itch sensation was based on VAS score and EASI (in patients with atopic dermatitis), both giving qualitative measures.

Another model that has been described in this chapter is the UV-B radiation model, which is used to induce pain stimulus in healthy volunteers. A couple of studies elucidates the occurrence of skin inflammation after UV-B radiation. However, no research has been done that focuses on skin inflammation in humans after using UV-B radiation.

The last model of this chapter triggering neo-antigen, is the KLH challenge model in healthy volunteers. KLH caused a delayed type IV immune response. An increase in cutaneous blood perfusion, erythema and swelling was observed after administration of KLH. This model could be used for proof-of-concept studies.

In general, all the challenge models that have been developed could be optimized by assessing pharmacodynamic endpoints focusing on the four pillars imaging, biophysical, clinical and cellular/molecular that together constitute a so-called 'dermatological toolbox'. For imaging, various tools can be used such as multispectral imaging, 2D/3D imaging, colorimetry and optical coherence tomography. Laser speckle contrast imaging, trans-epidermal water loss, thermography, transdermal analysis patch and microbiome analyses are able to provide objective information on biophysical condition of the skin. For completeness of the derma toolbox it is recommended to include the NRS pain/itch or VAS as well as the skin histology, immunohistochemistry and mRNA expression. This toolbox will allow us to develop and monitor advanced human skin challenge models that will provide a more holistic view and to move a step closer towards 'systems dermatology'.

Conflict of interest

No conflicts of interest.

Author details

Salma Assil[1], Robert Rissmann[1] and Martijn Bastiaan Adriaan van Doorn[2]*

1 Centre for Human Drug Research, Leiden, The Netherlands

2 Department of Dermatology, Erasmus University Medical Center, Rotterdam, The Netherlands

*Address all correspondence to: m.b.a.vandoorn@erasmusmc.nl

References

[1] Pocock SJ. Clinical Trials: A Practical Approach. Chichester: Wiley & Sons; 2013. pp. 1-263

[2] Rubio DM, Schoenbaum EE, Lee LS, Schteingart DE, Marantz PR, Anderson KE, et al. Defining translational research: Implications for training. Academic Medicine. 2010;**85**(3):470-475

[3] Sedgwick P. What are the four phases of clinical research trials? British Medical Journal. 2014;**348**:1-2

[4] Trials AC. Phases of clinical trials Australian Clinical Trials. 2015 Available from: https://www.australianclinicaltrials.gov.au/what-clinical-trial/phases-clinical-trials

[5] Umscheid CA, Margolis DJ, Grossman CE. Key concepts of clinical trials: A narrative review. Postgraduate Medicine. 2011;**123**(5):194-204

[6] Harris SA, Meyer J, Satti I, Marsay L, Poulton ID, Tanner R, et al. Evaluation of a human BCG challenge model to assess antimycobacterial immunity induced by BCG and a candidate tuberculosis vaccine, MVA85A, alone and in combination. The Journal of Infectious Diseases. 2014;**209**(8):1259-1268

[7] McShane H, Williams A. A review of preclinical animal models utilised for TB vaccine evaluation in the context of recent human efficacy data. Tuberculosis. 2014;**94**(2):105-110

[8] Talat Iqbal N, Hussain R. Non-specific immunity of BCG vaccine: A perspective of BCG immunotherapy. Trials in Vaccinology. 2014;**3**:143-149

[9] van der Kolk T, Assil S, Rijneveld R, Klaassen ES, Feiss G, Florencia E, et al. Comprehensive, multimodal characterization of an imiquimod-induced human skin inflammation model for drug development. Clinical and Translational Science. 2018;**11**(6):607-615

[10] Vinter H, Iversen L, Steiniche T, Kragballe K, Johansen C. Aldara®-induced skin inflammation: Studies of patients with psoriasis. The British Journal of Dermatology. 2015;**172**(2):345-353

[11] Hemmi H, Kaisho T, Takeuchi O, Sato S, Sanjo H, Hoshino K, et al. Small anti-viral compounds activate immune cells via the TLR7 MyD88-dependent signaling pathway. Nature Immunology. 2002;**3**(2):196-200

[12] Schon MP, Schon M. Imiquimod: Mode of action. British Journal of Dermatology. 2007;**157**:8-13

[13] van der Fits L, Mourits S, Voerman JSA, Kant M, Boon L, Laman JD, et al. Imiquimod-induced psoriasis-like skin inflammation in mice is mediated via the IL-23/IL-17 axis. Journal of Immunology. 2009;**182**(9):5836-5845

[14] Maini AA, George MJ, Motwani MP, Day RM, Gilroy DW, O'Brien AJA. Comparison of human neutrophils acquired from four experimental models of inflammation. PLoS ONE. 2016;**11**(10):e0165502

[15] Monnet E, Lapeyre G, Poelgeest EV, Jacqmin P, Graaf K, Reijers J, et al. Evidence of NI-0101 pharmacological activity, an anti-TLR4 antibody, in a randomized phase I dose escalation study in healthy volunteers receiving LPS. Clinical Pharmacology and Therapeutics. 2017;**101**(2):200-208

[16] Dinh PH, Corraza F, Mestdagh K, Kassengera Z, Doyen V, Michel O. Validation of the cantharidin-induced skin blister as an in vivo model of inflammation. British

Journal of Clinical Pharmacology. 2011;**72**(6):912-920

[17] Motwani MP, Flint JD, De Maeyer RP, Fullerton JN, Smith AM, Marks DJ, et al. Novel translational model of resolving inflammation triggered by UV-killed *E. coli*. The Journal of Pathology. Clinical Research. 2016;**2**(3):154-165

[18] Dickson MC, Dewit OE, Peters G, Norton N, McHugh S, Davis B, et al. Immunisation challenges with keyhole limpet haemocyanin (KLH) and bacteriophage PhiX174: Potential for modelling in vivo pharmacodynamic effects. Immunology. 2014;**143**:70

[19] Harris JR, Markl J. Keyhole limpet hemocyanin (KLH): A biomedical review. Micron. 1999;**30**(6):597-623

[20] Jurincic-Winkler CD, Metz KA, Beuth J, Klippel KF. Keyhole limpet hemocyanin for carcinoma in situ of the bladder: A long-term follow-up study. European Urology. 2000;**37** (Suppl 3):45-49

[21] Miller JS, Curtsinger J, Berthold M, Malvey K, Bliss RL, Le CT, et al. Diminished neo-antigen response to keyhole limpet hemocyanin (KLH) vaccines in patients after treatment with chemotherapy or hematopoietic cell transplantation. Clinical Immunology. 2005;**117**(2):144-151

[22] Spazierer D, Skvara H, Dawid M, Fallahi N, Gruber K, Rose K, et al. T helper 2 biased de novo immune response to keyhole limpet hemocyanin in humans. Clinical and Experimental Allergy. 2009;**39**(7):999-1008

[23] Bishop T, Ballard A, Holmes H, Young AR, McMahon SB. Ultraviolet-B induced inflammation of human skin: Characterisation and comparison with traditional models of hyperalgesia. European Journal of Pain. 2009;**13**(5):524-532

[24] Holst H, Arendt-Nielsen L, Mosbech H, Serup J, Elberling J. Capsaicin-induced neurogenic inflammation in the skin in patients with symptoms induced by odorous chemicals. Skin Research and Technology. 2011;**17**(1):82-90

[25] Mcmahon SB, Koltzenburg M. Itching for an explanation. Trends in Neurosciences. 1992;**15**(12):497-501

[26] Akiyama T, Lerner EA, Carstens E. Protease-activated receptors and itch. Handbook of Experimental Pharmacology. 2015;**226**:219-235

[27] Criado PR, Criado RF, Maruta CW, Machado Filho C. Histamine, histamine receptors and antihistamines: New concepts. Anais Brasileiros de Dermatologia. 2010;**85**(2):195-210

[28] De Benedetto A, Yoshida T, Fridy S, Park JES, Kuo IH, Beck LA. Histamine and skin barrier: Are histamine antagonists useful for the prevention or treatment of atopic dermatitis? Journal of Clinical Medicine Research. 2015;**4**(4):741-755

[29] Falcone D, Uzunbajakava N, Richters R, van de Kerkhof PCM, van Erp PEJ. Histamine iontophoresis as in vivo model to study human skin inflammation with minimal barrier impairment: Pilot study results of application of the model to a sensitive skin panel. Skin Pharmacology and Physiology. 2017;**30**(5):246-259

[30] Gutowska-Owsiak D, Greenwald L, Watson C, Selvakumar TA, Wang X, Ogg GS. The histamine-synthesizing enzyme histidine decarboxylase is upregulated by keratinocytes in atopic skin. British Journal of Dermatology. 2014;**171**(4):771-778

[31] Hanifin JM. The role of antihistamines in atopic-dermatitis. Journal of Allergy and Clinical Immunology. 1990;**86**(4):666-669

[32] Rossbach K, Nassenstein C, Gschwandtner M, Schnell D, Sander K, Seifert R, et al. Histamine H1, H3 and H4 receptors are involved in pruritus. Neuroscience. 2011;**190**:89-102

[33] Sandilands EA, Crowe J, Cuthbert H, Jenkins PJ, Johnston NR, Eddleston M, et al. Histamine-induced vasodilatation in the human forearm vasculature. British Journal of Clinical Pharmacology. 2013;**76**(5):699-707

[34] Papoiu ADP, Tey HL, Coghill RC, Wang H, Yosipovitch G. Cowhage-induced itch as an experimental model for pruritus. A comparative study with histamine-induced itch. PLoS ONE. 2011;**6**(3):1-5

[35] Schmelz M. Itch and pain. Neuroscience and Biobehavioral Reviews. 2010;**34**(2):171-176

[36] Assarsson M, Duvetorp A, Dienus O, Soderman J, Seifert O. Significant changes in the skin microbiome in patients with chronic plaque psoriasis after treatment with narrowband ultraviolet B. Acta Dermato-Venereologica. 2018;**98**(4):428-436

[37] Elwood JM, Diffey BL. A consideration of ambient solar ultraviolet-radiation in the interpretation of studies of the etiology of melanoma. Melanoma Research. 1993;**3**(2):113-122

[38] Frodin T, Molin L, Skogh M. Effects of single doses of UVA, UVB, and UVC on skin blood-flow, water-content, and barrier function measured by laser-doppler flowmetry, optothermal infrared spectrometry, and evaporimetry. Photodermatology. 1988;**5**(4):187-195

[39] Kim Y, Lee SK, Bae S, Kim H, Park Y, Chu NK, et al. The anti-inflammatory effect of alloferon on UVB-induced skin inflammation through the down-regulation of pro-inflammatory cytokines. Immunology Letters. 2013;**149**(1-2):110-118

[40] Matsumura Y, Ananthaswamy HN. Toxic effects of ultraviolet radiation on the skin. Toxicology and Applied Pharmacology. 2004;**195**(3):298-308

[41] Okkerse P, van Amerongen G, de Kam ML, Stevens J, Butt RP, Gurrell R, et al. The use of a battery of pain models to detect analgesic properties of compounds: A two-part four-way crossover study. British Journal of Clinical Pharmacology. 2017;**83**(5):976-990

[42] Drolet BC, Lorenzi NM. Translational research: Understanding the continuum from bench to bedside. Translational Research. 2011;**157**(1):1-5

[43] Guttman-Yassky E, Krueger JG. Psoriasis: Evolution of pathogenic concepts and new therapies through phases of translational research. The British Journal of Dermatology. 2007;**157**(6):1103-1115

[44] Krueger JG, Bowcock A. Psoriasis pathophysiology: Current concepts of pathogenesis. Annals of the Rheumatic Diseases. 2005;**64**:30-36

[45] Nickoloff BJ, Nestle FO. Recent insights into the immunopathogenesis of psoriasis provide new therapeutic opportunities. Journal of Clinical Investigation. 2004;**113**(12):1664-1675

[46] Wagner EF, Schonthaler HB, Guinea-Viniegra J, Tschachler E. Psoriasis: What we have learned from mouse models. Nature Reviews Rheumatology. 2010;**6**(12):704-714

[47] Gudjonsson JE, Johnston A, Dyson M, Valdimarsson H, Elder JT. Mouse models of psoriasis. Journal of Investigative Dermatology. 2007;**127**(6):1292-1308

[48] Schon MP. Animal models of psoriasis: A critical appraisal. Experimental Dermatology. 2008;**17**(8):703-712

[49] Suckling K. Animal research: Too much faith in models clouds judgement. Nature. 2008;**455**(7212):460

[50] Hartung T. Thoughts on limitations of animal models. Parkinsonism & Related Disorders. 2008;**14**(Suppl 2):S81-S83

[51] Schon MP, Detmar M, Parker CM. Murine psoriasis-like disorder induced by naive CD4+ T cells. Nature Medicine. 1997;**3**(2):183-188

[52] Leung DYM, Soter NA. Cellular and immunologic mechanisms in atopic dermatitis. Journal of the American Academy of Dermatology. 2001;**44**(1):S1-S12

[53] Grabbe S, Schwarz T. Immunoregulatory mechanisms involved in elicitation of allergic contact hypersensitivity. Immunology Today. 1998;**19**(1):37-44

[54] Tracy RP. The five cardinal signs of inflammation: Calor, dolor, rubor, tumor… and penuria (apologies to Aulus Cornelius Celsus, De medicina, c. AD 25). The Journals of Gerontology. Series A, Biological Sciences and Medical Sciences. 2006;**61**(10):1051-1052

[55] Bieber T. Mechanisms of disease: Atopic dermatitis. New England Journal of Medicine. 2008;**358**(14):1483-1494

[56] Pasparakis M, Haase I, Nestle FO. Mechanisms regulating skin immunity and inflammation. Nature Reviews. Immunology. 2014;**14**(5):289-301

[57] Dickson MC, Ludbrook Valerie J, Perry Hayley C, Wilson Paul A, Garthside Sam J, Binks MH. A model of skin inflammation in humans leads to a rapid and reproducible increase in the interferon response signature: A potential translational model for drug development. Inflammation Research. 2015;**64**(3-4):171-183

[58] Szeimies RM, Gerritsen MJ, Gupta G, Ortonne JP, Serresi S, Bichel J, et al. Imiquimod 5% cream for the treatment of actinic keratosis: Results from a phase III, randomized, double-blind, vehicle-controlled, clinical trial with histology. Journal of the American Academy of Dermatology. 2004;**51**(4):547-555

[59] Flutter B, Nestle FO. TLRs to cytokines: Mechanistic insights from the imiquimod mouse model of psoriasis. European Journal of Immunology. 2013;**43**(12):3138-3146

[60] Larange A, Antonios D, Pallardy M, Kerdine-Romer S. TLR7 and TLR8 agonists trigger different signaling pathways for human dendritic cell maturation. Journal of Leukocyte Biology. 2009;**85**(4):673-683

[61] Hawkes JE, Gudjonsson JE, Ward NL. The snowballing literature on imiquimod-induced skin inflammation in mice: A critical appraisal. Journal of Investigative Dermatology. 2017;**137**(3):546-549

[62] Beutner KR, Spruance SL, Hougham AJ, Fox TL, Owens ML, Douglas JM. Treatment of genital warts with an immune-response modifier (imiquimod). Journal of the American Academy of Dermatology. 1998;**38**(2):230-239

[63] van Seters M, van Beurden M, ten Kate FJW, Beckmann I, Ewing PC, Eijkemans MJC, et al. Treatment of vulvar intraepithelial neoplasia with topical imiquimod. New England Journal of Medicine. 2008;**358**(14):1465-1473

[64] Dowling JK, Mansell A. Toll-like receptors: The swiss army knife of

immunity and vaccine development. Clinical and Experimental Immunology. 2016;**5**(5):e85

[65] U.S. National Library of Medicine. Clinical trials, Toll-Like Receptor 7. 2019. Available from: https://clinicaltrials.gov/ct2/results?cond=&term=TLR7&cntry=&state=&city=&dist=

[66] Yosipovitch G, Greaves MW, Schmelz M. Itch. Lancet. 2003;**361**(9358):690-694

[67] Yosipovitch G, Samuel LS. Neuropathic and psychogenic itch. Dermatologic Therapy. 2008;**21**(1):32-41

[68] Binder A, Koroschetz J, Baron R. Disease mechanisms in neuropathic itch. Nature Clinical Practice Neurology. 2008;**4**:329

[69] Potenzieri C, Undem BJ. Basic mechanisms of itch. Clinical and Experimental Allergy. 2012;**42**(1):8-19

[70] Shim WS, Oh U. Histamine-induced itch and its relationship with pain. Molecular Pain. 2008;**4**

[71] Schmelz M, Schmidt R, Bickel A, Handwerker HO, Torebjork HE. Specific C-receptors for itch in human skin. The Journal of Neuroscience. 1997;**17**(20):8003-8008

[72] Yarbrough KB, Neuhaus KJ, Simpson EL. The effects of treatment on itch in atopic dermatitis. Dermatologic Therapy. 2013;**26**(2):110-119

[73] D'Orazio J, Jarrett S, Amaro-Ortiz A, Scott T. UV radiation and the skin. International Journal of Molecular Sciences. 2013;**14**(6):12222-12248

[74] Sayre RM, Desrochers DL, Wilson CJ, Marlowe E. Skin type, minimal erythema dose (MED), and sunlight acclimatization. Journal of the American Academy of Dermatology. 1981;**5**(4):439-443

[75] Oertel BG, Lotsch J. Clinical pharmacology of analgesics assessed with human experimental pain models: Bridging basic and clinical research. British Journal of Pharmacology. 2013;**168**(3):534-553

[76] Olofsen E, Romberg R, Bijl H, Mooren R, Engbers F, Kest B, et al. Alfentanil and placebo analgesia: No sex differences detected in models of experimental pain. Anesthesiology. 2005;**103**(1):130-139

[77] Chow S, Rizzo C, Ravitskiy L, Sinha AA. The role of T cells in cutaneous autoimmune disease. Autoimmunity. 2005;**38**(4):303-317

[78] Swaminathan A, Lucas RM, Dear K, McMichael AJ. Keyhole limpet haemocyanin—A model antigen for human immunotoxicological studies. British Journal of Clinical Pharmacology. 2014;**78**(5):1135-1142

[79] Curtis JE, Hersh EM, Harris JE, McBride C, Freireich EJ. The human primary immune response to keyhole limpet haemocyanin: Interrelationships of delayed hypersensitivity, antibody response and in vitro blast transformation. Clinical and Experimental Immunology. 1970;**6**(4):473-491

[80] Weigle WO. Immunochemical properties of hemocyanin. Immunochemistry. 1964;**1**:295-302

[81] Swanson MA, Schwartz RS. Immunosuppressive therapy. The relation between clinical response and immunologic competence. The New England Journal of Medicine. 1967;**277**(4):163-170

[82] Perabo FG, Muller SC. Current and new strategies in immunotherapy for superficial bladder cancer. Urology. 2004;**64**(3):409-421

[83] Grant RW, Mariani RA, Vieira VJ, Fleshner M, Smith TP, Keylock KT, et al.

Cardiovascular exercise intervention improves the primary antibody response to keyhole limpet hemocyanin (KLH) in previously sedentary older adults. Brain, Behavior, and Immunity. 2008;**22**(6):923-932

[84] Schuyler M, Lyons CR, Masten B, Bice D. Immunoglobulin response to intrapulmonary immunization of asthmatics. Immunology. 1997;**91**(2):167-175

[85] Kantele A, Hakkinen MP, Zivny J, Elson CO, Mestecky J, Kantele JM. Humoral immune response to keyhole limpet haemocyanin, the protein carrier in cancer vaccines. Clinical and Developmental Immunology. 2011;**2011**:614383

[86] Boelens PG, Fonk JCM, Houdijk APJ, Scheper RJ, Haarman HJTM, Meijer S, et al. Primary immune response to keyhole limpet haemocyanin following trauma in relation to low plasma glutamine. Clinical and Experimental Immunology. 2004;**136**(2):356-364

[87] Boulton C, Meiser K, David OJ, Schmouder R. Pharmacodynamic effects of steady-state fingolimod on antibody response in healthy volunteers: A 4-week, randomized, placebo-controlled, parallel-group, multiple-dose study. Journal of Clinical Pharmacology. 2012;**52**(12):1879-1890

[88] Bingham CO 3rd, Looney RJ, Deodhar A, Halsey N, Greenwald M, Codding C, et al. Immunization responses in rheumatoid arthritis patients treated with rituximab: Results from a controlled clinical trial. Arthritis and Rheumatism. 2010;**62**(1):64-74

[89] Saghari M, Ziagkos D, van Doorn MBA, Burggraaf J, Rissman R, Moerland M. Evaluation of delayed-type hypersensitivity (DTH) in healthy volunteers using innovative imaging techniques. Centre for Human Drug Research; 2019 [Unpublished]

Chapter 4

Sex Differences in Obesity-Induced Inflammation

Sari Terrazas, Lauren Brashear, Anna-Katherine Escoto, Shannon Lynch, Dylan Slaughter, Neena Xavier, Norman Robert Estes II and Samantha Giordano-Mooga

Abstract

Obesity is defined as a BMI greater than 25 kg/m^2. Once thought to simply be a nutritional disorder, obesity has become a major health concern characterized by a state of constant low-grade inflammation caused by chronic adiposity. This state of inflammation is characterized by circulating inflammatory mediators, such as IL-6, leptin, and TNF-α, as well as varying levels of glucose-regulating hormones produced by obese adipose tissue. When left untreated, obesity can lead to a number of diseases including, but not limited to, cardiovascular disease, metabolic syndrome, neurodegeneration, type II diabetes mellitus, chronic kidney disease, and infertility. The distribution of adiposity differs in men and women, and these differences, along with the differences in sex hormones and sex hormone levels, can exacerbate or attenuate the course of disease pathology. Obesity can also be exacerbated by stress, which can worsen disease pathogenesis. In this review, we will explore how obesity affects inflammation and disease and how sex can affect the course of these diseases.

Keywords: obesity, inflammation, sex differences, estrogen, testosterone

1. Introduction

Approximately 70% of the US adult population is considered overweight or obese [1]. Obesity has been associated with an elevated risk of type II diabetes, cancer, neurodegeneration, infertility and stress hypertension, and cardiovascular disease (CVD) [2, 3]. The increased risk for various health risks is due in part to the inflammatory adipokines produced by the adipose tissue itself. Clinically, body mass index (BMI) is the most widely used tool to measure adiposity. However, BMI measures total mass, including both fat and fat-free (lean) mass, so it is a poor indicator of adiposity [2]. Further, the different compartments of fat and different types of adipose tissue within these compartments play a major role in the overall increased health risks associated with increases in adiposity [4]. Lastly, the body composition differs between men and women; men have more lean mass than women, whereas women have more fat mass. In this book chapter, we help to unravel the differences in adipose-induced inflammation in men and women and how these differences may contribute to various pathophysiologies.

IntechOpen

2. Adipose tissue

Adipose tissue is composed of a variety of cells, including adipocytes, macrophages, leukocytes, endothelial cells, and fibroblasts. This metabolic tissue and the subsets of cells found within this tissue play a role in both the inflammatory and hormonal pathways. This has led many to believe that adipose tissue is a novel endocrine organ [5].

Classically adipocytes were believed to be either white or brown adipocytes. The white adipose tissue (WAT) is the adipose tissue which is often focused on in obesity research. The WAT is less metabolically active, is composed primarily of stored triglycerides, and produces adipokines which regulate hunger, satiation via leptin, breakdown of triglycerides via adiponectin, and insulin sensitivity via IL-1 and IL-6 [5]. WAT has also been associated with inflammatory adipokine production, including TNF-alpha, MCP-1, resistin, and IL-6 [5]. Interestingly, these adipokines become dysregulated in obese states which can further exacerbate cellular and systemic dysfunctions [6]. The increase in inflammatory cytokines is a contributing factor to the various pathophysiologies discussed within this chapter.

Brown adipose tissue (BAT) is colored brown due to the high mitochondrial content. This highly metabolically active tissue also plays a role in thermogenesis, classically in neonates, and in lipid breakdown [7]. Key features of BAT include the high levels of mitochondria and the presence of uncoupling protein 1 (UCP-1), which both play a role in the "extraction" of nutrients from free fatty acids and triglycerides [8, 9]. Recent studies have shown that BAT is not only found in neonates but can also be found in adults. A study conducted in males and females using PET-CT scans detected BAT tissue in the fascial plane in the ventral trunk and superficial and lateral sternocleidomastoid muscles [10]. Further, this study showed that there were differences in BAT mass in males and females, with females having more BAT than males. There was also an inverse correlation in BAT detection with age and BMI in older patients [10]. The data of this study suggest that shifting WAT to BAT also known as "beiging WAT" or increasing BAT production may be an effective treatment against obesity [11].

3. Sex differences in hormones and adipose tissue

The sex hormones, most notably testosterone (androgen) in males and estrogen and progesterone in females, play a role in fat deposition, metabolism, and energy balance within their respective sex. We will briefly discuss the specific roles of the sex hormones as they relate to adipose tissue. Estrogen has been shown to have both anti-inflammatory and antioxidant properties and can regulate metabolism [12]. Much of the data supporting estrogen as a protective factor comes from differences observed between pre- and postmenopausal women, where women in the premenopausal phase are protected against many cardiometabolic diseases, until they reach the menopausal period, where there is an increase in CVDs, inflammation, and weight gain [13]. Low testosterone levels in men have also been associated as a risk factor for pathophysiologies, including sexual dysfunction, CVD, insulin sensitivity, and type II diabetes [14].

Conversely, high levels of estrogen in men and high levels of testosterone in women have been shown to have negative effects on weight gain [15]. High levels of testosterone, seen in women with polycystic ovarian syndrome (PCOS), or low levels of estrogen seen in postmenopausal women have been linked to increased weight gain, specifically in the intra-abdominal fat [16]. Further, in men, testosterone replacement, when there are low levels of testosterone, has been shown to increase lean body mass and improve lipid and cholesterol levels [17, 18].

More recent studies have shown that while both estrogen and androgens are important for many physiological processes, the estrogen to androgen ratio is important in regulating adipose tissue deposition. Interestingly in a study looking at the effects of testosterone replacement therapy, men with the lowest levels of estrogen (<10 pg./mL) had the largest decrease in body fat reduction after 6 months of testosterone therapy [19]. An important step in the production of estrogen is the enzyme aromatase, which converts testosterone to estrogen. Both male and female aromatase null mice exhibited increased weight gain and obesity-related metabolic complications [20]. Together, these data suggest that both estrogen and testosterone play an important role in regulating obesity and adiposity.

As stated previously, the body composition differs between men and women. Men are more likely to accumulate adipose tissue around the trunk and abdomen, whereas women usually accumulate adipose tissue around the hips and thighs [21, 22]. Women have a higher percentage of body fat than lean fat when compared to men who have the same BMI. Therefore, the health consequences are different for each gender at the same BMI [21]. In addition, a higher portion of that fat is in the femoral-gluteal region as compared to the abdominal region for men [22]. Studies have shown that the relative distribution of fat has a greater impact on CVD risks than total excess body fat. The female pattern of fat distribution, around the femoral-gluteal area, is relatively protective, compared to the male pattern of abdominal fat accumulation [23–25].

Within the abdomen, fat can accumulate in the subcutaneous area, subcutaneous adipose tissue (SAT), or, in the deep abdomen, visceral adipose tissue (VAT). Both VAT and SAT, in the obese state, produce increased inflammatory cytokines, including TNF-α and IL-6, which produce increased levels of leptin and decreased levels of adiponectin [26, 27]. These changes can cause further inflammatory cascades, including inducing proinflammatory macrophages into the adipose tissue (**Figure 1**).

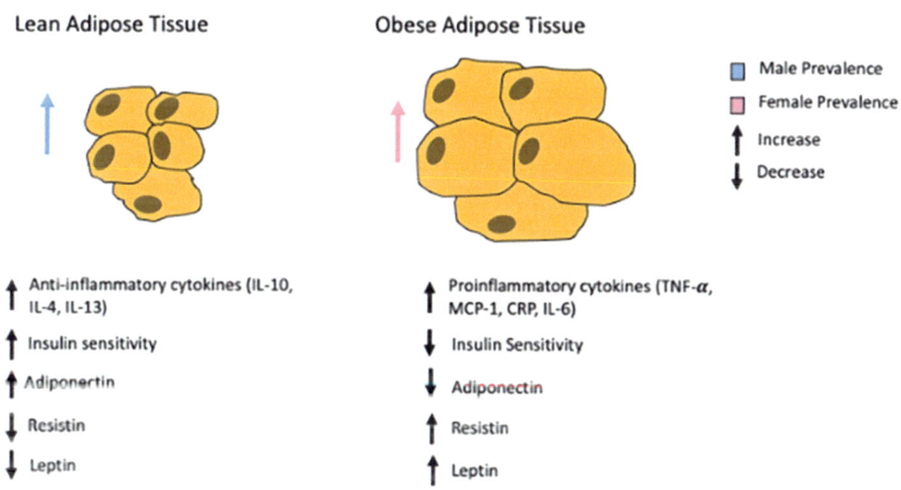

Figure 1.
The effects of lean vs. obese adipose tissue. A healthy diet and exercise are characterized by lean adipose tissue. Lean adipose tissue aids in regulating inflammation by secreting anti-inflammatory cytokines as well as secreting high levels of adiponectin which aids in insulin sensitivity [27]. Leaner adipose tissue also secretes low levels of leptin and resistin. Conversely, obese adipose tissue release high levels of resistin and leptin which promote insulin insensitivity. Obese adipose tissue also exhibits a proinflammatory cytokine profile which can lead to diseases such as diabetes and neurodegeneration. Men tend to have a greater ratio of lean to obese adipose tissue since they have greater muscle mass compared to women who have more obese adipose tissue [28].

These inflammatory cells exacerbate adipose tissue cytokine production or increase disease risks, which can further feed into this cycle.

Multiple studies have also shown that VAT is associated with a higher cardiovascular risk [24, 25]. Since the VAT has primarily been associated with the abdominal region, the VAT has historically played a more pathogenic role in male pathology. Because of the high rate of obesity in the United States, and the increased VAT deposition seen in both men and women, we understand that VAT deposition also increases risks in females. Therefore, more therapeutic interventions are needed to inhibit VAT deposition in both men and women.

4. Gender-specific differences in aging due to inflammation

Considerable amounts of data indicate that sex-specific differences in both acute and chronic inflammatory responses exist between males and females across multiple species and that these differences are altered with advancing age. Various studies suggest that these sex-specific variances include differences in multiple inflammatory biomarkers, including TNF-alpha, IL-6, IL-10, and C-reactive protein (CRP) [29]. While it appears clear that variations between the sexes do exist and these variations change with aging, the exact fluctuations in inflammatory biomarkers, both between sexes and with aging, are not fully elucidated.

Complicating matters is the established role of adipose tissue as a source of both pro- and anti-inflammatory cytokines. Leptin, adiponectin, and other cytokines synthesized and secreted by adipose tissue have been shown to play a profound role in modulating both systemic and localized inflammatory reactions. Adipose tissue likely plays a role as a source of pro- and anti-inflammatory cytokines and since, as previously described, males and females accumulate adipose tissue in different/store body fat in different locations, the adipose tissue plays an important role in the sex-specific differences in inflammatory responses, especially with aging.

Another complicating factor regarding inflammatory responses between males and females is the potential role of steroid hormones in various sex-specific physiological responses, including accumulation and storage of adipose tissue, and inflammation. Estrogen has been shown to have potent anti-inflammatory activity and cardioprotective effects in females, and as estrogen levels decline with age after the onset of menopause, these protective effects of estrogen are minimized [12, 30]. While much has been determined, further study into the sex-specific differences between males and females, how these levels change over time with aging in a sex-specific manner, and the role that these levels and their changes play in both acute and chronic diseases are warranted.

Many biomarkers of inflammation have been investigated regarding adiposity, age, sex, and ethnic variations. The most studied biomarkers include C-reactive protein (CRP), interleukin-6 (IL-6), interleukin-10 (IL-10), tumor necrosis factor alpha (TNF-alpha). Data from a meta-analysis investigating potential relationships between the adipose tissue-derived cytokines leptin and adiponectin and inflammatory biomarkers including CRP, IL-6, and TNF-alpha suggested a positive correlation between leptin and all three inflammatory biomarkers, whereas there was a negative correlation with respect to adiponectin and the biomarkers [31]. When adjusted for age, Grassman et al. observed that correlations weakened as the age of the participants increased. In contrast to other studies, the authors found no significant differences when looking at sex and inflammatory markers in relation to adipose tissue. In another study aimed at elucidating mechanisms responsible for differences in inflammatory responses across sexes, Wegner et al. found that proinflammatory responses to endotoxin in women were greater compared to men, with significantly higher increases in plasma TNF-alpha and IL-6 [32]. Interestingly, increases in circulating plasma cortisol levels were also found to be significantly elevated in women as compared to men, which could play a role in the heightened response.

In contrast Kuo et al. used endotoxin exposure in young (5–6 weeks) versus adult (9–10 weeks) male and female mice to investigate relationships in the inflammatory responses in these groups [33]. Older male mice showed significantly higher levels of pro-inflammatory markers IL-6, IL-10, and TNF-alpha than age-matched female mice upon stimulation with endotoxin. In younger mice, however, they did not find a gender-specific difference in these same biomarkers. An investigation of factors associated with biomarkers of systemic inflammation using age-, sex-, and body mass index (BMI)-adjusted linear regression found an age-related effect on the markers. They examined multiple factors in relation to inflammatory biomarkers including CRP, IL1β, IL6, IL8, and TNFα in adults between the ages of 50 and 76 years. The results of this study indicated that age influenced circulating concentrations of all biomarkers except IL1β, with increasing age being associated with higher concentrations of all other biomarkers tested [34]. When they looked at sex-specific differences, the results were varied, with CRP and IL-6 levels being lower among men.

In looking at sex-specific differences of oxidative stress and inflammation with regard to cardiovascular risk factors in Arab populations, Khadir et al. found that females had higher levels of reactive oxygen species (ROS) and CRP after adjustment for body mass index (BMI) and waist circumference [35]. Conversely, males had increased levels of IL-6, IL-8, and TNF-alpha. In order to look at the relative impact of central obesity versus general obesity, the authors adjusted for age, BMI, and gender and noted that the levels of IL-6, TNF-alpha, and ROS were associated with central obesity but not general obesity, further suggesting that sex-specific patterns of adipose distribution can potentially account for some of the observed sex-specific differences in males versus females. The authors concluded that the relative contribution of inflammation and oxidative stress to CVD in Arab populations was linked, at least in part, to gender-specific distributions of body fat [35].

5. Sex differences in obesity-induced inflammation in pathology

While it is well known that obesity is a risk factor for many diseases, it is important to understand that the chronic state of inflammation associated with obesity further exacerbates obesity itself. Therefore, in many cases, obesity and inflammation increase pathophysiology, and these pathophysiologies further exacerbate the inflammation and obesity in a continuous vicious cycle. It is important to understand the role of sex and the sex hormones in this vicious cycle in order for better/more effective treatments and treatment plans for obese patients with various pathophysiologies. Below we describe the role of the sex hormones on obesity-induced inflammation in metabolic syndrome, CVD, type II diabetes, chronic kidney disease (CKD), neurodegeneration, cancer, infertility, and stress.

5.1 Metabolic syndrome

Metabolic syndrome (MetS), also known as syndrome x, is a health condition characterized by insulin resistance, glucose intolerance, hypertension, high triglycerides, low HDL cholesterol, abdominal obesity, dyslipidemia, and inflammation [36]. The increased incidence of MetS has been linked to obesity and a lack of physical activity [37]. According to the Centers for Disease Control (CDC), a review of the NHANES data shows that as of 2012 more than one-third of US adults were considered to have MetS [38]. MetS affects over 30% of people by the time they reach age 65, and these statistics are expected to rise in the upcoming years [26]. By simply losing 5–10% of body weight, risk of developing metabolic syndrome, CVD, and type 2 diabetes is reduced significantly [26]. This emphasizes that prevention, rather than treatment, is the key to reducing the prevalence of metabolic syndrome in those at risk and those who are pre-symptomatic.

Diagnostic criteria for metabolic syndrome vary among organizations but typically include blood pressure, a large waist circumference, and the following: high levels of triglycerides and blood glucose and low levels of high-density lipoprotein cholesterol [26, 37, 39]. Previous diagnoses relied on body mass index; however, this has recently shifted to favor waist circumference because of its role in identifying central/abdominal obesity [36]. As previously described in this chapter, abdominal/central obesity, with increased VAT, has been associated with increased risks for disease and inflammation.

Interestingly, there is no difference in prevalence of MetS between men and women, but there are differences in symptoms among men and women; women are more likely to have abdominal obesity, whereas men have more varied symptoms [36]. As previously described, intra-abdominal obesity is not classically associated with women and, therefore, may play a more pronounced role in this gender. Further, it has been shown that women throughout their lives have consistently higher levels of adiponectin which increases insulin sensitivity and leptin, which signals fullness to the brain than males. This implies that the adipose tissue in women produces adipokines which play a role in female adipose deposition and regulation [40–43].

It is well known that brown adipose tissue (BAT) is characterized by the expression of UCP-1 which causes an increase in mitochondrial function and metabolism [44, 45]. UCP-1 has been linked to the "beiging of WAT" and a more metabolically active tissue. Further, in oxidative phosphorylation, genes, responsible for assisting in transcriptional activation in the mitochondria, have increased levels of expression in women [41]. The upregulation of this UCP-1 and increases in oxidative phosphorylation genes indicate that women express more metabolically active fat mass in comparison to men. Understanding that women have more metabolically active fat may help to explain the differing symptoms seen in MetS between men and women.

MetS and obesity can induce changes in gene expression. PPAR γ is one of the hormone receptors responsible for regulating adipocyte differentiation and lipolysis. Genetic SNP predispositions within this receptor, which are found in women, have been linked to increased susceptibility for obesity and insulin resistance [46] Estrogen can also activate a variety of metabolism genes, which play a role in the increased fat metabolism in humans and rodents [44, 47]. Women in the postmenopausal period, when estrogen levels have decreased, have a higher incidence in central adiposity and a higher risk for developing MetS [48]. Contrastingly, throughout life men have larger muscle mass and less free fat in organs that are highly metabolically active like the kidneys, liver, and brain. Males are more likely than women to experience an increase in incidence of diabetes due to decreases in insulin sensitivity [46]. Men also have lower expression of oxidative phosphorylation genes and brown adipose tissue, as indicated by UCP1, compared to women [49]. Taken together, these data support the idea that men and women present with different symptoms of metabolic syndrome and, therefore, may need different treatments for MetS consistent with these symptoms.

5.2 Cardiovascular disease

According to the American Heart Association, CVD is a term that encompasses many conditions including heart disease, heart valve issues, heart failure, and stroke. CVD is the leading cause of death for a variety of US ethnic populations [50]. Risk factors include metabolic syndrome, high blood lipid and glucose levels, high blood pressure, central/abdominal adiposity, low HDL, and high LDL cholesterol [46]. Further, there are differences in the prevalence of CVD among race, sex, and hormone levels [50]. Classically, men have higher levels of CVD than women, until women reach the postmenopausal period, the sixth decade of life, where women have similar or higher incidence of CVD than males of the same age [50].

Obesity, specifically abdominal adiposity, is a main risk factor for CVD. The Framingham Heart Study, a long-term observational study, determined that obesity increases cardiovascular disorders by 64% for women and 46% for men [51]. Further, Garcia et al. have shown that obesity more greatly impacts women's risk and incidence of CVD than men [52]. Therefore, reducing and preventing obesity could be a critical method for mitigating cardiovascular-related disorders in both men and women.

Fat accumulation of the neck has been found to be a strong predictor of CVD [53]. Fat accumulation is usually estimated via the measuring the neck circumference. In contrast to the well-defined and studied compartments and sex differences in accumulation with the abdominal fat deposition, less is known about these factors in the neck. In one retrospective study, overweight and obese women have more subcutaneous neck fat compared to men even after age and BMI matching. In the same study, subcutaneous neck fat was associated with higher incidence of metabolic risk than intermuscular fat deposits in both sexes [54]. This suggests that similar to abdominal fat, women have more subcutaneous fat and men more intermuscular fat in the neck.

Obesity creates an inflammatory state of the body that affects heart health. However, the overall effects may differ among the sexes based on sex hormone activity. Men have a higher overall incidence of death due to CVD [50]. The X chromosome in men upregulates the expression of genes responsible for functions of cell death mechanisms and cellular trafficking/migration, while the Y chromosome is responsible for genes involved in innate immunity activation. Activating the innate immune system, specifically the immune cell, the macrophages, induces inflammation and increases the risk for developing atherosclerosis [46]. Therefore, by inheriting a Y chromosome, men increase their genetic risk for developing CVD. Data suggests that testosterone does not confer any protection against obesity, inflammation, and CVD [46].

Levels of the sex hormone estrogen do not appear to affect men as severely as women [46]. It is hypothesized that the gender difference of varying estrogen levels only becomes evident in postmenopausal women who have lower levels of this sex hormone. Treatment and prevention methods using statins for CVD have been targeted more at men than women, as deemed appropriate by the American Heart Association. However, guidelines have recently been tailored to be more gender-inclusive based on cardiovascular risk factor assessments [52]. Sex differences attributed to genetic factors and lifestyle habits lead women to be more susceptible to CVD with elevated risk if preventative methods are not taken. Sex differences in CVD arise as the result of a combination of effects from various genetic and environmental factors.

Another important sex difference in CVD is the effect of the sex hormone estrogen. Circulating levels of estrogen fluctuate during a woman's life span and can regulate inflammation. Inflammation increases cardiovascular risk, as indicated by increased levels of C-reactive protein [52]. CRP is both an inflammatory protein and an important biomarker of cardiovascular damage. It is hypothesized that the higher levels of systemic estrogen, associated with pre-menopausal women, have been shown to have a cardioprotective effect and reduce inflammation. The Women's Health Initiative designed a study to determine the possible use of hormone therapy as a preventative measure against CVD in postmenopausal women. The initial trials were ended early due by the Data Safety Monitoring Board (DSMB) due to the increased incidence of stroke and breast cancer in the estrogen + progesterone arm of the trial [55]. Further analysis of this randomized control study ultimately provided evidence for a concept known as the "timing hypothesis." This hypothesis states that hormone replacement therapy near the onset of menopause, within 5 years, may lower the risk for CVD, while MHT treatment in women greater than 5 years from menopause is harmful [56]. The timing hypothesis has had an important impact in clinical settings [30].

Traditional CVD risk factors that are increased for women include lack of physical activity, smoking, diabetes, obesity, dyslipidemia, and hypertension. Many of these risk factors are highly prevalent in the United States, meaning comorbidities are associated with CVD. For example, every two in three adults are overweight or obese, highly increasing their risk to develop CVD as well as other conditions [52]. These risk factors are preventable and reducible by means of lifestyle changes such as eating a healthy diet and maintaining exercise. Some nontraditional risk factors for women CVD include the following: depression, autoimmune diseases, treatment for breast cancer, hypertensive pregnancy disorders, gestational diabetes, delivering a preterm child, and ischemic heart disease [52]. It is hypothesized that women with ischemic heart disease have higher mortality rates and worse CVD outcomes than men due to insufficient detection and treatment options.

One method to improve adipose deposition detection is through imaging, as advancements in technology have allowed for detailed assessment of subcutaneous and visceral fat compartments. Computed topography (CT) and magnetic resonance imaging (MRI) are considered the gold standard for detailed assessment of body composition. However, these tests are expensive, not readily available, and, in the case of CT, associated with a significant dose of radiation. Dual-energy X-ray absorptiometry (DXA) is a technique used for osteoporosis screening and more readily available and less expensive and has relatively minimal radiation exposure. Therefore, it is more often used as it is able to assess body composition, such as fat and lean mass, and can quantify VAT and SAT accurately in obese patients [57, 58]. Fox et al. examined over 3000 subjects from the Framingham Heart Cohort who underwent CT of the abdomen [59]. They demonstrated a significant association between abdominal SAT and VAT in men and women and increased risk of hypertension, diabetes mellitus type 2, and metabolic syndrome. There was a stronger correlation with VAT and most of the cardiovascular risk factors. Interestingly, there were significant sex interactions with increasing volumes of SAT and VAT. Increasing volumes of SAT and VAT were more strongly and consistently associated with higher cardiovascular risks in women than in men [59]. These findings suggest that women who accumulate more VAT have a higher cardiovascular risk than men with more VAT.

5.3 Type II diabetes mellitus

Type II diabetes mellitus (TIIDM) is also known as non-insulin-dependent or insulin-resistant diabetes and is characterized by high blood glucose, polyuria, and polydipsia. The most common risk factors attributed to TIIDM are poor diet and lack of exercise but have also been linked to obesity. TIIDM was traditionally been considered a disease of adulthood, but this is rapidly changing since there is an increased incidence of TIIDM in children and adolescents [60]. The common comorbidities of TIIDM include metabolic syndrome, increased adiposity, and inflammatory conditions [37].

Males and females exhibit sex-specific differences in total muscle mass and in distribution of muscle that becomes apparent in puberty. Males typically have greater total muscle mass and greater in the upper body compared to the lower body [61]. Janssen et al. performed whole body MRI in men and women 18–88 years of age, and the results of their study suggested that men had significantly higher skeletal muscle mass than women relative to total body mass (38% vs. 31%) and that the sex differences were greater in the upper body (40%) than lower body (33%) [62]. It further showed that with aging, there is an age-associated loss of muscle mass, with the greatest loss in the lower body [62].

Skeletal muscle plays an important role in determining glucose homeostasis as the muscle mass is responsible for the majority of basal and insulin-stimulated glucose uptake. In addition, impaired insulin activity at the level of the skeletal muscle is a central component to the clinical findings associated with TIIDM. The reported sex differences in muscle mass emphasize the differences of maintaining muscle during aging and could represent an important target in women who are at greater risk for sarcopenic obesity given their higher fat and lower muscle mass [63].

Studies have shown that exercise and fasting both present conditions that result in lower insulin levels with greater instances of insulin receptor binding. However, obese conditions result in greater levels of insulin with low insulin binding. A study conducted by Hotamisligil et al. suggests that TNF-a secretion by adipocytes decreases insulin-mediated glucose uptake by lowering the usage of glucose by fat and muscle tissues [64]. Insulin aids in glucose uptake in conjunction with the GLUT4 receptor. However, with the inability of insulin to properly interact with its receptor, GLUT4 is unable to take up glucose, and it continues to circulate throughout the blood [65]. The increased blood glucose and the increased inflammatory cytokines produced by the adipose tissue exacerbate TIIDM pathology.

If the levels of adipokines and free fatty acids rise, their presence will result in the recruitment of inflammatory cell types such as macrophages. When the inflammatory cells are recruited to the adipose tissue, they become activated and release additional cytokines such as TNF-alpha and IL-6 to recruit even more inflammatory cells. This results in a positive feedback loop that results in a chronic state of inflammation. Inflammation-resolving proteins such as annexin A1 are typically increased in obese patients but are inactivated by dysregulated cleavage [66]. Cleavage of annexin A1 deactivates the inflammation-resolving properties of the protein, leading the patient to maintain a chronic state of inflammation [66].

Various estrogen replacement therapy studies have shown that estrogen provides anti-inflammatory and antioxidant effects in women [67]. A meta-analysis of these studies investigated the effects of replacement therapy on women based on the age they start therapy and noted that when women began therapy within 10 years of entering the postmenopausal phase of life, estrogen provided protective anti-inflammatory and antioxidant effects [12]. When women present with TIIDM, the benefits of estrogen are also lost regardless of age of onset, and they begin to present with the same diseases that are typically more prevalent in postmenopausal women [68].

The loss of estrogen protection after TIIDM diagnosis causes the female body to be attacked more aggressively compared to men of the same age. Men diagnosed with TIIDM have significantly lower levels of testosterone compared to healthy men, while women have significantly higher levels of testosterone [69]. These data suggest that the sex hormones can regulate TIIDM severity in both men and women.

5.3.1 Chronic kidney disease in TIIDM

TIIDM diagnosis increases the risk of kidney stones and hypertension, both of which are precursors for CKD [70]. CKD is not usually diagnosed until the patient goes to the doctor for a physical, and they are diagnosed with high blood pressure, or protein is found in the urine. The Centers for Disease Control has estimated that as of 2015, 14% of the US population lives with CKD; of those that live with CKD, approximately 22% also have TIIDM.

Recent studies have shown parallels between the obesity epidemic and the onset of CKD. Obese patients with CKD are often seen with glomerular scarring, also known as glomerulosclerosis. This is now being termed obesity-related glomerulopathy due to its prevalence in obese patients [71]. Development of this condition has been related to lipid accumulation in the kidneys which may be a response to hyperfiltration if the patient also has TIIDM [71]. Under normal conditions glucose is not filtered through the glomerulus. However, if a patient has unregulated TIIDM, glucose is constantly being filtered out through the glomerulus, which becomes more permeable when blood glucose levels are high. When the glomerulus is constantly filtering glucose, the glomerular net becomes weak and more permeable to other large molecules such as proteins. This eventually leads to total dysregulation of the glomerulus and, ultimately, CKD [72]. Diabetic kidney disease is the leading cause of CKD worldwide and affects over 40% of patients diagnosed with TIIDM [73].

The overall increase in adiposity in obesity in patients with TIIDM is also correlated with an increase in kidney stone formation. Due to the increased levels of circulating adipokines released by the engorged adipocytes, these patients have an overall inflamed profile that results in higher levels of oxidative stress that can lead to the development of nephrolithiasis or kidney stones. Chronic kidney stone formation can also affect glomerular filtration rate and lead to CKD [70]. This increase in oxidative stress further upregulates inflammation in a positive feedback loop that can eventually lead to CKD and more serious pathology.

Advanced diabetes-related kidney disease is more prevalent in women than in men. However, men have a greater risk of onset. This difference may stem from how diabetes negates the protective qualities of estrogen. The effects of TIIDM on testosterone are unknown but do not appear to lead to progression of diabetes-related kidney disease. Women with TIIDM appear to have diabetic kidney disease more severely than men [74–76]. Obesity-related CKD that does not coincide with metabolic abnormalities is more prominent in men than women [77]. Estrogen may prevent kidney dysregulation in women, but these protective effects are negated in women with metabolic abnormalities.

5.4 Cancer

Approximately 14% of cancer deaths in men and 20% of cancer deaths in women can be attributed to obesity [78]. This can be related to the activation of signaling pathways in adipocytes which lead to secretion of low levels of inflammatory cytokines by the adipocytes, thereby leading to low-grade inflammatory responses throughout the body in locations where fat is most present [78]. Similarly, obesity increases endoplasmic reticulum stress resulting in oxidative stress, the unfolded protein response, and the upregulation of additional inflammatory cytokines [78]. These different inflammatory mechanisms can all contribute to the formation and progression of cancer, making obesity a deadly player in the onset of certain cancers.

The incidence of certain sex-linked cancers, such as breast cancer, may be upregulated in obese patients. In women specifically, the dysregulation of hormones that is linked with obesity can exacerbate the onset of breast cancer [79].

Non-sex-linked cancers, such as liver cancer, may also have an increased risk in relation to obesity [78]. The obesity-related development of nonalcoholic fatty liver disease (NAFLD), nonalcoholic steatohepatitis (NASH), and NASH-related cirrhosis are also associated with an increased risk of hepatocellular carcinoma [78]. By affecting both sex-linked and non-sex-linked cancers, obesity's wide range of potential effects on tumor initiation and progression could contribute to an increased prevalence of cancer in obese patients.

A meta-analysis of cohort studies done by Larsson and Wolk found that obese individuals had an 89% increased risk of liver cancer [80]. However, the relative risk for liver cancer was significantly higher in men than in women, indicating that there may be hormone-dependent mechanisms at play [80]. Secretion of proinflammatory cytokines including IL-6, IL-8, IL-10, and IL-17 by hypertrophic adipocytes triggers an inflammatory cascade in the liver [81]. Damage induced by these inflammatory mediators can cause carcinogenesis. Further, the AMPK-TORC1 pathway that regulates autophagy is decreased by obesity and hypernutrition [81]. The decrease in the autophagy pathway causes a decrease in the clearance of damaged cellular organelles which can further induce inflammation and carcinogenesis.

Obesity may be a driving force in sex-related cancers such as prostate cancer and breast cancers in men and women. In women, obesity is related to a higher incidence of pre-menopausal triple-negative breast cancers, while ER-positive breast cancers had a higher incidence among postmenopausal women [82]. This is suggested in that breast cancer progression in pre-menopausal obese women is not affected by high amounts of systemic estrogen. However, in postmenopausal women, with normally low circulating estrogen levels, the incidence in ER-positive breast cancer increases. Additionally, the obesity associated risk with triple-negative breast cancer in postmenopausal women is inversely associated with obesity [82]. Among men, obesity and BMI are strong risk factors for male breast cancer [83]. Studies have shown that male breast cancer tumors show an increase in the estrogen and progesterone receptors [84]. The hormone aromatase, produced by the adipose tissue, plays a role in increasing estrogen levels by converting testosterone into estrogen and can therefore exacerbate breast cancer in obese men.

In summary, studies have indicated that there are sex-related differences in relation to obesity and the onset of cancer, specifically in response to breast cancers. Low-grade inflammation as a result of obesity seems to be an underlying cause of the disruption of important protective pathways, contributing to the initiation and/or progression of cancer.

5.5 Neurodegeneration

Neurodegeneration involves the gradual breakdown of the nervous system and causes anxiety, dysphoria, apathy, disinhibition, and euphoria [85]. Alzheimer's disease, (AD) the most common neurodegenerative disease and the sixth leading cause of death in the United States, is the cause of death in one in three seniors living in the United States [86]. It is estimated that 5.7 million Americans are affected by Alzheimer's, two-thirds of which are women [86]. Currently AD is the only unpreventable, untreatable disease of the top 10 leading causes of death in the United States [86]. While the cause of Alzheimer's may be unknown, research has shown strong links between neurodegeneration and obesity.

AD and other dementias occur more commonly in women than in men worldwide suggesting that there may be some sex-specific hormonal influences to the progression of the disease [87]. Although the specific hormonal influences are not known, men may have a certain ability to protect themselves against the severity of neurodegeneration, or women may simply lose their ability to do so. As awareness increases, TIIDM is becoming recognized as a contributor to the risk of developing AD [88]. The widespread association between TIIDM and neurodegenerative diseases may eventually wind up providing a link between the two. With the expected population diagnosed with diabetes reaching 573 million within 12 years by the World Health Organization, research into the implications of diabetes and other overnutrition illness is becoming essential [89].

Neurodegeneration related to over nutrition has been shown to have profound implications on the functionality of the central nervous system and cerebral functions in particular. Recently, the IKK-beta/NF-kappaB pathway has been shown to be triggered by overnutrition, leading to inflammation of the hypothalamus and other CNS peripheral tissues [90]. This is critical because the hypothalamus is responsible for regulating functions such as energy balance as well as controlling some metabolic activities related to the sympathetic and parasympathetic nervous systems [90]. This inflammation due to overnutrition has been deemed "metabolic inflammation" [90].

A diet that is high in fat may contribute to the progression of neurodegeneration through increased fatty acid uptake. Saturated fatty acids cause activation of the immune system through Toll-like receptor 4 (TLR4), leading to the production of cytokines by astrocytes [91]. This thereby induces an inflammatory response that could lead to damage of the hypothalamus. Additionally, loss of normal function of the TLR4 increases and encourages diet-induced obesity [91]. This positive feedback loop would encourage inflammation while also sustaining the nutrient- and fat-rich environment in which it was produced. Microglia, macrophages in the brain, produce inflammasomes in diseased states such as obesity and TIIDM [91]. Therefore, any inflammation already pre-existing in the body due to obesity would only encourage self-damaging signaling cascades. These processes hijack the body's natural defense mechanisms to further the progression of neurodegeneration.

Advanced glycation end products, or AGEs, are markers of carbonyl stress due to oxidative stress, and their formation is irreversible and leads to protein deposits and amyloidosis [92]. Unnatural amyloid deposits in critical areas of the central nervous system can result in irregularities of normal functioning, and AGE formation seems to occur early in the stages of plaque formation in connection with AD [92]. AGE leads to a release of free radicals that are associated with the oxidation of sugars which eventually can lead to site-specific attacks of proteins and lipid peroxidation [92]. Additionally, when AGEs induce the expression of AGE cell surface receptors (RAGE), superoxide radicals and hydrogen peroxide are released, further contributing to cytotoxic effects on cells and inflammation [92]. The combination of these effects continues to incite an inflammatory response and furthers the progression of the neurodegenerative diseases and other neurological damages. These findings support the claim that hyperglycemia-derived AGEs constitute a crucial link between diabetes and AD [91].

Diabetes mellitus may serve as a very relevant risk factor for AD. This link may be due to the existence of insulin resistance in both patients affected by TIIDM and in neural cells [93]. Insulin receptors activate receptor tyrosine kinases which in turn phosphorylate insulin receptor subtypes 1 and 2 [93]. The interaction of these receptors with Src domains allows for several protective processes to occur and promote cellular division and longevity of healthy cells [93]. Cells that are deficient in this receptor, or that cannot express sufficient amounts, are subsequently at risk for diminished functioning capabilities. Furthermore, insulin specifically binds to the respective receptors to initiate different functions, so the expression of both receptors is vital to cellular functioning [93]. In the brain, the highest levels of insulin are found in the hypothalamus, temporal lobe, and cerebellum [93]. A lack of the protecting effects of insulin may explain why the hypothalamus is classically inflamed in conditions of obesity.

Obesity-associated low-grade inflammation seems to be an underlying cause in the progression of neurodegenerative diseases, specifically AD. While there seem to be sex-related differences in the relationship between neurodegeneration and obesity, more research is needed to identify what the exact cause is. Nevertheless, the correlation between neurodegeneration, TIIDM, and obesity is apparent, and further research is needed to elucidate this mechanism.

5.6 Infertility

Infertility is defined as the inability of a couple to conceive after 12 months or more of regular, unprotected sex [94]. There can be many causes of infertility, but an emerging comorbidity and risk factor is obesity. Obesity can affect reproduction and development by altering sex hormones, sex cells, and different genes within the sex cells. These alterations can be found in both men and women; however, the effects differ slightly. Both sexes exhibit an increase of the androgen sex hormone [95, 96]. Obese men and women are also shown to produce less sex cells overall [97]. A 2015 epidemiological study found that over 100 genes that were related to infertility were also related to obesity [95, 96]. Furthermore, genes that support sex cell maturation and function have been shown to be altered with an increase in adiposity [98]. Maintaining a healthy body weight can help normalize these factors of reproduction, while obesity can cause reproductive alterations that can result in infertility.

5.6.1 Males

Infertility in males is linked to decreased viable sperm count, sperm motility, or supporting sex hormones. When compared to men with a normal body mass index (BMI) of 20–25 kg/m^2, obese men with a BMI greater than 25 kg/m^2 showed a decrease in concentration of the number of sperm per milliliter of ejaculatory fluid, a decrease in total sperm count in millions, and a decrease in healthy sperm cells [97]. Successful conception rates have been directly related to sperm counts; greater sperm counts correlate to an increased chance of conception, and in addition to sperm count, obesity-induced epigenetic modifications play a role in sperm-egg interaction [97]. Increased obesity-induced DNA methylation and decreased DNA acetylation affect sperm cell gene expression [99]. This change can inhibit a successful fertilization by altering embryogenesis, and this can lead to a failed pregnancy or problems in embryo development.

In males, onset of obesity correlates with an increase in estrogen and a decrease in supporting sex hormones such as testosterone, sex hormone-binding globulin (SHBG), and inhibin B [97]. SHBG is mainly produced in the liver and primarily functions by binding to and transporting sex steroids throughout the blood. Decreased SHBG protein levels have been linked to metabolic and endocrine disorders and obesity [100]. Obesity has been correlated with low secretion levels of luteinizing hormone (LH) from the pituitary gland, which induces testosterone release from the Leydig cells. In a healthy male, after testosterone secretion, a majority of the steroid would bind to SHBG and then travel to various androgen receptors throughout the male body, with small levels being converted to estrogen via aromatase. However, obese patients tend to have a greater aromatase activity and therefore have higher levels of estrogen than nonobese men [99]. An increase in metabolism of free testosterone to estrogen can lead to decreased testicular sensitivity to LH, further leading to high estrogen and low testosterone levels [99]. This creates a negative feedback loop, ultimately leading to a decrease in sperm production.

Inhibin B is a glycoprotein produced by Sertoli cells that aids in regulating follicle-stimulating hormone (FSH) in a negative feedback manner [101]. When spermatogenesis appears to be elevated based on activity of the hypothalamic-pituitary-gonadal hormone (HPG), this indicates a high sperm count due to FSH secretions. Inhibin B will regulate FSH levels based on HPG status which modulates sperm concentration. An inhibin B study found that a negative correlation between sperm count and inhibin B was revealed [101]. Inhibin B activity is high when sperm count is concentrated; infertile men often have very low levels of inhibin B; this relationship indicates further exacerbation of infertility and low sperm count. Decreased gonadal function in obese men has been characterized by lower levels of inhibin B even though FSH levels remain similar before and after weight loss [102]. Therefore, while obese males have similar levels of FSH to nonobese males, the high aromatase activity converts much of the testosterone to estrogen, thereby inhibiting spermatogenesis and decreasing fertility [103].

Lastly, in healthy males, the scrotum usually is about 2–3°C lower than body temperature, which is essential for sperm storage, health, and motility [104]. Obesity can also result in increased scrotum temperatures which can lead to infertility [104]. The changes associated with obesity-induced infertility can be circumvented by weight loss [104]. Staying healthy and maintaining a moderate BMI can help regulate hormone and sex cell secretions and promote fertility.

5.6.2 Females

Obesity in females can lead to infertility by decreasing oocyte quality, altering ovulation, and affecting developmental factors. The mitochondria and mitochondrial oxidative phosphorylation are essential to oocyte maturation, fertilization, and implantation [105]. It has been shown that mice lacking the mitochondrial replication protein, TFAM, are embryonic lethal and reduced levels of TFAM cause decreased fertility [106]. The effects of high-fat diet (HFD) on obesity are summarized in Grindler et al. but briefly show that HFD-induced obesity alters mitochondrial function and mitochondrial membrane potential, increases reactive oxygen species, and decreases mitochondrial DNA copy number in oocytes which indicates damaged and unhealthy oocytes [105]. Regular diets with less fat would minimize mitochondrial dysfunction and oxidative damage to oocytes and keep them viable.

Menstrual abnormalities contributing to infertility like anovulation are seen in obese women [107]. SAT plays a role in regulating anovulation, whereas VAT plays more of a role in proinflammatory secretions [108]. Regulating fat intake can improve chances of conception by regulating menstrual cycles and oocyte development. Further, the proinflammatory secretions from VAT create a positive feedback loop causing more inflammation and more ovulation complications. The changes in ovulation and the increased levels of inflammatory cytokines exacerbate infertility in females.

Regulation of the follicular environment is necessary for oocyte development, and obesity changes the follicular environment and consequently the oocyte gene expression which contribute to infertility [109]. Leptin is typically elevated in obese patients and can cause negative changes to the follicular environment. Interestingly, women with higher BMI have higher levels of lactate, triglycerides, and CRP and decreased levels of SHGB in their follicular fluid, compared to normal-weight women, which can be linked to decreased oocyte viability and an inhospitable environment for oocyte development [109]. In addition, the same decrease in SHBG seen in obese men was seen in obese women [109]. This decrease in SHBG expression would lead to decreased transport of estrogen and thereby decreased oocyte development. This suggests that secretions from adipose tissues could be contributing to decreased oocyte function. Further, when oocytes were extracted from women of BMIs considered normal, overweight, and obese, fewer oocytes were obtained from the women in the obese category with a BMI of greater than 30 kg/m^2 [109]. Taken together this data indicates that obesity impairs oocyte development.

The increase in C-reactive protein suggests that systemic inflammation can also affect fertility and oocyte development [109]. High amounts of inflammatory secretions such as C-reactive protein seen in obese women contribute to decreased fertility. Obesity-induced inflammation presents damaging effects to oocytes and contributes to infertility. Obesity decreases chances of healthy oocyte fertilization and implantation. Couples will have a better chance at conception and successful pregnancy if a healthy weight is maintained.

5.7 Stress

Obesity and stress cause a vicious positive feedback loop to cause more obesity and stress. Outside stressors activate the sympathetic nervous system and the hypothalamic-pituitary-adrenal (HPA) axis. When these systems are dysregulated by continuous stress, the hyperactivity causes health issues, such as obesity [110]. Under normal conditions, the HPA axis is needed to maintain energy and metabolic homeostasis through modulating hormones such as insulin and leptin [111]. When activated, the sympathetic nervous system will cause secretion of epinephrine and norepinephrine from the adrenal gland, and the HPA axis will release cortisol. Negative feedback mechanisms inhibit the HPA axis from continuously secreting cortisol and maintaining alterations in metabolism [112]. Homeostatic fluctuation of the HPA axis controls metabolism; however, stress and inflammation alter this feedback loop and contribute to metabolic dysfunction.

Obesity-induced inflammation has also been correlated with an increase in the HPA axis function. Cortisol can increase leptin levels and inhibit leptin from suppressing appetite, or cortisol can induce neuropeptide Y release, which stimulates fat growth [110]. Therefore, cortisol can increase fat deposition. The origin of cortisol, from stress or normal homeostatic activation, and the obesity status play a role in fat deposition. For example, stress-induced increases in cortisol levels cause women to gain more weight compared to non-stressed women with the same cortisol levels. Further, elevated cortisol levels in overweight women cause increased weight gain at a faster pace than women with average weight and similar elevated cortisol levels [110]. The correlation between cortisol and weight gain in men appears to be related more to weight gain than to increases in cortisol levels, and the increased cortisol production seen in men could be further stimulated by the inflammatory cytokines secreted in fat tissues [110]. Together, this data suggests gender differences in cortisol-induced adiposity.

Stress can affect choice of food intake differently in males and females by modulating appetite. While most individuals were seen to eat less in high stress, individuals were seen to eat more in continuous low or moderate stress levels [113]. This suggests that prolonged moderate stress could contribute more to obesity than high stress in a shorter time period. Not only does stress increase appetite for some people, but it also affects food choice. Individuals under stress were seen to increase the intake of higher-calorie "comfort foods" in replacement of vegetables [111]. These findings support the role of stress-induced weight gain in chronically stressed people.

Ideas of self-image, ideal weight, or body shape also lead to increased stress. The ideas of normal or desired body image are found everywhere and are often unrealistic and idealized. The role of weight based stigmas and how they differ in males and females offer inconclusive results [114]. In a recent study by Sattler et al., weight-based stigmas in obese population caused weight gain and a decreased desire to exercise in females more than males [114]. Females with weight-associated stigmas had less motivation to participate in physical activities, while males had more motivation to exercise [114]. These stigmas can cause increases in stress levels and cortisol release and may actually have a negative impact on exercise and weight loss in obese patients. The idea that this weight stigma differentially affects males and females is important to understand, in order to effectively motivate overweight and obese males and females to exercise and to lose weight. This data suggests that the stress of ideal body image can also negatively affect stress-induced adiposity.

Stress and obesity combined contribute to fat growth, changes in appetite, and additional stress. The negative self-image, depression, or anxiety that obese people have provides the stress for prolonged HPA axis activation and increased adiposity.

6. Conclusion

Obesity plagues approximately 70% of US adults. Obese adipose tissue is responsible for releasing proinflammatory cytokines throughout the body as well as dysregulating glucose-regulating hormones. Chronic obese adiposity puts the body in a state of chronic inflammation which leads to numerous diseases including CVD, TIIDM, MetS, cancer, neurodegeneration, and infertility (**Figure 2**). Sex differences play a role in regulating the prevalence of disease, causing sexual dimorphism in diseases and disease pathogenesis in men than women. The role of the sex hormones, estrogen, and testosterone should be further explored in order to most effectively treat obese patients and their numerous pathophysiologies.

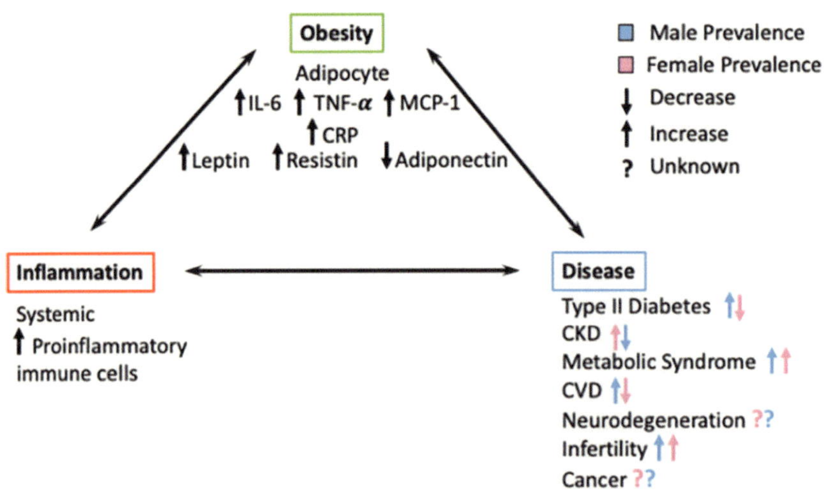

Figure 2.
The relationship between obesity, inflammation, and disease. Obesity, inflammation, and chronic diseases cause a vicious cycle, each exacerbating the other. Inflammatory cytokines and adipokines are produced systemically and by adipocytes, respectively, and play a role in exacerbating disease states. Prevalence of disease caused by inflammation and obesity varies between men and women, and sex differences may be due to the proposed protective nature of the primary female sex hormone, estrogen.

Acknowledgements

We would like to thank the UAB BMD faculty and staff for their support while writing this book chapter.

Author details

Sari Terrazas[1], Lauren Brashear[1], Anna-Katherine Escoto[1], Shannon Lynch[1], Dylan Slaughter[1], Neena Xavier[2], Norman Robert Estes II[1] and Samantha Giordano-Mooga[1]*

1 Biomedical Sciences Program, Department of Clinical and Diagnostic Sciences, University of Alabama at Birmingham, Birmingham, Alabama, USA

2 Physician's Assistant Program, Department of Clinical and Diagnostic Sciences, University of Alabama at Birmingham, Birmingham, Alabama, USA

*Address all correspondence to: sgiordan@uab.edu

References

[1] Ogden CL, Carroll MD, Flegal KM. Prevalence of obesity in the United States. Journal of the American Medical Association. 2014;**312**(2):189-190

[2] Gallagher D et al. Healthy percentage body fat ranges: An approach for developing guidelines based on body mass index. The American Journal of Clinical Nutrition. 2000;**72**(3):694-701

[3] Hamilton MT, Hamilton DG, Zderic TW. Role of low energy expenditure and sitting in obesity, metabolic syndrome, type 2 diabetes, and cardiovascular disease. Diabetes. 2007;**56**(11):2655-2667

[4] Krotkiewski M et al. Impact of obesity on metabolism in men and women. Importance of regional adipose tissue distribution. The Journal of Clinical Investigation. 1983;**72**(3):1150-1162

[5] Wozniak SE et al. Adipose tissue: The new endocrine organ? A review article. Digestive Diseases and Sciences. 2009;**54**(9):1847-1856

[6] Schoettl T, Fischer IP, Ussar S. Heterogeneity of adipose tissue in development and metabolic function. Journal of Experimental Biology. 2018;**221**(Pt Suppl 1):3-12

[7] Arbuthnott E. Brown adipose tissue: Structure and function. The Proceedings of the Nutrition Society. 1989;**48**(2):177-182

[8] Cannon B, Nedergaard J. Brown adipose tissue: Function and physiological significance. Physiological Reviews. 2004;**84**(1):277-359

[9] Rothwell NJ, Stock MJ. A role for brown adipose tissue in diet-induced thermogenesis. Nature. 1979;**281**(5726):31-35

[10] Cypess AM et al. Identification and importance of brown adipose tissue in adult humans. The New England Journal of Medicine. 2009;**360**(15):1509-1517

[11] Thyagarajan B, Foster MT. Beiging of white adipose tissue as a therapeutic strategy for weight loss in humans. Hormone Molecular Biology and Clinical Investigation. 2017;**31**(2):3-8

[12] Giordano S et al. Estrogen and cardiovascular disease: Is timing everything? The American Journal of the Medical Sciences. 2015;**350**(1): 27-35

[13] Fried LP et al. Association of comorbidity with disability in older women: Tthe Women's Health and Aging Study. Journal of Clinical Epidemiology. 1999;**52**(1):27-37

[14] Wang C et al. Low testosterone associated with obesity and the metabolic syndrome contributes to sexual dysfunction and cardiovascular disease risk in men with type 2 diabetes. Diabetes Care. 2011;**34**(7):1669-1675

[15] Quarta C et al. Role of sex hormones in modulation of brown adipose tissue activity. Journal of Molecular Endocrinology. 2012;**49**(1):R1-R7

[16] Lobo RA. Metabolic syndrome after menopause and the role of hormones. Maturitas. 2008;**60**(1):10-18

[17] Traish AM et al. Testosterone deficiency. The American Journal of Medicine. 2011;**124**(7):578-587

[18] Traish AM, Kypreos KE. Testosterone and cardiovascular disease: An old idea with modern clinical implications. Atherosclerosis. 2011;**214**(2):244-248

[19] Colleluori G et al. Fat mass follows a U-shaped distribution based on

estradiol levels in postmenopausal women. Frontiers in Endocrinology (Lausanne). 2018;**9**:315

[20] Jones ME et al. Aromatase-deficient (ArKO) mice accumulate excess adipose tissue. The Journal of Steroid Biochemistry and Molecular Biology. 2001;**79**(1-5):3-9

[21] Lemieux S et al. Are gender differences in cardiovascular disease risk factors explained by the level of visceral adipose tissue? Diabetologia. 1994;**37**(8):757-764

[22] Lemieux S et al. Sex differences in the relation of visceral adipose tissue accumulation to total body fatness. The American Journal of Clinical Nutrition. 1993;**58**(4):463-467

[23] Ohlson LO et al. The influence of body fat distribution on the incidence of diabetes mellitus. 13.5 years of follow-up of the participants in the study of men born in 1913. Diabetes. 1985;**34**(10):1055-1058

[24] Bjorntorp P, Rosmond R. Visceral obesity and diabetes. Drugs. 1999;**58**(Suppl 1):13-18; discussion 75-82

[25] Bjorntorp P. Metabolic abnormalities in visceral obesity. Annals of Medicine. 1992;**24**(1):3-5

[26] Han TS, Lean ME. A clinical perspective of obesity, metabolic syndrome and cardiovascular disease. JRSM Cardiovascular Disease. 2016;**5**:2048004016633371

[27] Nakamura K, Fuster JJ, Walsh K. Adipokines: A link between obesity and cardiovascular disease. Journal of Cardiology. 2014;**63**(4):250-259

[28] Manolopolos KN, Karpe F, Frayn KN. Gluteofemoral body fat as a determinant of metabolic health. International Journal of Obesity. 2010;**34**:949-959

[29] Thorand B et al. Association of cardiovascular risk factors with markers of endothelial dysfunction in middle-aged men and women. Results from the MONICA/KORA Augsburg Study. Thrombosis and Haemostasis. 2006;**95**(1):134-141

[30] Miller VM, Harman SM. An update on hormone therapy in postmenopausal women: Mini-review for the basic scientist. American Journal of Physiology. Heart and Circulatory Physiology. 2017;**313**(5):H1013-H1021

[31] Grassmann S et al. Association between peripheral adipokines and inflammation markers: A systematic review and meta-analysis. Obesity (Silver Spring). 2017;**25**(10):1776-1785

[32] Wegner A et al. Sex differences in the pro-inflammatory cytokine response to endotoxin unfold in vivo but not ex vivo in healthy humans. Innate Immunity. 2017;**23**(5):432-439

[33] Kuo SM. Gender difference in bacteria endotoxin-induced inflammatory and anorexic responses. PLoS One. 2016;**11**(9):e0162971

[34] Navarro SL et al. Factors associated with multiple biomarkers of systemic inflammation. Cancer Epidemiology, Biomarkers & Prevention. 2016;**25**(3): 521-531

[35] Khadir A et al. Gender-specific association of oxidative stress and inflammation with cardiovascular risk factors in Arab population. Mediators of Inflammation. 2015;**2015**:512603

[36] Pradhan AD. Sex differences in the metabolic syndrome: Implications for cardiovascular health in women. Clinical Chemistry. 2014;**60**(1):44-52

[37] Dandona P et al. Metabolic syndrome: A comprehensive perspective based on interactions between

obesity, diabetes, and inflammation. Circulation. 2005;**111**(11):1448-1454

[38] Moore JX, Chaudhary N, Akinyemiju T. Metabolic syndrome prevalence by race/ethnicity and sex in the United States, National Health and Nutrition Examination Survey, 1988-2012. Preventing Chronic Disease. 2017;**14**:E24

[39] WHO Collaborative Study of Cardiovascular Disease and Steroid Hormone Contraception. Haemorrhagic stroke, overall stroke risk, and combined oral contraceptives: Results of an international, multicentre, case-control study. Lancet. 1996;**348**(9026):505-510

[40] Nishizawa H et al. Androgens decrease plasma adiponectin, an insulin-sensitizing adipocyte-derived protein. Diabetes. 2002;**51**(9):2734-2741

[41] Mauvais-Jarvis F. Sex differences in metabolic homeostasis, diabetes, and obesity. Biology of Sex Differences. 2015;**6**:14

[42] Considine RV et al. Serum immunoreactive-leptin concentrations in normal-weight and obese humans. The New England Journal of Medicine. 1996;**334**(5):292-295

[43] Nookaew I et al. Adipose tissue resting energy expenditure and expression of genes involved in mitochondrial function are higher in women than in men. The Journal of Clinical Endocrinology and Metabolism. 2013;**98**(2):E370-E378

[44] Gonzalez-Granillo M et al. ERbeta activation in obesity improves whole body metabolism via adipose tissue function and enhanced mitochondria biogenesis. Molecular and Cellular Endocrinology. 2019;**479**:147-158

[45] Lo KA, Sun L. Turning WAT into BAT: A review on regulators controlling the browning of white adipocytes. Bioscience Reports. 2013;**33**(5):712-715

[46] Winham SJ, de Andrade M, Miller VM. Genetics of cardiovascular disease: Importance of sex and ethnicity. Atherosclerosis. 2015;**241**(1):219-228

[47] Klinge CM. Estrogenic control of mitochondrial function and biogenesis. Journal of Cellular Biochemistry. 2008;**105**(6):1342-1351

[48] Ziaei S, Mohseni H. Correlation between hormonal statuses and metabolic syndrome in postmenopausal women. Journal of Family & Reproductive Health. 2013;**7**(2):63-66

[49] van den Beukel JC et al. Women have more potential to induce browning of perirenal adipose tissue than men. Obesity (Silver Spring). 2015;**23**(8):1671-1679

[50] Benjamin EJ et al. Heart disease and stroke Statistics—2018 update: A report from the American Heart Association. Circulation. 2018;**137**(12):e67-e492

[51] Hajar R. Framingham contribution to cardiovascular disease. Heart Views. 2016;**17**(2):78-81

[52] Garcia M et al. Cardiovascular disease in women: Clinical perspectives. Circulation Research. 2016;**118**(8):1273-1293

[53] Preis SR et al. Neck circumference as a novel measure of cardiometabolic risk: The Framingham heart study. The Journal of Clinical Endocrinology and Metabolism. 2010;**95**(8):3701-3710

[54] Torriani M et al. Compartmental neck fat accumulation and its relation to cardiovascular risk and metabolic syndrome. The American Journal of Clinical Nutrition. 2014;**100**(5):1244-1251

[55] Rossouw JE et al. Risks and benefits of estrogen plus progestin in healthy

postmenopausal women: Principal results from the Women's Health Initiative randomized controlled trial. Journal of the American Medical Association. 2002;**288**(3):321-333

[56] Rossouw JE et al. Postmenopausal hormone therapy and risk of cardiovascular disease by age and years since menopause. Journal of the American Medical Association. 2007;**297**(13):1465-1477

[57] Micklesfield LK et al. Dual-energy X-ray performs as well as clinical computed tomography for the measurement of visceral fat. Obesity (Silver Spring). 2012;**20**(5): 1109-1114

[58] Bredella MA et al. Assessment of abdominal fat compartments using DXA in premenopausal women from anorexia nervosa to morbid obesity. Obesity (Silver Spring). 2013;**21**(12):2458-2464

[59] Fox CS et al. Abdominal visceral and subcutaneous adipose tissue compartments: Association with metabolic risk factors in the Framingham Heart Study. Circulation. 2007;**116**(1):39-48

[60] Reinehr T. Type 2 diabetes mellitus in children and adolescents. World Journal of Diabetes. 2013;**4**(6):270-281

[61] Kanehisa H et al. Cross-sectional areas of fat and muscle in limbs during growth and middle age. International Journal of Sports Medicine. 1994;**15**(7):420-425

[62] Janssen I et al. Skeletal muscle mass and distribution in 468 men and women aged 18-88 yr. Journal of Applied Physiology (1985). 2000;**89**(1):81-88

[63] DeFronzo RA, Tripathy D. Skeletal muscle insulin resistance is the primary defect in type 2 diabetes. Diabetes Care. 2009;**32**(Suppl 2):S157-S163

[64] Hotamisligil GS, Shargill NS, Spiegelman BM. Adipose expression of tumor necrosis factor-alpha: Direct role in obesity-linked insulin resistance. Science. 1993;**259**(5091):87-91

[65] Kanai F et al. Insulin-stimulated GLUT4 translocation is relevant to the phosphorylation of IRS-1 and the activity of PI3-kinase. Biochemical and Biophysical Research Communications. 1993;**195**(2):762-768

[66] Pietrani NT et al. Proresolving protein Annexin A1: The role in type 2 diabetes mellitus and obesity. Biomedicine & Pharmacotherapy. 2018;**103**:482-489

[67] Kautzky-Willer A, Harreiter J, Pacini G. Sex and gender differences in risk, pathophysiology and complications of type 2 diabetes mellitus. Endocrine Reviews. 2016;**37**(3):278-316

[68] Schrijnders D et al. Sex differences in obesity related cancer incidence in relation to type 2 diabetes diagnosis (ZODIAC-49). PLoS One. 2018;**13**(1):e0190870

[69] Ding EL et al. Sex differences of endogenous sex hormones and risk of type 2 diabetes: A systematic review and meta-analysis. Journal of the American Medical Association. 2006;**295**(11):1288-1299

[70] Lieske JC et al. Diabetes mellitus and the risk of urinary tract stones: A population-based case-control study. American Journal of Kidney Diseases. 2006;**48**(6):897-904

[71] de Vries AP et al. Fatty kidney: Emerging role of ectopic lipid in obesity-related renal disease. The Lancet Diabetes and Endocrinology. 2014;**2**(5):417-426

[72] Palatini P. Glomerular hyperfiltration: A marker of early renal damage in pre-diabetes and

pre-hypertension. Nephrology, Dialysis, Transplantation. 2012;**27**(5):1708-1714

[73] Alicic RZ, Rooney MT, Tuttle KR. Diabetic kidney disease: Challenges, Progress, and possibilities. Clinical Journal of the American Society of Nephrology. 2017;**12**(12):2032-2045

[74] Bowers JL et al. Resveratrol acts as a mixed agonist/ antagonist for estrogen receptors alpha and beta. Endocrinology. 2000;**141**(10):3657-3667

[75] Yu G, Traish AM. Induced testosterone deficiency: From clinical presentation of fatigue, erectile dysfunction and muscle atrophy to insulin resistance and diabetes. Hormone Molecular Biology and Clinical Investigation. 2011;**8**(1):425-430

[76] Yu MK et al. Risk factor, age and sex differences in chronic kidney disease prevalence in a diabetic cohort: The pathways study. American Journal of Nephrology. 2012;**36**(3):245-251

[77] Sakurai M et al. Sex differences in associations among obesity, metabolic abnormalities, and chronic kidney disease in Japanese men and women. Journal of Epidemiology. 2016;**26**(8):440-446

[78] Kolb R, Sutterwala FS, Zhang W. Obesity and cancer: Inflammation bridges the two. Current Opinion in Pharmacology. 2016;**29**:77-89

[79] Crespi E, Bottai G, Santarpia L. Role of inflammation in obesity-related breast cancer. Current Opinion in Pharmacology. 2016;**31**:114-122

[80] Larsson SC, Wolk A. Overweight, obesity and risk of liver cancer: A meta-analysis of cohort studies. British Journal of Cancer. 2007;**97**(7):1005-1008

[81] Sun B, Karin M. Obesity, inflammation, and liver cancer. Journal of Hepatology. 2012;**56**(3):704-713

[82] Picon-Ruiz M et al. Obesity and adverse breast cancer risk and outcome: Mechanistic insights and strategies for intervention. CA: A Cancer Journal for Clinicians. 2017;**67**(5):378-397

[83] Brinton LA et al. Anthropometric and hormonal risk factors for male breast cancer: Male breast cancer pooling project results. Journal of the National Cancer Institute. 2014;**106**(3):djt465

[84] Akosa A, Van Norden S, Tettey Y. Hormone receptor expression in male breast cancers. Ghana Medical Journal. 2005;**39**(1):14-18

[85] Levenson RW, Sturm VE, Haase CM. Emotional and behavioral symptoms in neurodegenerative disease: A model for studying the neural bases of psychopathology. Annual Review of Clinical Psychology. 2014;**10**:581-606

[86] Calderon-Garciduenas AL, Duyckaerts C. Alzheimer disease. Handbook of Clinical Neurology. 2017;**145**:325-337

[87] Mazure CM, Swendsen J. Sex differences in Alzheimer's disease and other dementias. Lancet Neurology. 2016;**15**(5):451-452

[88] Verdile G, Fuller SJ, Martins RN. The role of type 2 diabetes in neurodegeneration. Neurobiology of Disease. 2015;**84**:22-38

[89] Kelly T et al. Global burden of obesity in 2005 and projections to 2030. International Journal of Obesity. 2008;**32**(9):1431-1437

[90] Cai D. Neuroinflammation and neurodegeneration in overnutrition-induced diseases. Trends in Endocrinology and Metabolism. 2013;**24**(1):40-47

[91] Pugazhenthi S, Qin L, Reddy PH. Common neurodegenerative pathways in obesity, diabetes, and Alzheimer's disease. Biochimica et Biophysica Acta—Molecular Basis of Disease. 2017;**1863**(5):1037-1045

[92] Srikanth V et al. Advanced glycation endproducts and their receptor RAGE in Alzheimer's disease. Neurobiology of Aging. 2011;**32**(5):763-777

[93] de la Monte SM et al. Insulin resistance and neurodegeneration: Roles of obesity, type 2 diabetes mellitus and non-alcoholic steatohepatitis. Current Opinion in Investigational Drugs. 2009;**10**(10):1049-1060

[94] Mosher WD. Fecundity and infertility in the United States. American Journal of Public Health. 1988;**78**(2):181-182

[95] Butler MG, McGuire A, Manzardo AM. Clinically relevant known and candidate genes for obesity and their overlap with human infertility and reproduction. Journal of Assisted Reproduction and Genetics. 2015;**32**(4):495-508

[96] Butler MG et al. Currently recognized clinically relevant and known genes for human reproduction and related infertility with representation on high-resolution chromosome ideograms. Gene. 2016;**575**(1):149-159

[97] Jensen TK et al. Body mass index in relation to semen quality and reproductive hormones among 1,558 Danish men. Fertility and Sterility. 2004;**82**(4):863-870

[98] Ruebel ML et al. Obesity modulates inflammation and lipid metabolism oocyte gene expression: A single-cell transcriptome perspective. The Journal of Clinical Endocrinology and Metabolism. 2017;**102**(6):2029-2038

[99] Craig JR et al. Obesity, male infertility, and the sperm epigenome. Fertility and Sterility. 2017;**107**(4):848-859

[100] Goldstajn MS et al. Sex hormone binding globulin (SHBG) as a marker of clinical disorders. Collegium Antropologicum. 2016;**40**(3):211-218

[101] Manzoor SM et al. Serum inhibin B as a diagnostic marker of male infertility. Journal of Ayub Medical College, Abbottabad. 2012;**24**(3-4):113-116

[102] Globerman H et al. Inhibin B in men with severe obesity and after weight reduction following gastroplasty. Endocrine Research. 2005;**31**(1):17-26

[103] Huhtaniemi I. A short evolutionary history of FSH-stimulated spermatogenesis. Hormones (Athens, Greece). 2015;**14**(4):468-478

[104] Du Plessis SS et al. The effect of obesity on sperm disorders and male infertility. Nature Reviews. Urology. 2010;**7**(3):153-161

[105] Grindler NM, Moley KH. Maternal obesity, infertility and mitochondrial dysfunction: Potential mechanisms emerging from mouse model systems. Molecular Human Reproduction. 2013;**19**(8):486-494

[106] Wai T et al. The role of mitochondrial DNA copy number in mammalian fertility. Biology of Reproduction. 2010;**83**(1):52-62

[107] Hartz AJ et al. The association of obesity with infertility and related menstural abnormalities in women. International Journal of Obesity. 1979;**3**(1):57-73

[108] Kuchenbecker WK et al. The subcutaneous abdominal fat and not the intraabdominal fat compartment is associated with anovulation in

women with obesity and infertility. The Journal of Clinical Endocrinology and Metabolism. 2010;**95**(5):2107-2112

[109] Robker RL et al. Obese women exhibit differences in ovarian metabolites, hormones, and gene expression compared with moderate-weight women. The Journal of Clinical Endocrinology and Metabolism. 2009;**94**(5):1533-1540

[110] Foss B, Dyrstad SM. Stress in obesity: Cause or consequence? Medical Hypotheses. 2011;**77**(1):7-10

[111] Hryhorczuk C, Sharma S, Fulton SE. Metabolic disturbances connecting obesity and depression. Frontiers in Neuroscience. 2013;**7**:177

[112] Herman JP et al. Regulation of the hypothalamic-pituitary-adrenocortical stress response. Comprehensive Physiology. 2016;**6**(2):603-621

[113] Brownell AASKD. The stress-eating paradox: Multiple daily measurements in adult males and females. Psychology & Health. 1994;**9**:425-436

[114] Sattler KM et al. Gender differences in the relationship of weight-based stigmatisation with motivation to exercise and physical activity in overweight individuals. Health Psychology Open. 2018;**5**(1):2055102918759691

Chapter 5

The Wound-Healing Portal Hypertensive Response

Maria Angeles Aller, Javier Blanco-Rivero, Ana Arias and Jaime Arias

Abstract

Portal hypertensive inflammation is associated with chronic liver diseases. The three successive and overlapping systemic inflammatory phenotypes, i.e., neurogenic, immune, and endocrine, which characterize the wound-healing response, are expressed by the portal venous system upon liver injury. The diverse functions of hepatic stellate cells in homeostasis and inflammation indicate the versatile nature of these mesenchymal-derived cells, which could adopt numerous phenotypes according to the interstitial microenvironmental characteristics. Consequently, these inflammatory phenotypes could represent the reexpression of two extra-embryonic functional axis, i.e., coelomic-amniotic and trophoblastic-vitelline, whose coupling in the portal system would induce a gastrulation-related phenotype. Therefore, hepatic stellate cells and liver-specific mesenchymal cells could recapitulate and couple these abovementioned extra-embryonic phenotypes during portal hypertension. These hepatic cellular population, thanks to their potential ability to integrate and reexpress functions showing analogies to extra-embryonic functions, display characteristics of stem/progenitor cells. In this way, during the development of portal hypertension, hepatic stellate cells not only could reexpress extra-embryonic functions, but also could adapt themselves in order to induce a gastrulation-related process in the space of Disse. Hence, by understanding the ontogenic interactions between hepatic stellate cells and the host inflammatory response in portal hypertension, it is possible to design effective therapeutic and prophylactic strategies to avoid or reverse wound-like hypertensive response.

Keywords: liver fibrosis, extra-embryonic functions, inflammation, wound-healing, portal hypertension

1. Introduction

Portal hypertension is a frequent complication of chronic liver disease [1]. At the same time, cirrhosis represents the final stage of chronic liver disease due to any cause [2]. Cirrhosis can be defined as an advanced stage of fibrosis involving the formation of the regenerative nodule of the parenchyma surrounded and separated by fibrotic septa, a scenario also characterized by significant changes in hepatic angioarchitecture [3–5].

The cause-effect relationship existing between inflammation and fibrotic processes is so narrow that the term "inflammatory fibrosis" [6] appropriately describes multiple fibrotic diseases, including local conditions, such as wound healing [7] and liver cirrhosis [5]. Therefore, the chronic activation of the wound-healing response represents the driving force for progressive fibrosis, eventually leading to liver cirrhosis and hepatic failure [5].

2. The wound-healing response

Knowledge relating to wounding repair and healing comprises a significant fraction of the science of surgery and its specialties [8]. Wound healing is an obligatory sequence of events starting with inflammation due to a variety of stimuli [9]. In lower vertebrate tissues, regeneration can restore injured organs and even severe limbs or other body segments [10]. However, in higher vertebrates, tissue repair consists of a fibroproliferative response that usually results in a fibrotic scar [10, 11]. Regenerating vertebrates, such as zebrafish and salamanders, offer a unique example where wounds are not only resolved without the formation of a fibrotic scar, but also the wound tissue executes tissue patterning equivalent to the original process of embryonic development to restore lost tissue [11, 12].

Scarring is a frequent consequence of full-thickness mammalian wound healing [10, 13]. However, the mid-gestation fetus is capable of regenerative healing with wound healing indistinguishable from surrounding skin [14, 15]. Current therapies to minimize scarring in postnatal wound have attempted to recapitulate singular aspects of the fetal regenerative phenotype and have met with varying degrees of clinical success [14].

Cutaneous wound repair is an integration of dynamic interactive processes involving soluble mediators, formed blood elements, extracellular matrix, and parenchymal cells [10]. These processes follow a specific time sequence which is classically grouped into three interrelated phases: inflammation, proliferation with tissue formation, and tissue remodeling [16, 17]. In brief, coagulation and inflammatory cells are crucial to the initial inflammatory phase. Neutrophils and macrophages enter the fibrin-rich zone. In addition to phagocyte pathogens and tissue debris, these cells secrete a multitude of chemokines, cytokines, and growth factors. Granulation tissue—composed of macrophages, fibroblasts, and endothelial cells—is the hallmark of the proliferative phase. Reepithelization is essential for the reestablishment of tissue integrity [18]. During the remodeling phase, formation of granulation tissue ceases through apoptosis of the responsible cells. With maturation of the wound, the type III collagen deposited during the proliferative phase is slowly degraded and replaced with stronger type I collagen. Furthermore, the wound undergoes a contractile response and reduces the surface area of the scar [19].

3. The systemic wound-healing phenotypes

From a general point-of-view, the wound-healing response could be considered as a systemic inflammatory response in the body, which appears to develop through the expression of three successive and overlapping phenotypes, the neurogenic, immune, and endocrine [20]. The above-mentioned phenotypes, which characterize the evolution of the systemic inflammatory response to the injury, are focused and integrated within the interstitial space of the injured tissue or organ [7, 21, 22].

3.1 The neurogenic inflammatory phenotype

The systemic inflammatory response begins with an immediate pathological neuromuscular response that includes sensitive impairments like stress sensation, pain, analgesia, and motor alterations. In particular, these motor alterations are harmful to the skeletal muscle (fight-to-flight and withdrawal reflexes), myocardium (tachycardia), and vascular smooth muscle (vasoconstriction and vasodilation), which induces systemic and local hemodynamic impairments, including blood flow redistribution and ischemia-reperfusion [21, 22]. A common and basic pathogenic mechanism of this complex neuromuscular response would be sudden hydroelectrolytic alterations [20–22]. Consequently, there is increasing evidence that the systemic inflammatory response is actually associated with abnormal ion transport [23].

The ischemia-reperfusion phenomenon, which causes oxidative and nitrosative stress, could be responsible for exudation and the progression of interstitial edema in the injured tissues or organs [21]. While edema is being produced, the lymphatic circulation is activated [20, 22]. Since the inflammatory *interstitium* is initially hypoxic and shows metabolic anaerobic acidosis, mainly due to the accumulation of acid by-products including lactate, the hypoxic and acid environment could represent an ideal stem cell niche [24].

In the early evolutionary period of the neurogenic stress response, the hypothalamic-pituitary-adrenocortical, sympathetic-adrenal-medullary, and renin-angiotensin-aldosterone axes, with the secretion of catecholamines, glucocorticoids, and mineralocorticoids in the circulation, are activated [25, 26]. Chromaffin vesicles in adrenal medullary chromaffin cells also store granins, which can function as prohormones giving rise to bioactive peptides, some with potent antimicrobial activity [27]. Consequently, these substances are selectively accumulated in the interstitial space of the tissues suffering from ischemia-reperfusion because endothelial permeability is increased, especially in the post-capillary venules [7, 20–22] (**Table 1** and **Figure 1**).

3.2 The immune inflammatory phenotype

The immune inflammatory phenotype corresponds to the intermediate phase of systemic wound-healing response to injury. In this phase, the tissue or organ which has previously suffered ischemia-reperfusion is infiltrated by inflammatory cells and even by bacteria [22]. This infiltration occurs in an edematous oxygen-poor environment [7, 21].

Today, the inflammatory bone marrow-related response is considered both a key and complementary arm of the stress response [7, 22]. The inflammatory activation of the bone marrow stem cell niche indicates the stimulation of the hematopoietic stem cells (HSCs) and the mesenchymal stem cells (MSCs), which are both multipotent stem cells [28, 29]. HSCs are the progenitors of all blood and immune cells that infiltrate all the tissues and organs that have been previously primed by oxidative and nitrosative stress [22]. Inflammatory signaling molecules, including chemokines, interferons, tumor necrosis factor-alpha, and toll-like receptors appear to stimulate HSC proliferation in the short term [30]. In turn, interferon gamma mediates HSC stimulation in response to chronic inflammation [31].

This immune phenotype could be characterized by enzymatic stress related to intracellular digestion, i.e., autophagy [32], phagocytosis, and antigen presentation [21, 22]; and extracellular digestion, i.e., fermentation [20], all of which favor tissue tropism [7, 20]. In addition, macrophages and dendritic cells also take advantage of the lymphatic circulation activation. Macrophages migrate within the lymphatic circulation until reaching the lymph nodes where they activate lymphocytes [7, 33].

The cells that infiltrate the *interstitium* in the inflamed tissues and organs, thanks to the open microcirculatory system, acquire metabolic characteristics that transform them into tissues with great functional autonomy. Thus, leukocytes express adrenoceptors, catecholamines [34, 35], serotonin [36], pro-opiomelanocortin (POMC)

The neurogenic phenotype
Neuromuscular response
• Sensitive
○ Stress sensation, pain analgesia
• Motor
○ Skeletal muscle
○ Myocardium
○ Vascular smooth muscle
• Ischemia-reperfusion
• Oxidative and nitrosative stress
• Interstitial edema and storage of catecholamines, glucocorticoids, mineralocorticoid and granins
• Impairment of lymphatic pumping
• Increased lymphatic drainage
The immune phenotype
Inflammatory bone marrow-related response
• Hematopoietic stem cells
○ Leukocytes
• Mesenchymal stem cells
○ Resolution of the immune response
○ Enhance the regenerative potential of the tissues
Acute-phase reaction
• Positive acute-phase proteins
• Alteration in lipid metabolism
The endocrine phenotype
Proliferative inflammatory mesenchyma
• Granulation tissue
○ Angiogenesis
○ Fibrosis
• Reepithelization

Table 1.
The systemic wound-healing inflammatory phenotypes.

peptides [37], and cholinergic activity [38]. Perhaps, these are the reasons why the stress response axis can be retrieved by the immunocytes participating in the inflamed *interstitium* of tissues and organs, where the corticotrophin-releasing hormone (CRH), adrenocorticotrophin (ACTH)-like and biogenic amines are present [37].

MSCs are usually derived from bone marrow, but can also be isolated from adipose and other tissues [29]. MSCs act through complex interactions with the endogenous cells and tissues, and they may function in the multiple mechanisms of tissues [39]. MSCs in the wound bed contribute to the generation of a high-quality well-vascularized granulation tissue; they enhance reepithelialization of the wound and attenuate the formation of fibrotic scar tissue [39, 40]. Bone marrow-derived MSCs secrete molecules that inhibit the effector function of immune cells and are implicated in the resolution of inflammation [41, 42].

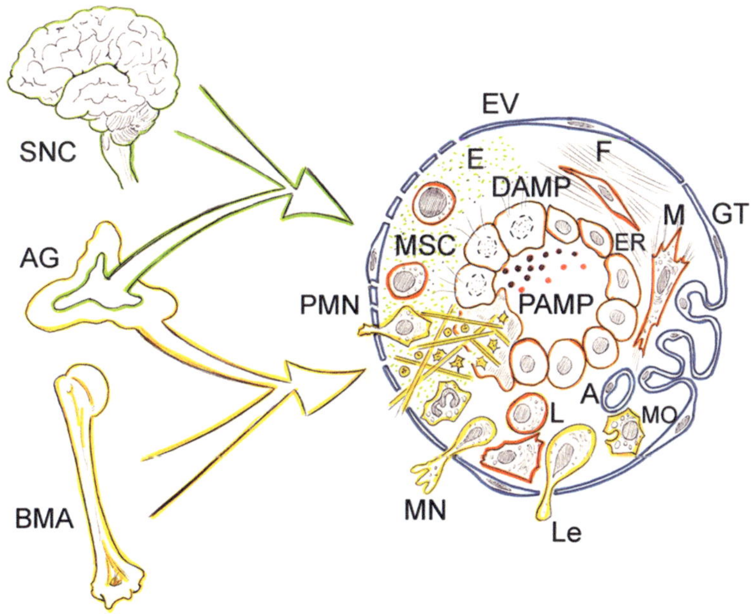

Figure 1.
The systemic wound-healing phenotypes. N: the neurogenic phenotype with sensitive and motor functions including ischemia-reperfusion and edema. A niche is created that can host stem cell-like cells. This interstitial niche accumulates molecules from the neuroendocrine stress response of the organism. I: the immune phenotype is associated with acute-phase response and an inflammatory bone marrow-related response, i.e., hematopoietic stem cells and mesenchymal stem cells. E: the endocrine phenotype. Formation of a new tissue that could execute a regenerative role or a reparative role through fibrosis. A: angiogenesis; AG: adrenal gland; BMA: bone marrow; CNS: central nervous system; DAMP: damage-associated molecular pattern; E: edema; ER: epithelial regeneration; EV: post-capillary vascular endothelium; F: fibrosis; GT: granulation tissue; L: lymphocyte; Le: leukocyte; Mo: macrophages; M: myofibroblast; MN: monocyte; MSC: mesenchymal stem cell; PAMP: pathogen-associated molecular pattern; PMN: polymorphonuclear neutrophil leukocyte; SC: stem cells.

During the expression of the immune phenotype, the acute-phase reaction becomes more prominent and exhibits diverse pathophysiological changes, including pyrexia, leukocytosis, and dramatic changes in the plasmatic concentrations of acute-phase proteins [43, 44]. Acute-phase proteins are circulating biomarkers of inflammation and are defined as either positive or negative, depending on whether they increase or decrease during the inflammatory response [43]. Positive acute-phase proteins are synthesized by hepatocytes in response to IL-6 as part of the innate immune response [45]. Positive acute-phase proteins include proteins of the coagulation-fibrinolysis system (fibrinogen, prothrombin, factor VIII, Von-Willebrand factor, complement factors plasminogen), protease inhibitors (alpha-1-antitrypsin, alpha-1-antichymotrypsin), transport proteins (ceruloplasmin, hemopexin, haptoglobin), and lipid transport proteins (serum amyloid A and serum amyloid P) [43, 44]. However, C-reactive protein is the main human acute-phase protein and one of the more sensitive markers of inflammation [44, 46].

Negative acute-phase proteins including albumin invade the *interstitium* of the injured tissues or organs through its plasmatic storage [21]. In turn, a pivotal function of the positive acute-phase proteins increases the availability of cellular free cholesterol. In particular, it has been suggested that acute-phase serum amyloid A is part of a systemic response to injury to recycle and reuse cholesterol from destroyed and damaged cells [47]. In this case, the recycling of cholesterol during serious injury could play an important role in survival [47]. In fact, the predominance of the lipid metabolism with accumulation of cholesterol in the inflamed tissue could be attributed to its role as a precursor molecule of many hormones, including aldosterone, corticoids, progesterone, androgens, and estrogens [48] and even vitamin D [49] (**Table 1** and **Figure 1**).

3.3 The endocrine inflammatory phenotype

It could be proposed that the expression of this inflammatory phenotype represents a metamorphosis through the creation of a pseudo-tissue made by a provisional parenchyma, with stem-like cells, and leukocytes, associated with a provisional stroma, i.e., coagulation and complement systems-related, which is finally transformed into a definitive tissue [50]. There is scattered evidence supporting the hypothesis that mononuclear phagocytes interact with cells with progenitor or "bona fide" stem cell properties, and that this interplay may contribute to repair and remodeling [51]. Even, it has been hypothesized that the immune system could create overriding signals that push the mesenchyme toward scarring rather than regeneration [52].

It has been proposed that the focus of the systemic phenotypes, neurogenic and immune, on the interstitial space of the injured tissue could be completed in two steps [7]. First, the upregulated neurogenic phenotype, characterized by systemic cardiovascular, hemodynamic, and hydroelectrolytic alterations, could favor the development of an interstitial niche with appropriate biochemical properties for the recruitment of cells with stem cell properties [7, 53]. In turn, the upregulated immune phenotype could mediate the inflammatory bone marrow response with an acute-phase reaction and a lipid metabolic switch linked to steroid synthesis [7]. Finally, the progressive polarization and integration of the functions that characterize both systemic inflammatory functions phenotypes, i.e., neurogenic and immune, in the injured tissue would condition the evolution of the tissue repair [7, 54].

The new tissue, a proliferative inflammatory mesenchyma, could execute a regenerative role or by default, repair through fibrosis [54, 55]. If so, several days after injury, a subset of wound fibroblasts can differentiate into myofibroblasts, which is responsible for repopulating the wounded area in parallel to angiogenesis, thus forming the granulation tissue [21]. Macrophages, fibroblasts, and blood vessels move into the wound space as a unit, suggesting an interdependence of these cells during the tissue repair [10, 51].

However, the dominating cell in this phase is the fibroblast, which fulfills different functions, such as the production of collagen and extracellular matrix substances, i.e., fibronectin, glycosaminoglycans, and proteoglycans [13]. Fibrosis is generally preceded by robust angiogenesis and vascular regression suggesting that the vascular apoptotic burden may be important to the fibrotic outcome [56, 57]. Recruited bone marrow mesenchymal cells could also transdifferentiate into epithelial cells [58] (**Figure 1**).

Therefore, the wound-healing response could be viewed as a successive and overlapping of systemic phenotypes, i.e., neurogenic and immune, which are coupled in the wounded area in order of reconstructing the injured tissue by regeneration or, by default, repairing it by fibrosis.

4. Inflammatory phenotypes and recapitulated ontogeny

Inflammation could recapitulate ontogeny by reexpressing two hypothetical extra-embryonic axes, i.e., exocoelomic-amniotic and trophoblastic-yolk sac in the interstitial space of the injured tissue [7, 22, 54]. If so, the inflammatory response could represent the postnatal debut of ancestral biochemical mechanisms that were used for normal embryonic development [22].

After fertilization, the first stage of embryogenesis is the zygote, which undergoes cleavage by mitosis. When the morula stage is reached, the embryo establishes polarity. The cells bind tightly to each other, forming a compact sphere or blastocyst, with two cell layers. The outermost layer becomes the trophoblast, giving rise to the placenta. The inner cells become the inner cell mass, giving rise to the embryo and the remaining structures, including the exocoelomic cavity, the amnion, yolk sac, and allantois [59]. The extra-embryonic coelom or exocoelomic cavity surrounds the blastocyst, which is composed of two structures, the amnion and the primary yolk sac. At the end of the fourth week of gestation, the developing exocoelomic cavity splits the extra-embryonic mesoderm into two layers, the somatic mesoderm, lining the trophoblast, and the splanchnic mesoderm, covering the secondary yolk sac and the embryo [60] (**Figure 2**).

The hypothetical recapitulation of these initial phases of the embryonic development during the early inflammatory response would imply the expression of functions similar to the extra-embryonic exocoelomic-amniotic and trophoblastic-yolk sac structures [22]. Accordingly, the exocoelomic-amniotic phenotype could be adopted by the inflamed *interstitium* that subsequently induces the accumulation of fluid with similar characteristics to coelomic and amniotic fluids in an environment with low pH and oxygen [60–62]. In essence, interstitial edema with high levels of proteins, in particular albumin, as well as electrolytes, metals, amino acids, antioxidants, cytokines, growth factors, and cholesterol-derived hormones would be produced in the inflammatory exudate [60–65]. In addition, the amnion is an embryonic functional axis with strong neural potential [66]. Amnion-derived multipotent progenitor cells secrete a unique combination of cytokines and growth factors, called the *amnion-derived cellular cytokine solution*, which establishes a connection between mesenchymal and epithelial cells during embryo development [67]. Furthermore, pluripotent stem cells within the amniotic fluid could be a new source for stem cell research [68] (**Figure 2**).

In turn, during trophoblast differentiation, trophoblast cells exhibit intense phagocytic activation leading to events as diverse as engulfment and destruction of extracellular material and the production of inflammatory mediators that may modulate both the immune response [69] and trophoblast invasiveness [70]. The wall of the secondary yolk sac in mammals is formed by an external mesothelial layer facing the exocoelomic cavity, a vascular mesenchyme and an endodermal layer facing the yolk sac cavity [60]. The formation of blood islands in the mesenchymal layer promotes the development of hematopoiesis and angiogenesis. Hemangioblasts found in these blood islands could generate blood cells through intermediate progenitors called hemogenic endothelial cells [71]. From the sixth week of gestation, the secondary yolk sac appears as a cystic structure covered by numerous superficial small vessels [60]. The mesothelial and endodermal layers have absorptive functions and are active in endocytosis/digestion [72]. In addition, the endodermal layer in the source of several proteins including acute-phase proteins, such as prealbumin, albumin, transferrin, and α_1-antitrypsin [73], as well as α-fetoprotein, which is produced by both the adult and fetal liver [60, 71]. A major function of the yolk sac is carbohydrate, protein, and lipid accumulation for embryo nutrition (*vitellum*) [74]. The yolk sac, therefore, provides lipids and lipid-soluble nutrients to embryos during the early phases of development [74].

It could be considered that the trophoblastic-yolk sac-related phenotype could favor the regulation of lipid metabolism genes [75], the hematopoietic-cell derived control with recruitment of immune cells and the induction of an angiogenic switch [71] to enable new tissue immunological tolerance during the inflammatory response [22]. In addition, through the synthesis and release of acute-phase

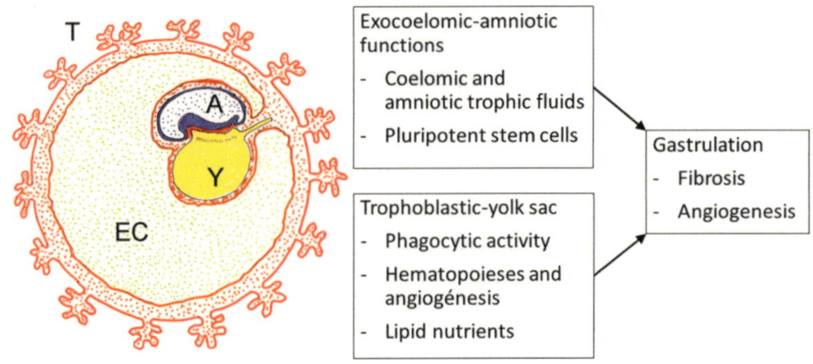

Figure 2.
The recapitulated extra-embryonic functions in the portal hypertensive inflammatory response. Inflammation could recapitulate ontogeny by reexpressing two hypothetical extra-embryonic axes: the exocoelomic-amniotic axis and the trophoblastic-yolk sac axis in the interstitial space of the injured tissue. The interstitial integration of both pathological axes into the injured tissues and organs could finally induce a gastrulation-like process, which contributes to develop a new tissue by regeneration and/or by scarring. A: amnion; EC: exocoelomic cavity; T: trophoblast; Y: yolk sac.

proteins, this extra-embryonic phenotype could reduce oxidative, nitrosative, and enzymatic stress, activate the complement-coagulation system, regulate the lipid metabolism [74], and favor phagocytosis [69, 70, 72], a specific form of endocytosis primarily associated with nutrition in unicellular organisms and with innate and adaptive immunity in mammals [69] (**Figure 2**).

The molecular and cellular contribution made by the above-mentioned extra-embryonic membranes, i.e., coelomic-amniotic and trophoblast-yolk sac to the intra-embryonic mesoderm, could be essential for embryo development and organogenesis [76]. Moreover, these primitive extra-embryonic structures can be internalized by the embryo at the early developmental stages [76]. Consequently, the hypothesized reexpression of the functions made by these extra-embryonic membranes during the postnatal life, when an inflammatory process is produced, could be a key process needed to repair the injured organism [7, 22, 54].

Both the coelomic-amniotic and trophoblast-yolk sac phenotypes reexpressed during the inflammatory response would therefore contribute to the formation of new tissue by regeneration and/or by scarring. Therefore, these two extra-embryonic phenotypes could act on the injured *interstitium* in a similar fashion as they act during embryonic development, using similar mechanisms [7, 22].

The hypothesized comparison between the coelomic-amniotic and trophoblastic-yolk sac phenotypes with the neurogenic and immune inflammatory phenotypes, respectively, would explain that the interstitial integration of both pathological axes in the injured tissues and organs could finally induce a gastrulation-like process [54] (**Figure 3**). It could be accepted that the above-mentioned extra-embryonic phenotypes are internalized during gastrulation to create the intra-embryonic mesoderm [76]. Gastrulation is the first major shape change of the developing embryo. In this development phase, the three embryogenic germ layers, i.e., ectoderm, mesoderm, and endoderm, are delineated [37]. Afterward, mesenchymal-epithelial transitions occur to create a secondary epithelium as part of somitogenesis. Then commitment and diversification of cells forming mesoendodermal structures are produced [77, 78]. The concept that fibroblasts are simple residual embryonic mesenchymal cells explains the incorrect and often interchangeable substitution of the term *fibroblast* for *mesenchymal cell* [78]. The vast arrangement of the mesenchyma, in the extra- and intra-embryonic structures, suggests an important role of the mesenchyma in orchestrating embryo development. In addition, mesenchymal stem cells are a versatile group of cells derived from mesodermal progenitors and can be found in several fetal and adult tissues [28–39].

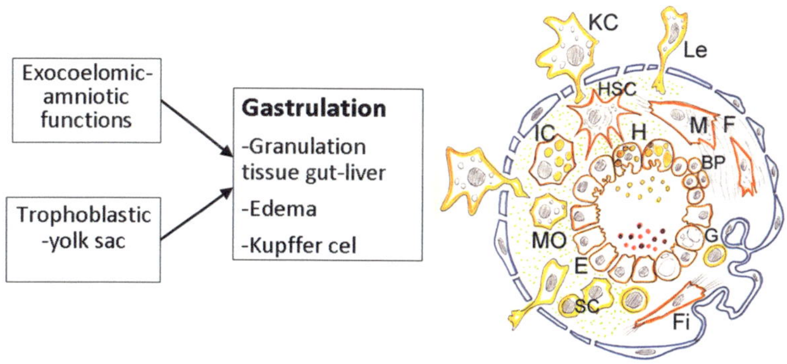

Figure 3.
The reexpression of the two hypothetical extra-embryonic axes. The exocoelomic-amniotic axis and the trophoblastic-yolk sac axis in the interstitial splanchnic space; i.e., the gut-liver axis. The interstitial activation of these two extra-embryonic axes induce a gastrulation-like process, which causes portal fibrosis and steatosis in the liver while in the gastrointestinal tract an excessive angiogenic response is produced. BP: biliary proliferation; E: enterocyte; F: fibrosis; Fi: fibroblasts; G: goblet cell; KC: Kupffer cell; H: hepatocyte; HSC: hepatic stellate cell; IC: Ito cell; Le: leukocyte; Mo: macrophages; MF: myofibroblasts; SC: stem cells.

5. The portal hypertensive inflammatory response: an ontogenic recapitulation

The portal venous system includes all veins that carry blood from the abdominal part of the alimentary tract, spleen, pancreas, and gallbladder to the liver [79]. The fetal architecture of the afferent portal venous circulation of the liver is acquired between the fourth and sixth week. At the end of this process, the portal venous system is formed from several distinct segments of the previous extra-embryonic vitelline veins. The efferent venous vessels of the liver also derive from the extra-embryonic vitelline veins [80].

The right and left paired vitelline veins transport blood from the yolk sac to the heart [80]. Hence, this type of circulation will be maintained and represented by the portal venous system; although, in this case, the blood transport is from the abdominal part of the alimentary tract, including the microbiome, spleen, pancreas, and gallbladder to the heart, but after passing through the liver [79]. Therefore, the portal venous system allows for the spatial distribution of different splanchnic functions and their coordinated integration that also is essential for the physiological functioning of the organism.

The existence of hyperpressure in the portal venous system induces the impairment of the splanchnic functions that, in addition are aggravated by the associated progression of the liver disease [81]. It could be hypothesized that chronic hemodynamic, vascular, and metabolic changes in portal hypertension could have an inflammatory origin, most probably subsequent to splanchnic inflammation [81–83]. Since, it has been proposed that the inflammatory response could recapitulate ontogeny by reexpressing the two hypothetical extra-embryonic axes, i.e., coelomic-amniotic and trophoblastic-yolk sac, in the interstitial space of the injured tissue [7, 22, 54], the splanchnic alterations related to portal hypertension could be also attributed to a recapitulation of the embryonic functions of the tissues and organs whose venous drainage is made for the portal system.

In this case, the splanchnic changes related to portal hypertension would represent the ontogenic recapitulation of the coelomic-amniotic-related (neurogenic inflammatory phenotype) and trophoblastic-yolk sac-related (immune inflammatory phenotype) functions. These functions would induce a gastrulation-like process (endocrine inflammatory phenotype), which would remodel it, since they are coupled into the *interstitium* of the splanchnic organs and tissues.

6. The reexpresion of the coelomic-amniotic-related phenotype in portal hypertension

Portal hypertension could evolve with the reexpression of the coelomic-amniotic phenotype, which begins with a pathological neuromuscular response that includes sensitive impairment, like unconscious stress sensation with autonomic dysfunction, and motor alterations including liver vasoconstriction (ischemia) and gut vasodilation (reperfusion) [1, 83]. It is noteworthy that although the mesenteric and the hepatic vascular beds share alterations in the same vasoactive pathways, they are not working in parallel [1]. Unlike the vasoconstriction in the intrahepatic vasculature, the alimentary tract vasculature undergoes a progressive vasodilation. In turn, the splanchnic vasodilation produces systemic hypotension, vascular underfilling, stimulation of endogenous vasoactive systems, including the renin-angiotensin-aldosterone system with save of Na^+ and water, plasma volume expansion, and increased cardiac index (hyperkinetic syndrome) [2, 79].

It is accepted that the hyperkinetic syndrome plays a key role in the pathogenesis of renal dysfunction and ascites in chronic liver disease [83]. Therefore, a basic pathogenic mechanism of this complex neurovascular response would be chronic hydroelectrolytic alterations [81].

The central nervous system has an initial and important influence in the evolution of portal hypertension. Chronic liver disease and portal hypertension can stimulate the hypothalamic-pituitary-adrenal axis and produce chronic secondary autonomic dysfunction [84] associated with a decreased response to vasoconstrictors, which may be caused by an increased concentration of vasodilators, including vasodilating peptides [85]. Chronic secondary autonomic dysfunction produces orthostatic hypotension, fatigue, gastrointestinal mobility disorders, with delayed gastric emptying, and prolonged transit times [84]. In addition, the central nervous system can influence immune function by stimulating the hypothalamic-pituitary-adrenal axis. It can also activate specific pathways within the sympathetic nervous system, which mainly damps down the immune phenotype triggered by the inflammatory splanchnic response [86].

The later evolution of the portal hypertensive syndrome is possibly determined by increased endothelial permeability in the gut-liver axis, which is secondary to a complex neurovascular response, that it also produces interstitial edema [81]. The increased hydrostatic pressure should preferentially drive fluid into the lymphatics, thus increasing mesenteric lymph flow [87, 88] and resulting in dilation of cistern chili [89]. It is accepted that when the high-output state of the mesenteric lymph circulation is overwhelmed, excess lymph is collected in the peritoneal cavity leading to ascites [87] and in 0.5–1% of cirrhotic patients even chylous ascites [90]. It has been proposed that decompensation related to severe hepatic insufficiency would induce an acute-on-chronic inflammatory response [81]. In this case, the splanchnic *interstitium*, the mesentery lymph, and the peritoneal mesothelium seem to create an inflammatory axis that produces ascites [91, 92].

Ascitic fluid formation is a not well-known pathogenic mechanism. However, ascitic fluid is a bioactive medium containing electrolytes, with high levels of sodium and proteins including albumin and enzymes, as well as cells including leukocytes [93]. Some of these characteristics make it similar to another bioactive medium, the amniotic fluid [94, 95]. Amniotic fluid, the protecting liquid contained in the amnion cavity, is an essential component for fetal development and maturation during pregnancy [95–97]. The hypothetical comparison of amniotic and ascitic fluid characteristics would make it worthwhile to reapproach the role of peritoneal mesothelial cells in the etiopathogeny of ascites in the portal hypertensive syndrome [81]. The functional comparison of amniotic and ascitic fluids would imply that in the decompensated portal hypertensive syndrome, the abdominal mesothelium acquires properties of the amniotic membrane or amnion. This hypothesis would imply several suggestions. For example, the intestine and, by extension, the liver, could not benefit from the supposed trophic properties of the ascitic fluid, given that peritoneal cavity-gastrointestinal tract pathway does not exist [91, 92]. In this way, the ascitic fluid could have therapeutic actions if it is administered by the enteral route in the cirrhotic patients [91, 92].

The interstitial edema in the gut-liver axis could be considered as the space where the battle of inflammation develops. In particular, during the intestinal inflammatory response secondary to portal hypertension the interstitial space increases in size as a consequence of successive infiltration suffered by plasmatic molecules, blood cells, and bacteria. The impairment of the lymph pumping and lymphangiectasia also collaborate in producing splanchnic edema [98, 99]. There is increased intestinal epithelial permeability associated with the endothelial post-capillary permeability in patients with chronic liver disease [100]. Findings of increased endotoxin and bacterial DNA in blood in patients with cirrhosis support the relevance of the increased intestinal epithelial permeability observed in these patients with portal hypertension [99, 100].

Liver and biliary tract diseases are common extra-intestinal manifestations for inflammatory bowel diseases, including gut microbiota alterations [101–105]. This is why the etiopathogenic participation of the intestinal inflammatory response cannot be excluded from the pathology produced in the hepatic parenchyma in the cases of portal hypertension. In particular, this pathophysiological mechanism occurs when portal hypertension leads to increased permeability of the sinusoidal endothelium that, in turn, causes edema in the interstitial space of Disse [106]. It is evident that the space of Disse has a connection to the interstitial space of the portal tract or space of Mall [98]. Therefore, it is likely that fluid filtered out of the inflamed sinusoids into the space of Disse flows through the channel traversing the limiting plate to reach the interstitial space of the portal tracts [98]. Interestingly enough, it was found that superphysiological or pathological levels of interstitial flow could induce fibroblast motility as well as drive myofibroblast differentiation and matrix alignment [106]. Hence, fibroblasts appear to be highly sensitive to interstitial flow and heightened flow could drive myofibroblast differentiation and extracellular matrix remodeling that recapitulates certain pathological features of cirrhosis [107]. Besides, in cases of endotoxemia, this increased interstitial flow would collaborate in the production of edema in the space of Disse. In addition, endotoxemia favors the intrahepatic lymph stasis, which may be caused by a reduction in the pumping activity of the extra-hepatic and the intrahepatic large lymph vessels [108]. In turn, the edematous interstitial space of Disse could show analogies to typical stem cell niches to retain mesenchymal stem cells or stem-like cells as well as to influence their cellular fate [109]. In this sense, the edematous space of Disse could serve as a niche of the hepatic stellate cells because of their mesodermal origin [109].

7. The reexpression of the trophoblastic-yolk sac-related phenotype in portal hypertension

An array of functions made up by the secondary yolk sac seems to be expressed by the organism when it suffers portal hypertension. In rats with prehepatic portal hypertension, the reexpression of this extra-embryonic phenotype by the splanchnic tissues and organs is coupled with the upregulation of the immune cells [2, 110, 111], as well as with the development of dyslipidemia and hepatic steatosis [112, 113].

Prehepatic portal hypertension is one factor determining bacterial intestinal translocation to mesenteric lymph nodes [111, 114]. In addition, the increased presence of mast cells in the hypertrophied mesenteric lymph nodes [115] would not only collaborate in the production of mesenteric adenitis [111], but also would constitute a source of inflammatory mediators located between the intestine and systemic blood circulation [116]. The mesenteric lymph nodes are key structures involved in the gut-associated lymphoid tissue (GALT) [117]. GALT constitutes the largest lymphoid organ of the body, and its activation in portal hypertensive enteropathy results in the release of several inflammatory mediators. These mediators would be transported by the intestinal lymph nodes to the pulmonary circulation inducing an inflammatory phenotype and later to the systemic circulation [91, 118, 119].

In response to bacterial translocation, gut epithelial cells release chemokines that induce the recruitment of dendritic cells to the mucosae [100, 114]. Once activated, mature intestinal dendritic cells can induce and prime mucosal and mesenteric lymph nodes, B and T cells [100, 114]. After maturation, these B and T cells are released into the blood stream and, due to surface expression of the specific homing markers, home back to reside within the lamina propria [114]. In addition, aberrant intestinal T lymphocytes homing to the liver may contribute to trigger immune hepatic damage [100]. Moreover, data from the literature indicate a relationship between the gut microbiota and the intestinal stem cells. Thus, lipopolysaccharide-sensitive cell types can be seen within bone marrow-derived cells which are involved in the development of inflammation in the adipose tissue of obese and type 2-diabetic mice [120]. Intestinal epithelial cells not only produce and release mediators affecting immune cells, but they also respond to factors produced by the subjacent immune cells [121]. In addition to the damage of intestinal epithelial cells, intestinal epithelial barrier dysfunction can result from loss of junctional complex integrity with increased paracellular permeability [100].

Nowadays, there have been various reports suggesting the role of gut flora and bacterial translocation in the pathogenesis of portal hypertension and chronic liver disease [101, 102, 122]. Translocated bacterial products could activate Kupffer cells through pattern recognition receptors such as toll-like receptors (TLRs) and NOD-like receptors (NLRs). Recent studies suggested that TLR4 signaling can be activated not only by pathogen-associated molecular patterns (PAMPs), but also by some endogenous ligands or damage-associated molecular patterns (DAMPs), which are released from damaged cells [123, 124]. In turn, activated Kupffer cells significantly increase their release of oxidative and nitrosative stress species and proinflammatory cytokines, including chemokines [101].

Chemokine expression by Kupffer cells, hepatic stellate cells, and sinusoidal endothelial cells drive the migration of immune cells populations [125]. In particular, CXCL12 (SDF-1α), which binds to the CXCR4 receptor, regulates several pathological responses. CXCL12 is crucial in early embryogenesis, hematopoiesis, and angiogenesis, as well as maintenance of the bone marrow stem cell niche [125]. In addition, the liver with its dual arterial and venous blood supply has a low oxygen tension, which has worsened during portal hypertension leading to hypoxic environment that could stimulate CXCL12 production with recruitment of immune cells [125].

Hepatic macrophages hold a central position in the pathogenesis of chronic liver injury. Resident hepatic macrophages or self-renewing embryo-derived local macrophages, i.e., Kupffer cells, appear essential for initiating inflammatory response while infiltrating bone marrow-derived macrophages originated from circulating monocytes are linked to chronic inflammation and fibrogénesis [126]. However, after local differentiation into resident macrophages they could restore liver integrity and then are termed restorative macrophages [126].

In the yolk sac, the blood islands are generated by mesodermal cell aggregates that differentiate into both hematopoietic and endothelial cells [127]. The simultaneous appearance of these two lineages suggests the existence of a common ancestral precursor for endothelial and hematopoietic cells: the hemangioblast [128]. In addition, the embryo could generate their definitive hematopoiesis from a hemogenic endothelium derived from a transient mesenchymal population [126, 127]. This close physiological ontogenic association between hematopoiesis and angiogenesis could persist during the pathophysiological response that produces portal hypertension. In this case, during the evolution of portal hypertensive pathology, the gut-liver axis could recapitulate the functions derived from the mesenchymal-angiogenic-hematopoietic axis that form the blood islands in the yolk sac [125, 127].

It has been suggested that mast cells could mediate the pathogenic relationship between portal hypertension and the angiogenic hyperactivity that occurs in experimental portal hypertension, particularly in the alimentary tract [110, 115]. The formation of new blood vessels is a key mechanism in the pathogenesis of portal hypertension [129]. Although the precise mechanisms by which the angiogenesis-associated response in portal hypertension is modulated remain to be defined, several mediators produced by mast cells are involved in angiogenesis [110]. This is the reason why it has been proposed that the angiogenic hyperactivity occurring in portal hypertension could mainly be mediated by mast cells [110, 115]. In addition, the exceeding angiogenesis through the neoformed collateral circulation allows portal blood flow to directly reach the systemic circulation [79]. However, the morphological vascular alterations stand out in the chronic portal hypertensive enteropathy [130]. The exacerbated angiogenesis produced in the intestinal wall during the evolution of portal hypertension is similar to the process of vasculogenesis that occurs in the extra-embryonic membranes [131]. More explicitly, the endothelial cells of the blood islands expand to cover the entire yolk sac creating a vascular network known as the capillary plexus [131], the precursor of the vitelline veins which, in turn, are the embryonic origin of the portal system [80].

From an ontogenic point of view, vitellogenesis plays a vital role in providing lipids and lipid-soluble nutrients to embryos [132]. The ability to transport fat in the form of lipoproteins through the circulatory system by eukaryotes is one of the most significant functions right from the beginning of existence [133]. Thus, the evolutionary advancement of storing energy in the form of fat has provided organisms with enormous advantages for adapting to environmental and developmental changes [134].

We have previously shown that prehepatic portal hypertension in the rat induces liver steatosis and causes changes in lipid and carbohydrate metabolisms similar to those produced in chronic inflammatory conditions described in metabolic syndrome in humans [112, 113, 135]. It has been suggested that in experimental prehepatic portal hypertension, the liver could constitute a kind of yolk sac in which the animal carries out a pathological deposit of lipids [81, 92]. Prehepatic portal hypertension in the rat, both in short- (1 month) and in the long-term (1 year), produces hepatic accumulation of triglycerides and cholesterol [112, 113]. Nonetheless, the mechanisms by which portal hypertension could induce liver steatosis are not finally understood [135] (**Figure 4**).

Inflammation, and the concomitant acute-phase response, induces marked changes in the lipoprotein profile [136]. Thus, in the prehepatic portal hypertensive rat, liver steatosis is associated with the plasmatic increase of low density lipoprotein (LDL) and lipopolysaccharide binding protein (LBP) as well as a reduction of high-density lipoproteins (HDL) [135]. In turn, hepatic steatosis might play a key role in the pathogenesis of cardiovascular disease through the systemic release of several inflammatory mediators and/or through the production of insulin resistance and atherogenic dyslipidemia [137, 138].

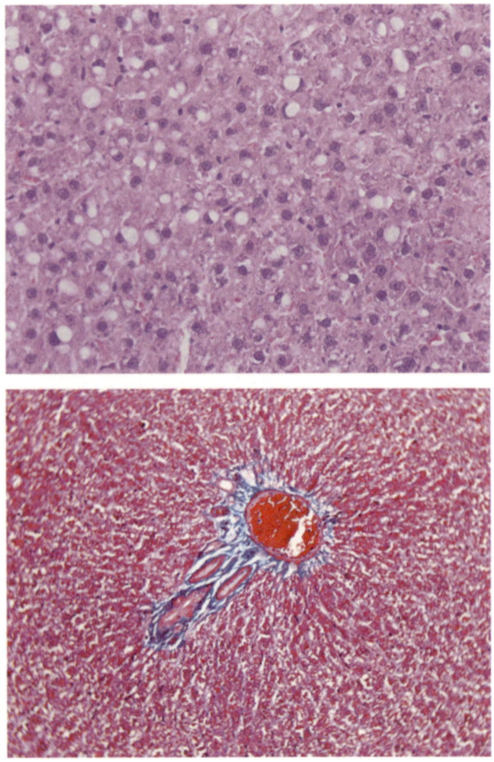

Figure 4.
Histopathological images of rat liver with long-term portal hypertension (3 months). The liver presents diffuse steatosis (superior) and portal fibrosis (inferior) as the result of splanchnic and systemic inflammatory responses. This inflammatory process could be proposed as the representation of the recapitulated extra-embryonic functions in the splanchnic area when portal hypertension is developed.

Gut microbiota could alter nutrient absorption, energy homeostasis, and intestinal permeability, with a translocation of bacteria-derived products to the liver. It could also cause hepatocellular inflammation and nonalcoholic fatty liver disease (NAFLD) [105, 139]. Western diet seems to cause dysbiosis, i.e., vitellogenic microbiome, which affects host gastrointestinal metabolism and contributes to higher incidences of metabolic syndrome, including NAFLD [139, 140]. Genetics might also modulate the spectrum of liver disease and its progression [141]. In turn, when portal hypertension coexists, the factors previously mentioned would represent an associated risk factor for the development of NAFLD and metabolic syndrome.

In portal hypertension, cholesterol synthesis could play a key role during the hypothesized reexpression of the vitellogenic phenotype. The liver plays a central role in cholesterol metabolism. Hepatocytes not only express a number of different lipoprotein receptors that enable them to take up cholesterol, but also synthesized cholesterol *de novo* within the liver [142, 143]. In addition, to these input pathways, the liver secretes cholesterol by two routes, the first, within triglyceride-rich very low density lipoprotein (VLDL) to supplying peripheral cells with fatty acids, fat soluble vitamins, and cholesterol. And, secondly, the liver releases cholesterol into bile, either directly as free cholesterol or after conversion into bile acids [142].

Cholesterol is used locally to synthesize glucocorticoids and mineralocorticoids, which could regulate microcirculatory functions and immune cell activation [144]. Perhaps, the ability of local corticosteroid synthesis is upregulated in the inflamed tissue due to the metabolic and functional needs of the neoformed tissue including angiogenesis in portal hypertension [7, 22]. Moreover, the pro-inflammatory and anti-inflammatory functions of androgens and estrogens and progesterone, respectively, suggest that endogenous sex steroids may influence immune functions [145–147] and, therefore, the evolution of the portal inflammatory response. In particular, estrogen has been shown to be effective in animal models of portal hypertension with cirrhosis by suppressing hepatic fibrosis and relaxing the hepatic sinusoid, and could reverse the severity of hyperdynamic circulation and the vascular hyporeactivity of the mesenteric arteries in portal hypertensive rats without cirrhosis [148].

Hence, it could be proposed that within the splanchnic impairments related to portal hypertension, the stimulation of the angiogenic-hematopoietic axis, the cellular and bacterial interstitial infiltration of the tissues and organs and the acute-phase-response, including dyslipidemia and hepatic steatosis (vitellogenic phenotype), seem to recall the functions characteristic of the secondary yolk sac during embryo development.

In this sense, the microvesicles, released from practically all cells including mesenchymal stem cells [149], would collaborate in inducing the recapitulation of extra-embryonic functions during the evolution of portal hypertension. Microvesicles contain lipids, proteins, RNA, and micro-RNAs and could act as vectors of information that regulate the function of target cells [150]. Microvesicles from inflammatory cells are suspected to be involved in various diseases. In particular, microvesicles probably enhance portal hypertension by contributing to splanchnic vasomotor alterations and angiogenesis [151].

8. Coupling extra-embryonic phenotypes to induce a gastrulation-like liver phenotype

In the current review, we propose that during the evolution of portal hypertension different extra-embryonic functions, such as the coelomic-amniotic and the trophoblastic-yolk sac or vitelline function, would be successively recapitulated. If so, the inflammatory conditions that characterize portal hypertension could actually represent the reexpression of extra-embryonic mechanisms that have been already used during the early phases of embryonic development. In this way, the pathophysiological mechanisms involved in the above-mentioned inflammatory response could represent the recapitulation of the extra-embryonic functions, which collaborate together to make an embryo-like tissue from gastrulation [7, 54] (**Figure 3**).

The liver stands out among other organs since its persistent injury usually results in the chronic activation of inflammation and the wound-healing response [7, 152]. Development of the liver during early embryogenesis may share similarities with pathophysiological processes seen in adulthood, such as acute liver injury and liver regeneration, but also in liver fibrosis [152–154]. The increasing knowledge of the extra hepatic involvement typical of this fibrotic liver disease, however, suggests that this wound healing process is associated with a complex systemic pathogenesis [155]. Portal hypertension is the major hemodynamic complication of a variety of diseases that obstruct portal blood flow, including liver cirrhosis [79]. Portal hypertension in the cirrhotic patient could be associated with hyperkinetic syndrome, increased total blood volume by sodium and water retention [155], endothelial dysfunction [81, 83, 156] in the splanchnic and systemic circulation [81, 83, 119], esophageal varices, ascites, encephalopathy, and hepatorenal syndrome [157].

The severe systemic complications of the portal hypertension syndrome accompanying the wound-healing liver reaction could be based on some metabolic similarities that can be established with the extra-embryonic coelomic-amniotic and trophoblastic-yolk sac functions playing the leading role during embryonic development [7]. Thus, the confluence of these two extra-embryonic axes in the injured liver could favor a gastrulation-like response in which fibrogenesis could predominate [7, 22, 54]. Therefore, the wound-healing liver reaction that characterizes the cirrhotic process could have properties comparable to an embryo and, in particular, with its initial evolutive phase, namely gastrulation [22]. If so, the gastrulation-related process with neoformation of a reparative tissue could be based on the recapitulation of the developmental process of the intra-embryonic mesenchyme [158].

The interstitial space of Disse could be schematically represented like an area fundamentally surrounded by a sinusoidal endothelium. Inside this endothelium, an inflammatory response is developed, which is made up by the hepatic stellate cell. In turn, the liver interstitial inflammation would be activated by means of the reexpression of extra-embryonic functions by the host organism, which provides molecules and cells selectively to the inflamed interstitial space through the sinusoidal endothelium [22] (**Figures 3** and **5**).

Hepatic stellate cells are liver-specific mesenchymal cells located in the space of Disse between the sinusoidal endothelial cells and hepatic epithelial cells [159]. Hepatic stellate cells also known as Ito cells, fat-storing cells, vitamin A-storing cells, or lipocytes, store excess vitamin A as retinyl esters in lipid droplets within their cytoplasm [159, 160]. In pathological conditions, hepatic stellate cells upon activation lose the vitamin A-containing lipid droplets and produce large amounts of collagen [160]. Therefore, modulation of vitamin A-containing lipid droplets has been suggested to have a therapeutic impact on the development of liver fibrosis [160] (**Table 2**). Hepatic stellate cells are known to express both mesenchymal and neural lineage markers [161, 162]. Moreover, during

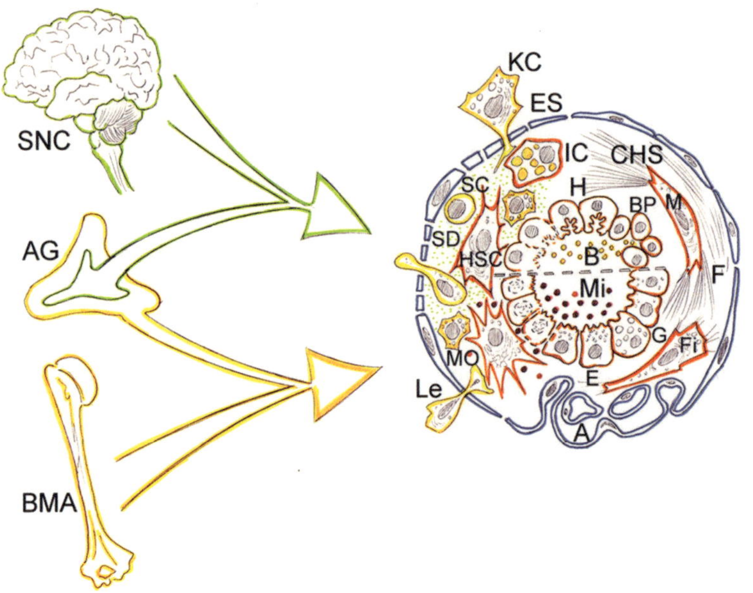

Figure 5.
Schematic representation of the systemic inflammatory response in portal hypertension in order to produce a systemic wound-healing phenotype. By means of two inflammatory phenotypes expression; i.e., neurogenic (CNS and AG) and immune (BMA), into the interstitial injured splanchnic area, an endocrine phenotype could be induced, that ultimately would causes a wound-like response. Thus, fibrosis and angiogenesis will be produced in the splanchnic area. A: angiogenesis; AG: adrenal gland; B: bile; BMA: bone marrow; BP: biliary proliferation; CHS: cholestasis; CNS: central nervous system; E: enterocyte; ES: endothelial sinusoid; G: goblet cell; HSC: hepatic stellate cell; IC: Ito cell; KC: Kupffer cell; Le: leukocyte; Mo: macrophages; M: myofibroblast; Mi: microbiome; SC: stem cells; SD: space of Disse.

The coelomic-amniotic phenotype
• Hyperkinetic syndrome
• Stimulation of the hypothalamo-pituitary-adrenal axis and the sympathetic nervous system
• Interstitial splanchnic edema
• Increased mesenteric lymph circulation
• Ascitic fluid
The trophoblastic-yolk sac (vitelline) phenotype
• Acute-phase response
• Dyslipidemia
• Local metabolism of cholesterol (steroid hormones)
• Hepatic steatosis
• Recapitulated mesenchymal-angiogenic-hematopoietic axis
• Portal hypertensive enteropathy
• Dysbiosis and intestinal bacterial translocation
• Splanchnic microvesicles
The gastrulation-like phenotype
• Hepatic stellate cell activation
• Fat-storing cells
• Myofibroblast
• Hepatic fibrosis

Table 2.
Portal hypertensive inflammatory phenotypes.

liver injury, stellate cells activate into alpha smooth muscle actin-expressing contractile myofibroblasts, which increase vascular resistance thereby promoting portal hypertension [163, 164]. Mesodermal mesenchymal cells including hepatic stellate cells are the major source of myofibroblasts [164]. In this sense, activated-hepatic stellate cells also strengthen the immune response through the production of a wide array of cytokines and chemokines [4]. Finally, hepatic stellate cells are able to adopt a fibrogenic phenotype and participate in extracellular matrix remodeling [163] (**Figure 4**).

Kupffer cells activate hepatic stellate cells via paracrine mechanisms, likely involving the profibrotic and mitogenic cytokines TGF-β and PDGF [165, 166]. Early deposition of an extracellular matrix in the subendothelial space of Disse causes *capillarization* of the sinusoid, diminished liver function, and contributes to the perpetuation of hepatic stellate cell activation [159, 160, 167]. Liver fibrogenesis is not only sustained by a heterogenic population of profibrogenic hepatic myofibroblasts [3, 4], but also includes mesothelial-related capsular fibrosis [167]. Mesothelial cells have a phenotype intermediate between epithelial cells and mesenchymal cells and these both type of cells could then undergo myofibroblastic transdifferentiation. Upon liver injury, it has been demonstrated that mesothelial cells participate in capsular fibrosis of the liver surface via differentiation to hepatic stellate cells and myofibroblasts [167]. In portal hypertension, the formation of a fibrotic scar tissue in the liver is associated with the development of an excessive gastrointestinal angiogenic response [110]. Therefore, the two principal components for creating granulation tissue, i.e., fibroplasia and angiogenesis, are distributed along the portal axis. In essence, the portal venous system continues playing a key role as a spatial delivery of functions in pathological situations.

9. Conclusion

The diverse functions of hepatic stellate cells in homeostasis and inflammation indicate the versatile nature of these mesenchymal-derived cells, which could adopt numerous phenotypes according to the interstitial microenvironmental characteristics [163]. Therefore, these hepatic cellular population, thanks to their potential ability to integrate and reexpress functions showing analogies to extra-embryonic functions, display characteristics of stem/progenitor cells [109]. In this way, during the development of portal hypertension, hepatic stellate cells not only could reexpress extra-embryonic functions but also could adapt themselves in order to induce a gastrulation-related process in the space of Disse. Therefore, by understanding the ontogenic interactions between hepatic stellate cells and the host inflammatory response in portal hypertension, it is possible to design effective therapeutic and prophylactic strategies to avoid or reverse wound-like hypertensive response.

Acknowledgements

The authors would like to thank Maria Elena Vicente for preparing the manuscript, Elizabeth Mascola for translating it into English, and Maria Jose Valdemoro, Head of Processes and Specialized Information of the Complutense University Medical School Library. This study was supported, in part, by a grant from Mutua Madrileña Foundation (Ref. No. AP6977/2009).

Author details

Maria Angeles Aller[1], Javier Blanco-Rivero[2,3,4], Ana Arias[5] and Jaime Arias[1*]

1 Department of Surgery, School of Medicine, Complutense University of Madrid, Madrid, Spain

2 Department of Physiology, School of Medicine, Autonomous University of Madrid, Madrid, Spain

3 Instituto de Investigación Biomédica La Paz (IdIPAZ), Madrid, España

4 Centro de Investigación Biomédica en Red (Ciber) de Enfermedades Cardiovasculares, Madrid, España

5 Department of Internal Medicine, Puerta de Hierro Hospital, School of Medicine, Autonoma University of Madrid, Madrid, Spain

*Address all correspondence to: jarias@med.ucm.es

References

[1] Garcia-Pagan JC, Gracia-Sancho J, Bosch J. Functional aspects on the pathophysiology of portal hypertension in cirrhosis. Journal of Hepatology. 2012;**57**:458-426. DOI: 10.1016/j.jhep.2012.03.007

[2] Loo NM-M, Fernandes Souza F, Garcia-Tsao G. Non-hemorrhagic acute complications associated with cirrhosis and portal hypertension. Best Practice & Research. Clinical Gastroenterology. 2013;**27**:665-678. DOI: 10.1016/j.bpg.2013.08.005

[3] Pinzani M, Rombouts K. Liver fibrosis from the bench to clinical targets. Digestive and Liver Disease. 2004;**36**:231-242. DOI: 10.1016/j.dld.2004.01.003

[4] Lee YA, Wallace MC, Friedman SL. Pathobiology of liver fibrosis: A translational success story. Gut. 2015;**64**:830-841. DOI: 10.1136/gutjnl-2014-306842

[5] Parola M, Pinzani M. Hepatic wound repair. Fibrogenesis & Tissue Repair. 2009;**2**:4. DOI: 10.1186/1755-1536-2-4

[6] Hunt TK, Andrew WWS, Halliday B, Greenburg G, Knighton D, Clark RA, et al. Chapter 1: Coagulation and macrophage stimulationof angiogenesis and wound healing. In: Dineen P, Hildick-Smith G, editors. The Surgical Wound. Philadelphia: Lea and Febiger; 1981. pp. 1-18. DOI: 10.1016/S0065-230X(08)60946-X

[7] Aller MA, Blanco-Rivero J, Arias JI, Balfagon G, Arias J. The wound-healing response and upregulated embryonic mechanisms: Brothers-in-arms forever. Experimental Dermatology. 2012;**21**:497-503. DOI: 10.1111/j.1600-0625.2012.01525.x

[8] Schilling JA. Advances in knowledge related to wounding, repair and healing: 1985-1984. Annals of Surgery. 1985;**201**:268-277. PMID: 3883919

[9] Hunt TK. Disorders of wound healing. World Journal of Surgery. 1980;**4**:271-277

[10] Clark RAF. Basics of cutaneous wound repair. The Journal of Dermatologic Surgery and Oncology. 1993;**19**:693-706. PMID: 8349909

[11] Galliot B, Crescenzi M, Jacinto A, Tajbakhsh S. Trends in tissue repair and regeneration. Development. 2017;**144**: 357-364. DOI: 10.1242/dev.144279

[12] Poss KD. Advances in understanding tissue regenerative capacity and mechanisms in animals. Nature Reviews. Genetics. 2010;**11**:710-722. DOI: 10.1038/nrg2879

[13] Reinke JM, Sorg H. Wound repair and regeneration. European Surgical Research. 2012;**49**:35-43. DOI: 10.1159/000339613

[14] Leung A, Crombleholme TM, Keswani SG. Fetal wound healing: Implications for minimal scar formation. Current Opinion in Pediatrics. 2012;**24**:371-278. DOI: 10.1097/MOP.0b013e3283535790

[15] Rolfe KJ, Grobbelaar AO. A review of fetal scarless healing. ISRN Dermatology. 2012;**2012**:698034. DOI: 10.5402/2012/698034

[16] Eming SA, Krieg T, Davidson JM. Inflammation in wound repair: Molecular and cellular mechanisms. The Journal of Investigative Dermatology. 2007;**127**:514-425. DOI: 10.1038/sj.jid.5700701

[17] Gurtner GC, Werner S, Barrandon Y, Longaker MT. Wound repair and regeneration. Nature. 2008;**453**:314-321. DOI: 10.1038/nature07039

[18] Ben Amar M, Wu M. Re-epithelialization advancing epithelium frontier during wound healing. Journal of The Royal Society Interface. 2014;**11**:20131038. DOI: 10.1098/rsif.2013.1038

[19] Profyris C, Tziotzios C, Do Vale I. Cutaneous scarring: Pathophysiology, molecular mechanisms, and scar reduction therapeutics. Journal of the American Academy of Dermatology. 2012;**66**:1-10. DOI: 10.1016/j.jaad 2011.05.055

[20] Aller MA, Arias JL, Nava MP, Arias J. Post-traumatic inflammation is a complex response based on the pathological expression of the nervous, immune and endocrine functional systems. Experimental Biology and Medicine (Maywood, N.J.). 2004;**229**:170-181. PMID: 14734796

[21] Aller MA, Prieto I, Blanco-Rivero J, Arias JI, Balfagon G, Arias J. The wound healing reaction. In: Arias J, Aller MA, Arias JI, editors. Surgical Inflammation. Vol. 5. Sharjah, the United Arab Emirates: Bentham ebook; 2013. pp. 129-153. DOI: 10.2174/97816080578561130101

[22] Aller MA, Arias JI, Prieto I, Gilsanz C, Arias A, Yang H, et al. Surgical inflammatory stress: The embryo takes hold of the reins again. Theoretical Biology & Medical Modelling. 2013;**10**:6. DOI: 10.1186/1742-4682-10-6

[23] Eisenhut M. Changes in ion transport in inflammatory disease. Journal of Inflammation. 2006;**3**:5. DOI: 10.1186/1476-9255-3-5

[24] Scadden DT. The stem-cell niches as an entity of action. Nature. 2006;**441**:1075-1079. DOI: 10.1038/nature04957

[25] Aguilera G. HPA axis responsiveness to stress: Implications for health aging. Experimental Gerontology. 2011;**46**: 90-95. DOI: 10.1016/j.exger.2010.08.023

[26] Groeneweg FL, Karst H, De Kloet ER, Jöels H. Rapid non-genomic effects of corticosteroids and their role in the central stress response. The Journal of Endocrinology. 2011;**209**:157-167. DOI: 10.1530/JOE-10-0472

[27] Crivellato E, Nico B, Ribatti D. The chromaffin vesicle: Advances in understanding the composition of a versatile, multifunctional secretory organelle. Anatomical Record (Hoboken, NJ). 2008;**291**:1587-1602. DOI: 10.1002/ar.20763

[28] Ehninger A, Trumpp A. The bone marrow stem cell niche grows up: Mesenchymal stem cells and macrophages move. The Journal of Experimental Medicine. 2011;**208**: 421-428. DOI: 10.1084/jem.20110132

[29] Burclaff J, Mills JC. Plasticity of differentiated cells in wound repair and tumorigenesis, part II: Skin and intestine. Disease Models & Mechanisms. 2018;**11**. DOI: 10.1242/dmm.035071. pii: dmm035071

[30] Balbridge MT, King KY, Goodell MA. Inflammatory signals regulate hematopoietic stem cells. Trends in Immunology. 2011;**32**:57-64. DOI: 10.1016/j.it.2010.12.003

[31] Balbridge MT, King KY, Boles NC, Weksberg DC, Goodell MA. Quiescent haematopoietic stem cells are activated by IFN-gamma in response to chronic infection. Nature. 2010;**465**:793-797. DOI: 10.1038/nature09135

[32] Choi AMK, Ryter SW, Levine B. Autophagy in human health and disease. The New England Journal of Medicine. 2013;**368**:651-661. DOI: 10.1056/NEJMra1205406

[33] Aller MA, Arias JI, Giner M, Losada M, Cruz A, Alonso-Poza A, et al. Oxygen-related inflammatory wound phenotypes. In: Middelton JE, editor. Wound Healing: Process, Phases and

Promoting. Huntington, New York: Nova Sciences Publishers; 2011. pp. 1-26. DOI: 10.1186/1742-4682-10-6

[34] Grisanti LA, Evanson J, Marchus E, Jorissen H, Woster AP, DeKrey W, et al. Pro-inflammatory responses in human monocytes are β_1-adrenergic receptor subtype dependent. Molecular Immunology. 2010;**47**:1244-1254. DOI: 10.1016/j.molimm.2009.12.013

[35] Flierl MA, Rittirsch D, Huber-Lang M, Sarma JV, Ward PA. Catecholamines-crafty weapons in the inflammatory arsenal of immune/inflammatory cells or opening Pandora's box. Molecular Medicine. 2008;**14**:195-204. DOI: 10.2119/2007-00105.Flierl

[36] Marazzitti D, Consoli G, Masala L, Catena Dell'Osso M, Baroni S. Latest advancements on serotonin and dopamine transporters in lymphocytes. Mini Reviews in Medicinal Chemistry. 2010;**10**:32-40. DOI: 10.2174/138955710791112587

[37] Smith EM. Neuropeptides as signal molecules in common with leukocytes and the hypothalamic-pituitary-adrenal axis. Brain, Behavior, and Immunity. 2008;**22**:3-14. DOI: 10.1016/j.bbi.2007.08.005

[38] Czura CJ, Tracey KJ. Autonomic neural regulation of immunity. Journal of Internal Medicine. 2005;**257**:156-166. DOI: 10.1111/j.1365-2796.2004.01442.x

[39] Jackson WM, Nesti LJ, Tuan RS. Clinical translation of wound healing therapies based on mesenchymal stem cells. Stem Cells Translational Medicine. 2012;**1**:44-50. DOI: 10.5966/sctm.2011-0024

[40] Li Y, Zheng L, Xu X, Song L, Li Y, Li W, et al. Mesenchymal stem cells modified with angiopoietin-1 gen promote wound healing. Stem Cell Research & Therapy. 2013;**4**:113. DOI: 10.1186/scrt324

[41] Aggarwal S, Pittenger MF. Human mesenchymal stem cells modulate allogenic immune cell response. Blood. 2005;**105**:1815-1822. DOI: 10.1182/blood-2004-04-1559

[42] Elman JS, Li M, Wang F, Gimble JM, Parekkadan B. A comparison of adipose and bone marrow-derived mesenchymal stromal cell secreted factors in the treatment of systemic inflammation. Journal of Inflammation. 2014;**11**:1. DOI: 10.1186/1476-9255-11-1

[43] Gabay C, Kushner I. Acute-phase proteins and other systemic responses to inflammation. The New England Journal of Medicine. 1999;**340**:448-454. DOI: 10.1056/NEJM199902113400607

[44] Jain S, Gautam V, Naseem S. Acute-phase proteins: As diagnostic tool. Journal of Pharmacy & Bioallied Sciences. 2011;**31**:18-27. DOI: 10.4103/0975-7406.76489

[45] Mihara M, Hashizume M, Yoshida H, Suzuki M, Shiina M. IL-6/IL-6 receptor system and its role in physiological and pathological conditions. Clinical Science (London, England). 2012;**122**:143-159. DOI: 10.1042/CS20110340

[46] Pepys MB, Hirschfield G. C-reactive protein: A critical update. The Journal of Clinical Investigation. 2003;**111**: 1805-1812. DOI: 10.1172/JCI200318921

[47] Kisilevsky R, Manley PN. Acute-phase serum amyloid A: Perspectives on its physiological and pathological roles. Amyloid. 2012;**19**:5-14. DOI: 10.3109/13506129.2011.654294

[48] Miller WL, Bose HS. Early steps in steroidogenesis: Intracellular cholesterol trafficking. Journal of Lipid Research. 2011;**5**:2111-2135. DOI: 10.1194/jlr.R016675

[49] Sassi F, Tamone C, D'Amelio P. Vitamin D: Nutrient, hormone, and

immuno-modulator. Nutrients. 2018;**10**. DOI: 10.3390/nu10111656. pii: E1656

[50] Aller MA, Arias JL, Nava MP, Arias J. Evolutive trophic phases of the systemic acute inflammatory response, oxygen use mechanisms and metamorphosis. Psicothema. 2004;**16**:369-372

[51] Mantovani A, Biswas SK, Galdiero MR, Sica A, Locati M. Macrophage plasticity and polarization in tissue repair and remodeling. The Journal of Pathology. 2013;**229**:176-185. DOI: 10.1002/path.4133

[52] Murawala P, Tanaka EM, Currie JD. Regeneration: The ultimate example of wound healing. Seminars in Cell & Developmental Biology. 2012;**23**:954-962. DOI: 10.1016/j.semcdb.2012.09.013

[53] Wong VW, Gurtner GC, Longaker MT. Wound healing: A paradigm for regeneration. Mayo Clinic Proceedings. 2013;**88**:1022-1031. DOI: 10.1016/j.mayocp.2013.04.012

[54] Aller MA, Arias JI, Arias J. Pathological axes of wound repair: Gastrulation revisited. Theoretical Biology & Medical Modelling. 2010;**7**:37. DOI: 10.1186/1742-4682-7-37

[55] Kapetanaki MG, Mora AL, Rojas M. Influence of age on wound healing and fibrosis. The Journal of Pathology. 2013;**229**:310-322. DOI: 10.1002/path.4122

[56] Segura I, Serrano A, Gonzalez De Buitrago G, Gonzalez MA, Abad JL, Claveria C, et al. Inhibition of programmed cell death impairs in vitro vascular-like structure formation and reduces in vivo angiogenesis. The FASEB Journal. 2002;**16**:833-841. DOI: 10.1096/fj.01-0819com

[57] Johnson A, Di Prieto LA. Apoptosis and angiogenesis: An evolving mechanism for fibrosis. The FASEB Journal. 2013;**27**:3893-3901. DOI: 10.1096/fj.12-214189

[58] Plikus MV, Gay DL, Treffeisen E, Wang A, Supapannachart RJ, Cotsarelis G. Epithelial stem cells and implications for wound repair. Seminars in Cell & Developmental Biology. 2012;**23**:946-953. DOI: 10.1016/j.semcdb.2012.10.001

[59] De Miguel MP, Arnalich-Montiel P, Lopez-Iglesias A, Blazquez Martinez A, Nistal M. Epiblast-derived stem cells in embryonic and adult tissues. The International Journal of Developmental Biology. 2009;**53**:1529-1540. DOI: 10.1387/ijdb.072413md

[60] Jauniaux E, Gulbis B. Fluid compartments of the embryonic environment. Human Reproduction Update. 2000;**6**:268-278. DOI: 10.1093/humupd/6.3.268

[61] Jauniaux E, Gulbis B, Jurkovic D. Relationship between protein concentrations in embryological fluids and maternal serum and yolk sac size during human pregnancy. Human Reproduction. 1994;**9**:161-166. PMID: 8195341

[62] Burton GJ, Hempstock J, Jauniaux E. Nutrition of the human fetus during the first trimester—A review. Placenta. 2001;**22**:570-577. DOI: 10.1053/plac.2001.0639

[63] Jauniaux E, Sherwood RA, Jurkovic D, Boa FG, Campbell S. Amino acid concentrations in human embryological fluids. Human Reproduction. 1994;**9**:1175-1179. PMID: 7962397

[64] Wathen NC, Delves HT, Campbell DJ, Chard T. The coelomic cavity: A reservoir for metals. American Journal of Obstetrics and Gynecology. 1995;**173**:1884-1888. DOI: 10.1016/0002-9378(95)90446-8

[65] Calleja-Agius J, Jauniaux E, Muttukrishna S. Inflammatory

cytokines in maternal circulation and placenta of chromosomally abnormal first trimester miscarriages. Clinical & Developmental Immunology. 2012;**2012**:175041. DOI: 10.1155/2012/175041

[66] Chang YJ, Huang SH, Tseng CP, Huang SH, Hsu LF, Hsu LW, et al. Isolation of mesenchymal stem cells with neurogenic potentials from the mesoderm of the amniotic membrane. Cells, Tissues, Organs. 2010;**192**:93-105. DOI: 10.1159/000295774

[67] Uberti HG, Pierpont YN, Ko F, Wright TE, Smith CA, Cruse CW, et al. Amnion-derived cellular cytokine solution (ACCS) promotes migration of keratinocytes and fibroblasts. Annals of Plastic Surgery. 2010;**64**:632-635. DOI: 10.1097/SAP.0b013e3181c39351

[68] Shaw SW, David AL, De Coppi P. Clinical applications of prenatal and postnatal therapy using stem cells retrieved from amniotic fluid. Current Opinion in Obstetrics & Gynecology. 2011;**23**:109-116. DOI: 10.1097/GCO.0b013e32834457b1

[69] Bevilacqua E, Hoshida M-S, Amarante-Paffaro A, Albieri-Borges A, Gomes SZ. Trophoblast phagocytic program: Roles in different placental systems. The International Journal of Developmental Biology. 2010;**54**:495-505. DOI: 10.1387/ijdb.082761eb

[70] Knöfler M. Critical growth factors and signaling pathways controlling human trophoblast invasion. The International Journal of Developmental Biology. 2010;**54**:269-280. DOI: 10.1387/ijdb.082769mk

[71] Ueno H, Weisman IL. The origin and fate of yolk sac hematopoiesis: Application of chimer analysis to developmental studies. The International Journal of Developmental Biology. 2010;**54**:1019-1031. DOI: 10.1387/ijdb.093039hu

[72] Gulbis B, Jauniaux E, Cotton F, Stordeur P. Protein and enzyme patterns in the fluid cavities of the first trimester gestational sac: Relevance to the absorptive role of secondary yolk sac. Molecular Human Reproduction. 1998;**4**:857-862. DOI: 10.1093/molehr/4.9.857

[73] Siegel N, Rosner M, Hanneder M, Freilinger A, Hengstschlager M. Human amniotic fluid stem cells: A new perspective. Amino Acids. 2008;**35**:291-293. DOI: 10.1007/s00726-007-0593-1

[74] Yoshida S, Wada T. Transfer of maternal cholesterol to embryo and fetus in pregnant mice. Journal of Lipid Research. 2005;**46**:2168-2174. DOI: 10.1194/jlr.M500096-JLR200

[75] Nakazawa F, Alev C, Jakt LM, Sheng G. Yolk sac endoderm is the major source for serum proteins and lipids and is involved in the regulation of vascular integrity in early chick development. Developmental Dynamics. 2011;**240**:2002-2010. DOI: 10.1002/dvdy.22690

[76] Rohen JW, Lütjen-Drecoll E. Embriologia funtional. In: Una Perspectiva Desde la Biología del Desarrollo. 3ª Edicion ed. Vol. 8008. Madrid, Spain: Médica Panamericana S.A. pp. 1-166. ISBN-13: 978-8498351552

[77] Acloque H, Adams MS, Fishwick K, Bronner-Fraser M, Nieto MA. Epithelial-mesenchymal transitions: The importance of changing cell state in development and disease. The Journal of Clinical Investigation. 2009;**119**:1438-1449. DOI: 10.1172/JCI38019

[78] Kalluri R, Neilson EG. Epithelial-mesenchymal transition and its implications for fibrosis. The Journal of Clinical Investigation. 2003;**112**: 1776-1782. DOI: 10.1172/JCI200320530

[79] Sherlock S. The portal venous system and portal hypertension. In: Sherlock S, editor. Diseases of the Liver and Biliary System. 8ª ed. Vol. 10. London: Blackwell Scientific Publications; 1989. pp. 151-207

[80] Collardeau-Frachon S, Scoazec J-Y. Vascular development and differentiation during human liver organogenesis. The Anatomical Record. 2008;**291**:614-627. DOI: 10.1002/ar.20679

[81] Aller MA, Arias JL, Cruz A, Arias J. Inflammation: A way to understanding the evolution of portal hypertension. Theoretical Biology & Medical Modelling. 2007;**4**:44. DOI: 10.1186/1742-4682-4-44

[82] Palma MD, Aller MA, Vara E, Nava MP, Garcia C, Arias-Diaz J, et al. Portal hypertension produces an evolutive hepato-intestinal pro- and anti-inflammatory response in the rat. Cytokine. 2005;**31**:213-226. DOI: 10.1016/j.cyto.2005.04.008

[83] Iwakiri Y, Groszmann RJ. The hyperdynamic circulation of chronic liver disease: From the patient to the molecule. Hepatology. 2006;**43**:S121-S131. DOI: 10.1002/hep.20993. PMID: 16447289

[84] Frith J, Newton JL. Autonomic dysfunction in chronic liver disease. Hepatic Medicine : Evidence And Research. 2011;**3**:81-87. DOI: 10.1111/j.1478-3231.2009.01985.x. PMID: 19323779

[85] Kimer N, Goetze JP, Bendtsen F, MØller S. New vasoactive peptides in cirrhosis: Organ extraction and relation to the vasodilatory state. European Journal of Clinical Investigation. 2014;**44**:441-452. DOI: 10.1111/eci.12249

[86] Tracey KJ. The inflammatory reflex. Nature. 2002;**420**:853-859. DOI: 10.1038/nature01321

[87] Witte CL, Witte MH, Dumont AE. Lymph imbalance in the genesis and perpetuation of the ascites syndrome in hepatic cirrhosis. Gastroenterology. 1980;**78**:1059-1068. PMID: 7380179

[88] Kvietys PR, Granger DN. Role of intestinal lymphatics in interstitial volume regulation and transmucosal water transport. Annals of the New York Academy of Sciences. 2010;**207**:E29-E43. DOI: 10.1111/j.1749-6632.2010.05709.x

[89] Ito K, Shimizu A, Tanabe M, Matsunaga N. *Cisterna chyli* in patients with portal hypertension: Evaluation with MR imaging. Journal of Magnetic Resonance Imaging. 2012;**35**:624-628. DOI: 10.1002/jmri.22875

[90] Steinemann DC, Dindo D, Clavien PA, Nocito A. Atraumatic chylous ascites: Systematic review on symptons and causes. Journal of the American College of Surgeons. 2011;**212**:899-905. DOI: 10.1016/j.jamcollsurg.2011.01.010

[91] Aller MA, Prieto I, Argudo S, De Vicente F, Santamaria L, De Miguel MP, et al. The interstitial lymphatic peritoneal mesothelium axis in portal hypertensive ascites: When in danger, go back to the sea. International Journal of Inflammation. 2010;**2010**:1486. DOI: 10.4061/2010/148689

[92] Aller MA, De las Heras N, Blanco-Rivero J, Arias JI, Lahera V, Balfagon G, et al. Portal hypertensive cardiovascular pathology: The rescue of ancestral survival mechanisms? Clinics and Research in Hepatology and Gastroenterology. 2012;**36**:35-46. DOI: 10.1016/j.clinre.2011.07.017

[93] Kim SU, Kim do Y, Lee CK, Park JY, Kim SH, Kim HM, et al. Ascitic fluid infection in patients with hepatitis B virus-related liver cirrhosis: Culture-negative neutrocytic ascites versus spontaneous bacterial peritonitis. Journal of Gastroenterology and

Hepatology. 2010;**25**:122-128. DOI: 10.1111/j.1440-1746.2009.05970.x

[94] Cho C-KJ, Shan SJ, Winsor EJ, Diamandis EP. Proteomics analysis of human amniotic fluid. Molecular & Cellular Proteomics. 2007;**6**:1406-1415. DOI: 10.1074/mcp.M700090-MCP200

[95] Tong XL, Wang L, Gao TB, Qin YG, Qi Y, Xu YP. Potential function of amniotic fluid in fetal development-novel insights by comparing the composition of human amniotic fluid with umbilical cord and maternal serum at mind and later gestation. Journal of Clinical Medicine. 2009;**72**:368-373. DOI: 10.1016/S1726-4901(09)70389-2

[96] Schmidt W. The amniotic fluid compartment: The fetal habitat. Advances in Anatomy, Embryology, and Cell Biology. 1992;**127**:1-100. PMID: 1514435

[97] Brace RA. Physiology of amniotic fluid volume regulation. Clinical Obstetrics and Gynecology. 1997;**40**:280-289. PMID: 9199840

[98] Ohtani O, Ohtani Y. Lymph circulation in the liver. Anatomical Record (Hoboken, NJ). 2008;**291**:643-652. DOI: 10.1002/ar.20681

[99] Takahashi Y, Fujimori S, Narahara Y, Gudis K, Ensaka Y, Kosugi Y, et al. Small intestinal edema had the strongest correlation with portal venous pressure amongst capsule endoscopy findings. Digestion. 2012;**86**:48-54. DOI: 10.1159/000338180

[100] Pijls KE, Jonkers DMAE, Elamin EE, Masclee AAM, Koek GH. Intestinal epithelial barrier function in liver cirrhosis: An extensive review of the literature. Liver International. 2013;**33**:1457-1469. DOI: 10.1111/liv.12271

[101] Frasinariu OE, Ceccarelli S, Alisi A, Moraru E, Nobili V. Gut-liver axis and fibrosis in nonalcoholic fatty liver disease: An input for novel therapies. Digestive and Liver Disease. 2013;**45**:543-551. DOI: 10.1016/j.dld.2012.11.010

[102] Rojas-Feria M, Castro M, Suarez E, Ampuero J, Romero-Gomez M. Hepatobiliary manifestations in inflammatory bowel disease: The gut, the drugs and the liver. World Journal of Gastroenterology. 2013;**19**:7327-7340. DOI: 10.3748/wjg.v19.i42.7327

[103] Visschers RG, Luyer MD, Schaap FG, Olde Damink SW, Soeters P. The gut-liver axis. Current Opinion in Clinical Nutrition and Metabolic Care. 2013;**16**:576-581. DOI: 10.1097/MCO.0b013e32836410a4

[104] Volta O, Caio G, Tovoli F, De Giorgio R. Gut-liver axis: An immune link between celiac disease and primary biliary cirrhosis. Expert Review of Gastroenterology & Hepatology. 2013;**7**:253-261. DOI: 10.1586/egh.13.5

[105] Chassaing B, Etienne-Mesmin L, Gewirtz AT. Microbiota-liver axis hepatic disease. Hepatology. 2014;**59**:328-339. DOI: 10.1002/hep.26494

[106] Wiig H, Swartz MA. Interstitial fluid and lymph formation and transport: Physiological regulation and roles in inflammation and cancer. Physiological Reviews. 2012;**92**:1005-1060. DOI: 10.1152/physrev.00037.2011

[107] Ng CP, Hinz B, Swartz MA. Interstitial fluid flow induces myofibroblast differentiation and collagen alignment in vitro. Journal of Cell Science. 2005;**118**:4731-4739. DOI: 10.1242/jcs.02605

[108] Shibayama Y, Urano T, Nakata K. Changes in hepatic lymph vessels in endotoxaemia. The Journal of Pathology. 1992;**168**:325-330. DOI: 10.1002/path.1711680313

[109] Sawitza I, Kordes C, Reister S, Haüssinger D. The niche of stellate cells within the liver. Hepatology. 2009;**50**:1617-1624. DOI: 10.1002/hep.23184

[110] Aller MA, Arias JI, Arias J. The mast cell integrates the splanchnic and systemic inflammatory response in portal hypertension. Journal of Translational Medicine. 2007;**5**:44. DOI: 10.1186/1479-5876-5-44

[111] Llamas MA, Aller MA, Marquina D, Nava MP, Arias J. Bacterial translocation to mesenteric lymph nodes increases in chronic portal hypertensive rats. Digestive Diseases and Sciences. 2010;**55**:2244-2254. DOI: 10.1007/s10620-009-1001-3

[112] Alonso MJ, Aller MA, Corcuera MT, Nava MP, Gomez F, Angulo A, et al. Progressive hepatic fatty infiltration in rats with prehepatic portal hypertension. Hepato-Gastroenterology. 2005;**52**:541-546. PMID: 15816474

[113] Aller MA, Vara E, Garcia C, Nava MP, Angulo A, Sanchez-Patan F, et al. Hepatic lipid metabolism changes in short- and long-term prehepatic portal hypertension rats. World Journal of Gastroenterology. 2006;**12**:6828-6834. DOI: 10.3748/wjg.v12.i42.6828

[114] Ponziani FR, Zocco MA, Cerrito L, Gasbarrini A, Pompili M. Bacterial translocation in patients with liver cirrhosis: Physiology, clinical consequences, and practical implications. Expert Review of Gastroenterology & Hepatology. 2018;**12**:641-656. DOI: 10.1080/17474124.2018.1481747

[115] Moquillaza LM, Aller MA, Nava MP, Santamaria L, Vergara P, Arias J. Partial hepatectomy, partial portal vein stenosis and mesenteric lymphadenectomy increases splanchnic mast cell infiltration in the rat. Acta Histochemica. 2010;**112**:372-382. DOI: 10.1016/j.acthis.2009.03.002

[116] Kunder CA, St. John AL, Li G, Leong KW, Berwin B, Staats HF, et al. Mast cell-derived particles deliver pheripheral signals to remote lymph nodes. The Journal of Experimental Medicine. 2009;**206**:2455-2467. DOI: 10.1084/jem.20090805

[117] Dever JB, Sheikh MY. Review article: Spontaneous bacterial peritonitis—Bacteriology, diagnosis, treatment, risk factors and prevention. Alimentary Pharmacology & Therapeutics. 2015;**41**:1116-1131. DOI: 10.1111/apt.13172

[118] Yang D, Xie Y, Pan H, Huang Y, Dai Y, Tong Y, et al. Clinical characteristics and prognostic factors of liver cirrhosis patients with systemic inflammatory response syndrome. Hepatology Research. 2017;**47**:1174-1185. DOI: 10.1111/hepr.12886

[119] Serino M, Blasco-Baque V, Nicolas S, Burcelin R. Managing the manager: Gut microbiotes, stem cells and metabolism. Diabetes & Metabolism. 2014;**40**:186-190. DOI: 10.1016/diabet.2013.12.004

[120] Wittkopf N, Neurath MF, Becker C. Immune-epithelial crosstalk at the intestinal surface. Journal of Gastroenterology. 2014;**49**:375-387. DOI: 10.1007/s00535-013-0929-4

[121] Seo YS, Shah VH. The role of gut-liver axis in the pathogenesis of liver cirrhosis and portal hypertension. Clinical and Molecular Hepatology. 2012;**18**:337-346. DOI: 10.3350/cmh.2012.18.4.337

[122] Van Bossuyt H, Wisse E. Structural changes produced in Kupffer cells of the rat liver by injection of lipopolysaccharide. Cell and Tissue Research. 1988;**251**:205-214. DOI: 10.1007/BF00215466

[123] Huang H, Evankovich J, Yan W, Nace G, Zhang L, Ross M, et al. Endogenous histones function as alarmins in sterile inflammatory liver injury through toll-like receptor 9 in mice. Hepatology. 2011;**54**:999-1008. DOI: 10.1002/hep.24501

[124] Saiman Y, Friedman SL. The role of chemokines in acute liver injury. Frontiers in Physiology. 2012;**3**:213. DOI: 10.3389/fphys.2012.00213

[125] Tacke F, Zimmermann HW. Macrophage heterogeneity in liver injury and fibrosis. Journal of Hepatology. 2014;**60**:1090-1096. DOI: 10.1016/j.jhep.2013.12.025

[126] Uberti MG, Lufkin AE, Pierpont YN, Ko F, Smith CA, Robson MC, et al. Amnion-derived cellular cytokine solution promotes macrophage activity. Annals of Plastic Surgery. 2011;**66**:575-580. DOI: 10.1097/SAP.0b013e318212f1d0

[127] Zovein AC, Hofmann JJ, Lynch M, French WJ, Turlo KA, Yang Y, et al. Fate tracing reveals the endothelial origin of hematopoietic stem cells. Cell Stem Cell. 2008;**3**:625-636. DOI: 10.1016/j.stem.2008.09.018

[128] Coulon S, Heindryckx F, Geerts A, Van Steenkiste C, Colle I, Van Vlierberghe H. Angiogenesis in chronic liver disease and its complications. Liver International. 2011;**31**:146-162. DOI: 10.1111/j.1478-3231.2010.02369.x

[129] Viggiano TR, Gostout CJ. Portal hypertensive intestinal vasculopathy: A review of the clinical, endoscopic and histopathological features. The American Journal of Gastroenterology. 1992;**87**:944-954. PMID: 1642217

[130] Jones EAV, Le Noble F, Eichmann A. What determines blood vessel structure? Genetic prespecification vs hemodynamics. Physiology (Bethesda). 2006;**21**:388-395. DOI: 10.1152/physiol.00020.2006

[131] Zohn IE, Sarkar AA. The visceral yolk sac endoderm provides for absorption of nutrients to the embryo during neurulation. Birth Defects Research. Part A, Clinical and Molecular Teratology. 2010;**88**:593-600. DOI: 10.1002/bdra.20705

[132] Tufail M, Takeda M. Molecular characteristics of insect vitellogenins. Journal of Insect Physiology. 2008;**54**:1447-1458. DOI: 10.1016/j.jinsphys.2008.08.007

[133] Arukwe A, GoksØyr A. Eggshell and egg yolk proteins in fish: Hepatic proteins for the next generation: Oogenetic population and evolutionary implications of endocrine disruption. Comparative Hepatology. 2003;**2**:4. DOI: 10.1186/1476-5926-2-4

[134] Sanchez-Patan F, Anchuelo R, Aller MA, Vara E, Garcia C, Nava MP, et al. Chronic prehepatic portal hypertension in the rat: Is it a type of metabolic inflammatory syndrome? Lipids in Health and Disease. 2008;**7**:4. DOI: 10.1186/1476-511X-7-4

[135] Jahangiri A. High-density lipoprotein and the acute phase response. Current Opinion in Endocrinology, Diabetes and Obesity. 2010;**17**:156-160. DOI: 10.1097/MED.0b013e328337278b

[136] Targher G, Day CP, Bonora E. Risk of cardiovascular disease in patients with nonalcoholic fatty liver disease. The New England Journal of Medicine. 2010;**363**:1341-1350. DOI: 10.1056/NEJMra0912063

[137] Aller MA, De las Heras N, Nava MP, Regadera J, Arias J, Lahera V. Splanchnic-aortic inflammatory axis in experimental portal hypertension. World Journal of Gastroenterology.

2013;**19**:7992-7999. DOI: 10.3748/wjg.v19.i44.7992

[138] Del Chierico F, Gnani D, Vernocchi P, Petrucca A, Alisi A, Dallapiccola B, et al. Meta-omic platforms to assist in the understanding of NAFLD gut microbiota alterations: Tools and applications. International Journal of Molecular Sciences. 2014;**15**:684-711. DOI: 10.3390/ijms15010684

[139] Wang Y, Li YY, Nie YQ, Zhou YJ, Cao CY, Xu L. Association between metabolic syndrome and the development of nonalcoholic fatty liver disease. Experimental and Therapeutic Medicine. 2013;**6**:77-84. DOI: 10.3892/etm.2013.1090

[140] Petta S, Miele L, Bugianesi E, Camma C, Rosso C, Boccia S, et al. Glucokinase regulatory protein gene polymorphism affects liver fibrosis in non-alcoholic fatty liver disease. PLoS One. 2014;**9**(2):e87523. DOI: 10.1371/journal.pone.0087523

[141] Dikkers A, Tietge UJF. Biliary cholesterol secretion: More than a simple ABC. World Journal of Gastroenterology. 2010;**16**:5936-5945. DOI: 10.3748/wjg.v16.i47.5936

[142] Trapani L, Segatto M, Pallottini V. Regulation and deregulation of cholesterol homeostasis: The liver as a metabolic "power station". World Journal of Hepatology. 2012;**4**:184-190. DOI: 10.4254/wjh.v4.i6.184

[143] Taves MD, Gomez-Sanchez CE, Soma KK. Extra-adrenal glucocorticoids and mineralocorticoids: Evidence for local synthesis, regulation and function. American Journal of Physiology. Endocrinology and Metabolism. 2011;**301**:E11-E24. DOI: 10.1152/ajpendo.00100.2011

[144] Gilliver SC. Sex steroids as inflammatory regulators. The Journal of Steroid Biochemistry and Molecular Biology. 2010;**120**:105-115. DOI: 10.1016/j.jsbmb.2009.12.015

[145] Cunningham M, Gilkeson G. Estrogen receptors in immunity and autoimmunity. Clinical Reviews in Allergy and Immunology. 2011;**40**:66-73. DOI: 10.1007/s12016-010-8203-5

[146] Nikolaenko L, Jia Y, Wang C, Diaz-Arjonilla M, Yee JK, French SW, et al. Testosterone replacement ameliorates non-alcoholic fatty liver disease in castrated rats. Endocrinology. 2013;**155**:417-428. DOI: 10.1210/en.2013-1648

[147] Zhang B, Zhang C-G, Zhou Q-B, Chen W, Wu Z-Y. Estrogen improves the hyperdynamic circulation and hyporeactivity of mesenteric arteries by alleviating oxidative stress in partial vein ligated rats. World Journal of Gastroenterology. 2013;**19**:6863-6868. DOI: 10.3748/wjg.v19.i40.6863

[148] Cocucci E, Racchetti G, Meldolesi J. Shedding microvesicles: Artefacts no more. Trends in Cell Biology. 2008;**19**:43-51. DOI: 10.1016/j.tcb.2008.11.003

[149] Tetta C, Bruno S, Fonsato V, Deregibus MC, Camussi G. The role of microvesicles in tissue repair. Organogenesis. 2011;7:105-115. DOI: 10.4161/org.7.2.15782

[150] Lemoinne S, Thabut D, Housset C, Moreau R, Valla D, Boulanger CM, et al. The emerging roles of microvesicles in liver diseases. Nature Reviews Gastroenterology & Hepatology. 2014;**11**:350-361. DOI: 10.1038/nrgastro.2014.7

[151] Aller MA, Arias JL, Garcia-Dominguez J, Arias JI, Duran M, Arias J. Experimental obstructive cholestasis: The wound-like inflammatory liver

response. Fibrogenesis & Tissue Repair. 2008;**1**:6. DOI: 10.1186/1755-1536-1-6

[152] Wasmuth HE, Tacke F, Trautwein C. Chemokines in liver inflammation and fibrosis. Seminars in Liver Disease. 2010;**30**:215-225. DOI: 10.1055/s-0030-1255351

[153] Pinzani M. Liver cirrhosis. Best Practice & Research. Clinical Gastroenterology. 2011;**25**:281-290. DOI: 10.1016/j.bpg.2011.02.009

[154] Iwakiri Y. Endothelial dysfunction in the regulation of cirrhosis and portal hypertension. Liver International. 2012;**32**:199-213. DOI: 10.1111/j.1478-3231.2011.02579.x

[155] Pasarin M, La Mura V, Gracia-Sancho J, Garcia-Caldero H, Rodriguez-Vilarrupla A, Garcia-Pagan JC, et al. Sinusoidal endothelial dysfunction precedes inflammation and fibrosis in a model of NAFLD. PLoS One. 2012;**7**(4):e32785. DOI: 10.1371/journal.pone.0032785

[156] Mahl TC, Groszmann RJ. Pathophysiology of portal hypertension and variceal bleeding. The Surgical Clinics of North America. 1990;**70**:251-266. PMID: 2181704

[157] Mikawa T, Poh AM, Kelly KA, Shii Y, Reese DE. Induction and patterning of the primitive streak, an organizing center of gastrulation in the amniote. Developmental Dynamics. 2004;**229**:422-432. DOI: 10.1002/dvdy.10458

[158] Hellerbrand C. Hepatic stellate cells—The pericytes in the liver. Pflügers Archiv - European Journal of Physiology. 2013;**465**:775-778. DOI: 10.1007/s00424-012-1209-5

[159] Friedman SL. Molecular regulation of hepatic fibrosis, an integrated cellular response to tissue injury. The Journal of Biological Chemistry. 2000;**275**:2247-2250. DOI: 10.1074/jbc.275.4.2247

[160] Asahina K, Tsai SY, Li P, Ishii M, Maxson RE, Sucov HM, et al. Mesenchymal origin of hepatic stellate cells, submesothelial cells, and perivascular mesenchymal cells during mouse liver development. Hepatology. 2009;**49**:998-1011. DOI: 10.1002/hep.22721

[161] Berardis S, Lombard C, Evraerts J, El Taghdouini A, Rosseels V, Sancho-Bru P, et al. Gene expression profiling and secretome analysis differentiate adult-derived human liver stem/progenitor cells and human hepatic stellate cells. PLoS One. 2014;**9**:e86137. DOI: 10.1371/journal.pone.0086137

[162] Higashi T, Friedman SL, Hoshida Y. Hepatic stellate cells as key target in liver fibrosis. Advanced Drug Delivery Reviews. 2017;**121**:27-42. DOI: 10.1016/j.addr.2017.05.007

[163] Lua I, James D, Wang J, Wang KS, Asahina K. Mesodermal mesenchymal cells give rise to myofibroblasts, but not epithelial cells, in mouse liver injury. Hepatology. 2014;**60**:311-322. DOI: 10.1002/hep.27035

[164] Tacke F, Weiskirchen R. Uptake on hepatic stellate cells: Pathogenic role in liver fibrosis and novel isolation techniques. Expert Review of Gastroenterology & Hepatology. 2012;**1**:67-80. DOI: 10.1586/egh.11.92

[165] Yin C, Evason KJ, Asahina K, Stainier DYR. Hepatic stellate cells in liver development, regeneration and cancer. The Journal of Clinical Investigation. 2013;**123**:1902-1909. DOI: 10.1172/JCI66369

[166] Urashima S, Tsutsumi M, Nakase K, Wang JS, Takada A. Studies on capillarization of the hepatic sinusoids in alcoholic liver disease. Alcohol and Alcoholism. Supplement.

1993;**1B**:77-84. DOI: 10.1093/alcalc/28.Supplement_1B.77

[167] Li Y, Wang J, Asahina K. Mesothelial cells give rise to hepatic stellate cells and myofibroblasts via mesothelial-mesenchymal transition in liver injury. PNAS. 2013;**110**:2324-2329. DOI: 10.1073/pnas.1214136110

Chapter 6

Review and Implications of Traditional Indian Medicine for Inflammatory Bowel Disease

Uma Ranjan Lal and Inder Pal Singh

Abstract

Inflammatory bowel disease (IBD) is a group of intestinal disorders that cause prolonged inflammation of digestive tract. Chronic inflammation results in Crohn's disease (CD) and ulcerative colitis (UC). There is a disruption of homeostasis of various regulatory factors, for example, cohesive functioning of intestinal epithelial barrier, macrophages, and cellular mediators such as cytokines and chemokines. Natural products derived from plants based on traditional system of medicine have exhibited efficacy for UC and CD in experimental models and clinical trials. In the present review, current developments of natural products and herbs for the treatment of IBD in the context of Indian traditional medicine have been highlighted. Two classes of Ayurvedic formulation, fermented preparations (*Asava* and *Arishta*) and *Ghrita* (preparations involving butter), are employed for the maintenance of intestinal disorders. Here, we discuss mainly about the fermented preparations, their main constituents, and correlations with modern findings. The way these fermented formulations are processed also affects the extraction of constituents in them. So, the correlation between the chemistry of the plant material (their constituents as well) with the IBD was done. These correlations may serve as a step forward to reduce the gap between modern system of medicine and traditional system of medicine.

Keywords: inflammatory bowel disease, traditional system of medicine, fermented preparations, gallotannins, ellagitannins

1. Introduction

Inflammatory bowel disease (IBD) is the intestinal disorder induced by chronic gastrointestinal inflammation. Crohn's disease (CD) and ulcerative colitis (UC) are global health problems, with the highest incidence and a prevalence rate of 0.5–1.0% in Europe [1]. The incidence of IBD is increasing dramatically in Asian countries, especially in China. There is rising incidence and prevalence of inflammatory bowel disease in India, topping the Southeast Asian (SEA) countries [2]. IBD is relatively complex disease that involves numerous factors such as commensal flora, genetic factors, immune system dysfunction, and environmental risk factors [3]. The human gastrointestinal tract serves as the first-line sensor, and defense against external environment stimuli is exposed to the external environment, particularly to bacterial antigens released from resident microbiota. It is the chronic inflammation in the intestinal surface that first leads to the development of UC, which can progress into CD and/or colon cancer [3]. Advances have been achieved in understanding the pathogenesis of IBD in the past few years, yet exact mechanisms remain to be elucidated. Patients usually suffer from severe pain, diarrhea, abscesses, fistulas, abdominal pain, and stenosis. Thus the development of effective treatments and/or reducing the symptoms of patients with IBD is urgently needed. The current mainstream management of IBD includes antibiotics, corticosteroids, thiopurines, anti-tumor necrosis factor (TNF) antibodies, and aminosalicylates [2]. They have severe side effects such as diarrhea, nausea, vomiting, headache, and osteoporosis when used for the long term. One-third of CD patients undergo surgery after long-term use of these mainstream treatments [4].

The Indian System of Medicine which mainly comprises of Ayurveda (meaning the *science of life*) is one of the oldest systems of medicine in India. This system of using natural resources for better health was developed through the experimentation and experiences of day-to-day lifestyle of Indian people. Evolution of Ayurveda and plant-based remedies for health care through day-to-day life experiences is a part of cultural heritage of India. There is class of Ayurveda fermented preparations called *Asava* and *Arishta* mainly intended for intestinal disorders. These weak alcoholic preparations are more appreciated because of their quick action and high preserving qualities. These preparations are made by soaking the drugs, either powder form or in the form of decoction in a solution of sugar or *jaggery*, as the case may be for a specified period of time, during which it undergoes fermentation. It facilitates dissolution of active principles and acts as a preservative. For *Arishta* preparation, the drugs mentioned in the text are coarsely powdered, and the decoction is prepared by boiling the plant material in a specified volume of water till it is reduced to one-fourth of the original volume. The decoction is filtered using muslin cloth. *Jaggery* as prescribed in formula is added and dissolved. Drugs indicated as *prakshepa dravyas* (plant material added after preparing decoction) are finely powdered and added. At the end *Woodfordia fruticosa* (*Dhataki pushpa*) if mentioned is added. The container is then sealed and kept for fermentation and monitored regularly. After the fermentation is over, the fluid is decanted without disturbing the sediment. The decanted preparation is then kept for maturation for 2 weeks. The fine particles in the decanted preparation settle down (**Figure 1**) [5, 6].

The present review mainly discusses the fermented preparations used in *Ayurveda* for the intestinal disorders and correlates the constituents used for the same. For the preparation of formulations in ancient times, mainly decoctions were used, and then they were preserved by some processing methods, as fermentation in the case of *Asava* and *Arishta*. During the making of formulations, it is the water-soluble ingredients that are mainly extracted to water, and during fermentation they are transformed fit for the body to be absorbed and are medicinally active. The formulations (*Parthadyarishta, Abhayarishta*, *and Jirakadyarishta*) have shown certain chemical changes during fermentation due to which the desired marker constituents in the decoction are transformed: polyphenolics to their monomeric counterparts and glycosides to their respective aglycones [7–9]. HPLC analysis of the selected formulations revealed that it is the polyphenolics which are easily decocted into water and they form the major constituent of these liquid oral formulations. There is also a breakdown of high molecular weight polyphenolics into the low molecular weight phenolics as evident from the quantitative analysis of the formulations. The changes in marker concentrations during fermentation also affect the antioxidant activity of the decoction and formulation [7–9]. Major constituents in these formulations based on their analysis have revealed the presence of polyphenolics (gallotannins and ellagitannins), flavonoids, 5- HMF, and phenolic glycosides, and constituents of jaggery formed the major constituents in the formulation. These constituents are correlated with modern finding in next section.

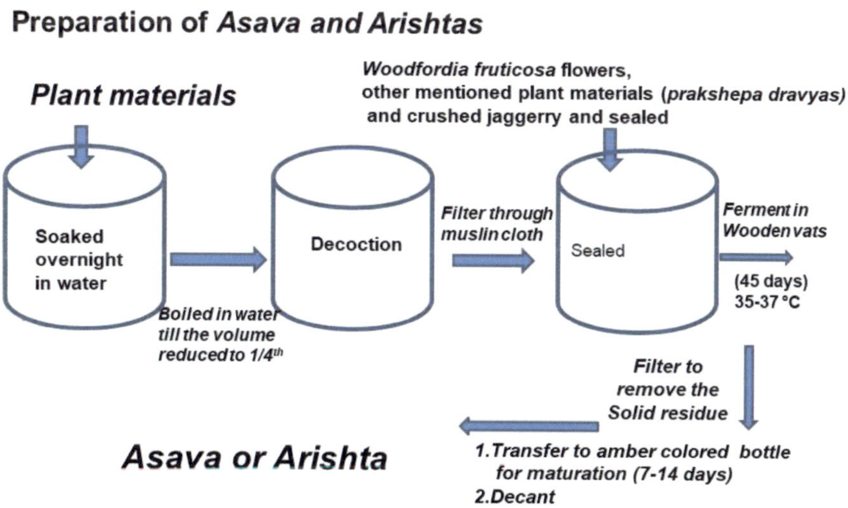

Figure 1.
Method of preparation of fermented preparations in Ayurveda.

2. Major constituents present in fermented preparations and correlation with inflammatory bowel disease

2.1 Gallotannins

Gallotannins are a major constituent of plant materials used for the preparation of fermented preparation *Abhayarishta*. The pericarp of *Terminalia chebula* fruit is used in the preparation which is rich in hydrolyzable tannins and is reported to contain the following constituents: chebulic acid (**1**), gallic acid (**2**), ethyl gallate (**3**), polygalloyl derivatives (**4–6**), chebulinic acid (7), chebulanin (7**a**), chebulagic acid (**8**), terchebin (**9**), and terchebulin (**10**). During the making of formulation, pericarp powder is boiled in water till the volume is reduced to one- fourth, and this process mainly decocts the hydrolyzable tannins. During fermentation these gallotannins are fermented to their monogalloyl and digalloyl derivatives (5) and other counterparts (chebulic acid (**1**) in case of *T. chebula*). The fermented counterparts in case of their preparations have shown more antioxidant activity [7]. They may have very good effect on IBD also as have shown to good inflammatory agents. For example, chebulic acid (**1**) inhibits TNF-α, TNF-α, IL-1β, and IL-6 as well as enhances antioxidant detoxification defensing mediators such as HO-1 and NQO1 expression, through ERK/Nrf2 signaling in HUVEC [10, 11]. It may be noted that tannins in case of *T. chebula* are of chebuloyl derivative [12], and during fermentation 7, 7**a**, and **8** will be hydrolyzed in acidic conditions to chebulic acid (**1**). It is also one of the major constituents in the formulation *Abhayarishta* [7]. Other constituents formed in final processed formulation during fermentation were monogalloyl derivatives and digalloyl derivative. This could be attributed to the presence of free galloyl group at anomeric carbon that makes chebulinic acid (7) and chebulagic acid (**8**) susceptible for cleavage [13]. Moreover, the amount of chebulinic acid (7) in decoction was found to be less (which is normally 2–4% of total dry weight of plant material). The reason for this may be the possible hydrolysis of the chebulinic acid (7) during boiling (as simple boiling resulted in hydrolysis) or less extraction of the same due to its hydrophobic properties resulting from free galloyl groups [13]. Ethyl gallate (**3**) and gallic acid (**1**) were formed as hydrolytic products and ethanolysis of tannic acid (**Figures 2** and **3**). These fermentation products had better radical scavenging activity [7], and among them gallic acid (**1**) has shown to induce ROS-dependent apoptosis and inhibited the growth of colon cancer cells [14]. These formulations are used as nutraceuticals in the Indian subcontinent [15], and the constituents present in the formulation (or formed during the fermentation) have good anti-inflammatory properties as discussed above.

2.2 Ellagitannins

Ellagitannins are the other major phytoconstituents that are extracted during the boiling/maceration with water. This is mainly due to the presence of hexahydroxy-diphenic (HHDP) moiety in ellagitannins [13]. Their extractability in water is more than the gallotannins. Terchebulin (**9**), punicalagin (**10**), and punicalin (**11**) are the major ellagitannins present in decoction and are fermented to increase concentration of ellagic acid in the final formulation [7, 12]. Studies have shown that there is formation

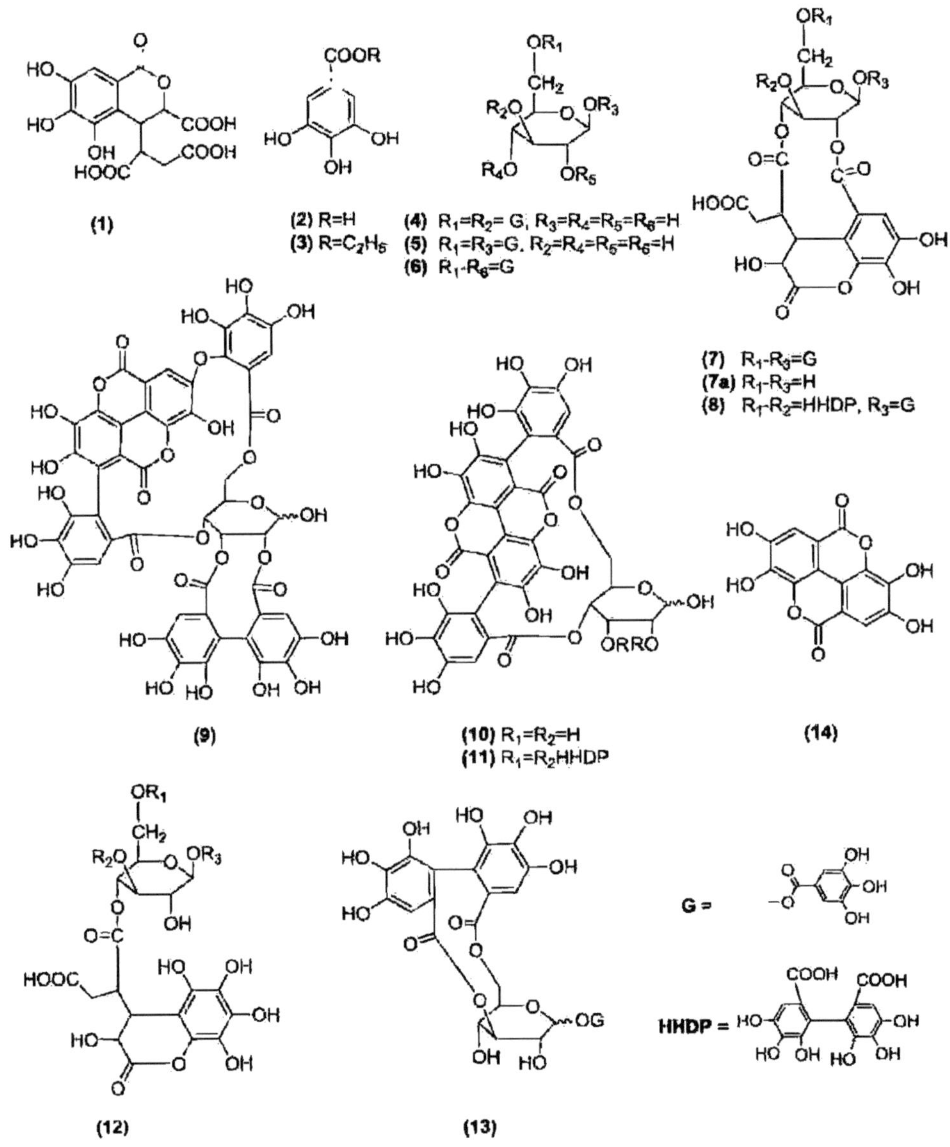

Figure 2.
Structures of compound present in T. chebula *(1–14).*

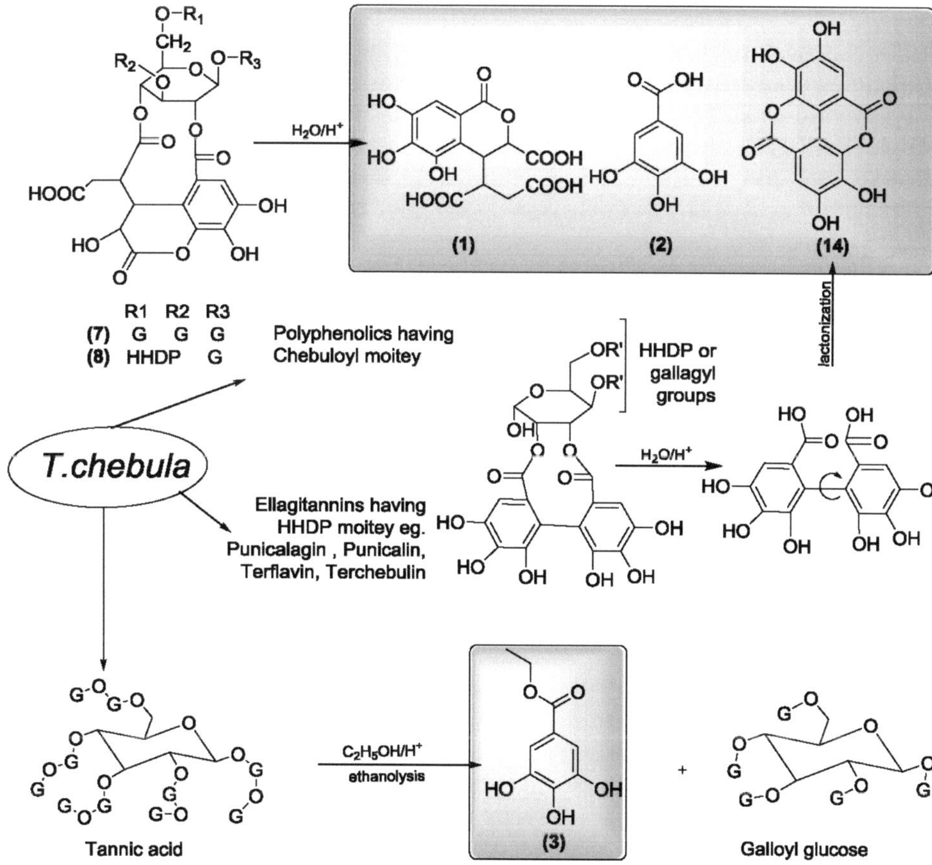

Figure 3.
Possible changes during fermentation in Abhayarishta.

of urolithin A, B, and C by human gut microbiota when an ellagitannin-rich diet was given, and also these urolithins significantly inhibited TNF-α production. The most potent urolithin A inhibition was observed at nanomolar concentrations (at 0.625 μM 29.2 ± 6.4% of inhibition). Urolithin C was the only compound inhibiting IL-6 production (at 0.625 μM 13.9 ± 2.2% of inhibition) [16]. These studies clearly indicate that ellagitannin-rich plant material extract has a good effect on gut microbiota. A combination of the ellagitannin metabolites found in the colon, urolithins and ellagic acid, at concentrations achievable in the intestine after the consumption of pomegranate, was able to moderately improve the inflammatory response of colon fibroblasts and suggest that consumption of ellagitannin-containing foods has potential beneficial effects on gut inflammatory diseases [17]. Effectiveness of polyphenols in dysbiosis and colon-related diseases mainly depends on their stability, absorption, and bioavailability and the gut microbiota composition [18]. Encapsulation technologies could be promising tools to improve bioavailability and bio-accessibility of polyphenols. In recent studies, several micro- and nano-encapsulation systems have been proposed for specific delivery of individual polyphenols or mixtures of polyphenols (food ingredients) in the gut [19].

2.3 Flavonoid glycosides and aglycones

Flavonoid glycosides and phenolic glycosides are the other class of phytoconstituents that are extracted in substantial amount during the boiling of plants during preparation of formulation. These were evident when formulations like

Jirakadyarishta and *Parthadyarishta* were analyzed for standardization purpose [8, 9]. The chemical constituents that are present in cumin seeds (major plant material in *Jirakadyarista*) are water-soluble flavonoid glycosides luteolin 4′-O-glucoside 7-O-galacturonoside (**15**), apigenin-7′-digalactouronoside (**16**), luteolin 7-O-glucoside (**17**), apigenin 7-O-glucoside (**18**), flavonoid aglycones luteolin (**19**), apigenin (**20**), sesquiterpene lactone glucosides, cuminoside A (**21**) and cuminoside B (**22**), cumic acid (**23**), cuminyl alcohol (**24**), glycosides of 2-C-methyl-D erythritol, alkyl glucosides, and various monoterpene glycosides [20–25].

RP-HPLC analysis of the decoction and the final processed formulation revealed that luteolin 4′-*O*-glucoside 7-*O*-galactouronoside (**15**) and luteolin 4′-O-glucoside 7-O-galactouronoside (**16a**) were the two major constituents of the decoction of *C. cyminum*. Selective hydrolysis of 7-O-glucosides of luteolin and apigenin during fermentation resulted in an increase in the amount of luteolin and apigenin in the final processed formulation. The 4′-O-glucoside-7-O-galacturonide of luteolin and galacturonide derivative of apigenin was not hydrolyzed during fermentation [9]. An increase in luteolin and apigenin concentration is also good for the gut health as recent studies have shown that flavonoids participate in the regulation of intestinal tight junction barrier integrity and that this regulation may partially contribute to the flavonoid-mediated biological effects on our health [26]. Dietary flavonoids are often transformed before absorption, and this transformation modulates their biological activity. Health benefits from this aglycone consumption should be attributed to their bioactive metabolites and also to the modulation of the intestinal bacterial population [27]. Flavonoids are the major constituents in the formulation, and various beneficial actions of flavonoids at the GI have been demonstrated through various reports, for example, (i) protection of the intestinal epithelium against pharmacological insults and food toxins and (ii) modulation of the activity of enzymes involved in lipid and carbohydrate absorption. Thus, they maintain the intestinal barrier integrity and modulate the secretion of gut hormones and finally modulate the GI tract immune system. They also have been shown to exert potential anti-colorectal cancer activity by shaping microbiota composition and function. The understanding of the mechanisms mediating the effects of flavonoids on the intestine (and its microbiota) is further required for the widespread recommendations of increasing the intake of plant bioactives [28].

Further, the addition of *Woodfordia fruticosa* for augmenting fermentation also adds flavonoid glycosides to the formulation in major quantity, as evident in the studies done on *Parthadyarishta,* where flavonoid aglycones quercetin and kaempferol were produced as fermentation products from flavonoid glycosides of *Woodfordia fruticosa* [8]. Thus these flavonoid glycosides and aglycones are present in substantial quantity in these formulations and have well-reported protective actions against the IBD through various mechanisms.

2.4 5-Hydroxymethyl furfuraldehyde (5-HMF)

5-Hydroxymethyl furfuraldehyde, 5-HMF (**25**), is another major constituent which is ought to be present in this class of formulation as per the analysis done for the selected formulations. 5-HMF is also present in decoction of fruits and flowers (*V. vinifera and M. indica*) used for preparation of fermented preparations. Another source for **25** in final processed formulation is jaggery and honey which is added in a substantial amount to augment fermentation (**Figures 1** and **4**). 5 -HMF is the major compound extracted during boiling and forms the major constituent in the formulation and is also reportedly formed under acidic conditions from fructose [29]. There was an enormous increase in amount of 5-HMF (**25**) in formulation as compared with decoction. The concentration of **25** needs proper monitoring in this class of formulations as recent reports suggest it to be genotoxic and cytotoxic [30].

Further, Maillard reaction product components, namely, 5-hydroxymethyl furfural and 5-hydroxymethyl-2-furoic acid (HMFA), were shown to have bioactive potential, especially in regard to suppressing oxidative stress and inflammation in IFN-γ- and PMA-induced Caco-2 cells [31]. 5-Hydroxymethyl furfural (HMF)–cysteine adduct, 1-dicysteinethioacetal–5-hydroxymethyl furfural (DCH), promoted the growth of *Lactobacillus*, *Tyzzerella*, *Enterobacter*, and *Streptococcus* and also increased

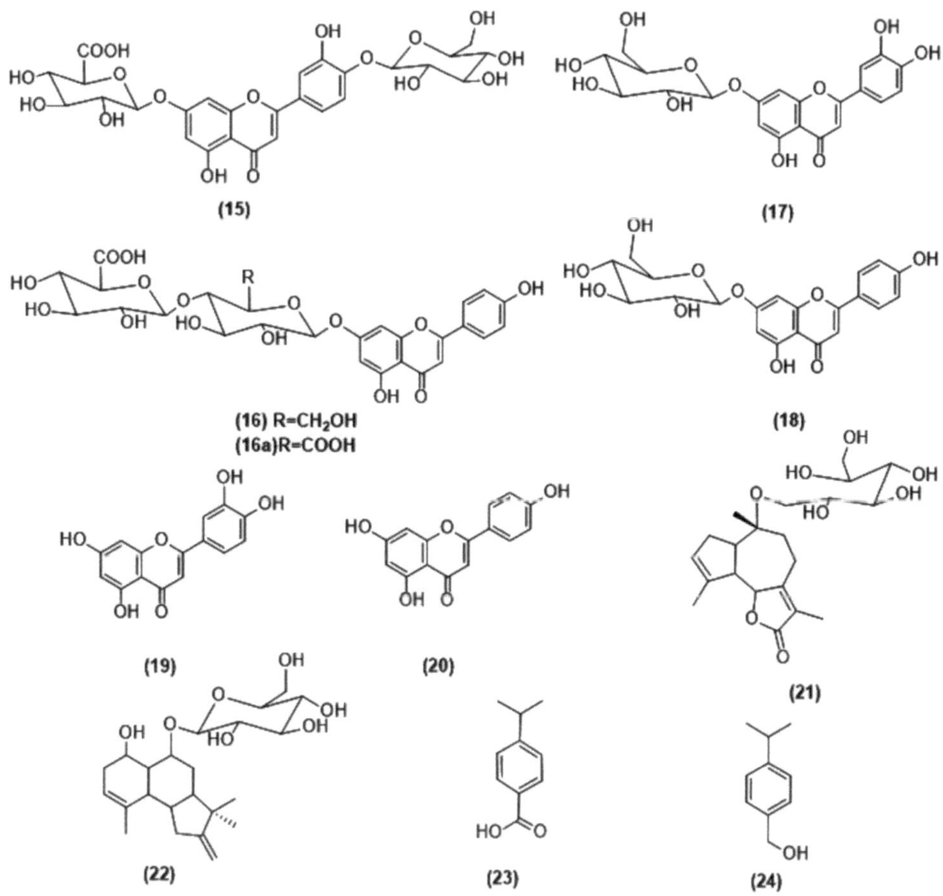

Figure 4.
Water-soluble constituents in cumin Cuminum cyminum *seeds.*

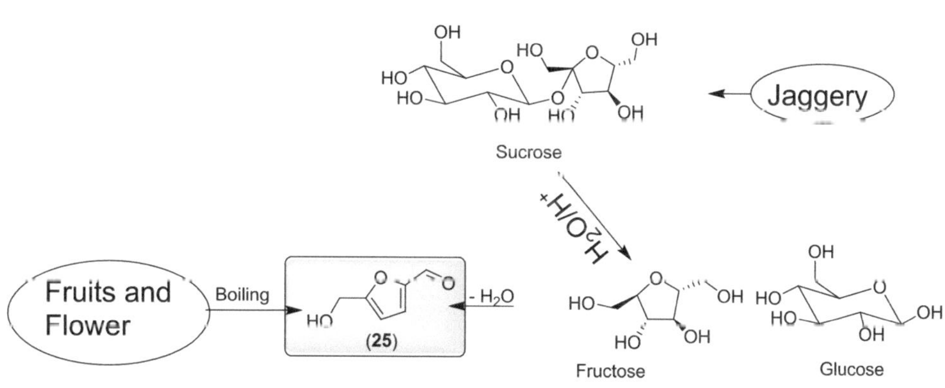

Figure 5.
5-HMF(25) as major constituent in fermented preparation.

the ratio of *Firmicutes/Bacteroidetes* and promoted the growth of *Akkermansia*, *Shigella*, and *Escherichia* while inhibiting the growth of *Lactobacillus* [32]. Thus these reports are suggestive of their usage in controlling IBD (**Figure 5**).

2.5 Bioactives present in jaggery

Jaggery constitutes a major part in this class of formulation. It is also used very frequently in other class of Ayurvedic formulations. Jaggery is traditionally made

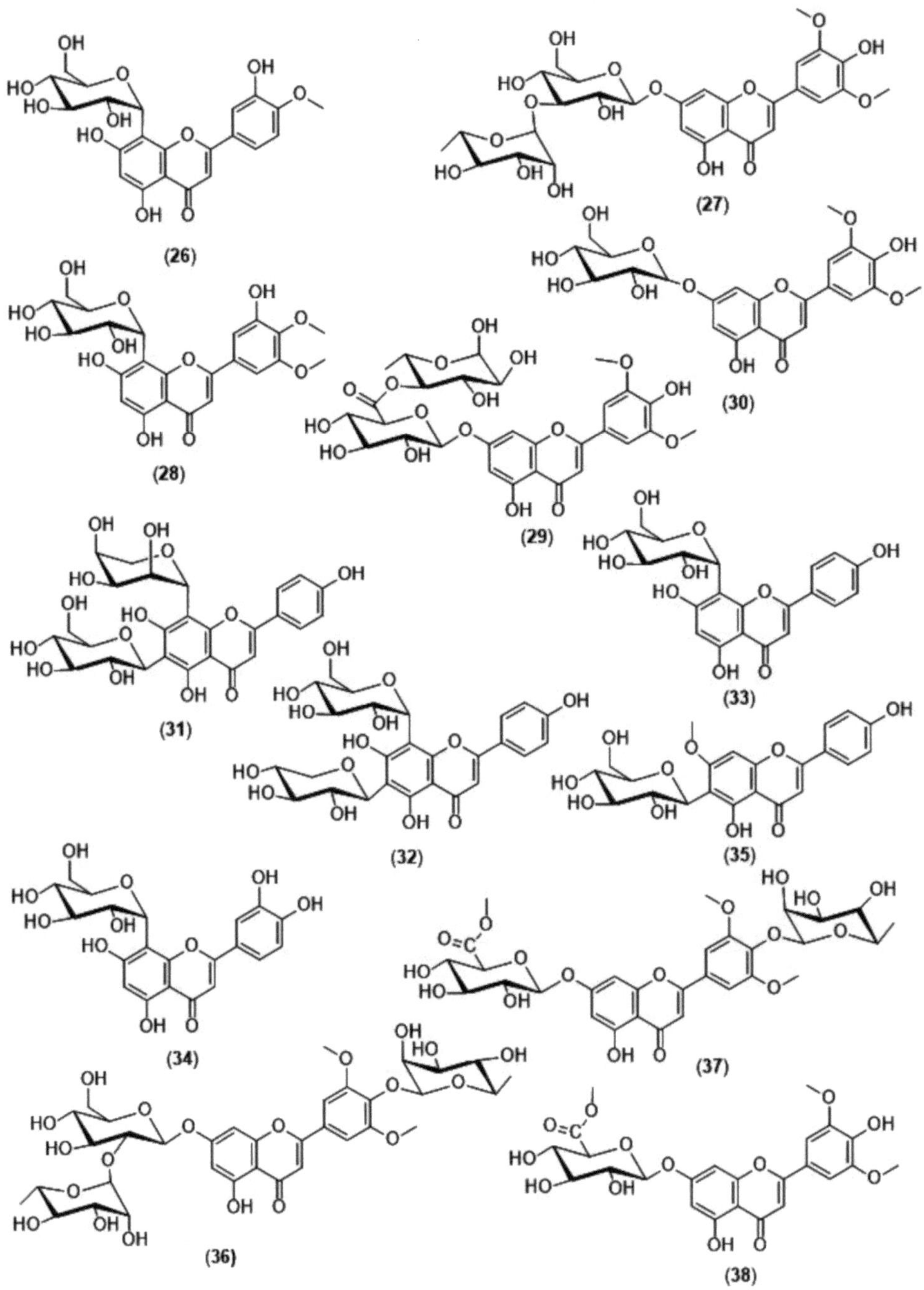

Figure 6.
Flavonoid glycosides in sugarcane juice: (27–38).

by boiling sugarcane juice to solid [33]. A review of chemistry of sugarcane juice and its products reveals that they are rich in phenolics, phenolic glycosides, and flavonoid glycosides (**Figure 6**), namely, diosmetin-8-*C*-glucoside (**26**), tricin-7-*O*-neohesperidoside (**27**), 4′,5′-dimethoxy-luteoline-8-*C*-glucoside (**28**), tricin-7-*O*-rhamnosylgalacturonide (**29**), tricin-7-*O*-glucoside (**30**), schaftoside (**31**), isoschaftoside (**32**), vitexin (**33**), and orientin (**34**). Four minor flavones swertisin (**35**), tricin-7-*O*-neohesperoside-4'-*O*-rhamnoside (**36**), tricin-7-*O*-methylglucuronate-4'-*O*-rhamnoside (**37**), and tricin-7-*O*-methylglucuronide (**38**) were isolated and identified from sugarcane juice [34–39]. There are health benefits from phenolic consumption, mainly attributed to their bioactive metabolites and also to the modulation of the intestinal bacterial population. Phenolic contents of the herbal preparation can be increased as a consequence of fermentation, and a positive correlation between polyphenols and the antioxidant activities of herbs has been well demonstrated. This is in agreement with evidence showing fermentation-mediated enhancement of the pharmacological properties and therapeutic efficacies of herbal formulations against a number of diseases including obesity and inflammation [27].

3. Conclusions

From the evidences cited above, it is very clear that herbal formulations and their analysis for the presence of bioactive constituents are important as far as their efficacy is concerned. Three formulations have been cited, and major constituents present in them have proven to be good agents for IBD. Natural products and herbal medicine formulas have exhibited efficacy in preclinical evaluation, improved symptoms, and decreased medical costs for IBD patients. The components of natural products and herbs are complex and have multiple mechanisms of action that may synergize to produce their overall efficacy. Intensive studies based on murine models of IBD and human studies are required for evaluating the efficacy of natural products and herbal medicine as an alternative treatment for IBD. Thus identification of the active component(s) and optimization of the dosage and development of treatment protocol(s) are of primary importance. The modern hyphenated techniques having high-throughput technologies shall enable the identification of the effective ingredient(s) and reveal the mechanisms of action of natural products and herbs in treating IBD. Natural products and herbal formulations (as co-adjuvants) with existing medications may also provide new therapy options for IBD patients.

Conflict of interest

Authors declare no conflict of interest.

Author details

Uma Ranjan Lal[1]* and Inder Pal Singh[2]

1 Department of Natural Products, National Institute of Pharmaceutical Education and Research, Ahmedabad, Palaj, Gandhinagar, Gujarat, India

2 Department of Natural Products, National Institute of Pharmaceutical Education and Research, Mohali, Punjab, India

*Address all correspondence to: urlalvv@yahoo.com

References

[1] Loddo I, Romano C. Inflammatory bowel disease: Genetics, epigenetics, and pathogenesis. Frontiers in Immunology. 2015;**6**:551

[2] Ray G. Inflammatory bowel disease in India—Past, present and future. World Journal of Gastroenterology. 2016;**22**(36):8123-8136. DOI: 10.3748/wjg.v22.i36.8123

[3] Chen X, Nie Y, Xiao H, et al. TNFR2 expression by CD4 effector T cells is required to induce full-fledged experimental colitis. Scientific Reports. 2016;**6**:328-334

[4] Chan HC, Ng SC. Emerging biologics in inflammatory bowel disease. Journal of Gastroenterology. 2017;**52**:141-150

[5] Anonymous. Ayurvedic Formulary of India—Part I. 2nd ed. New Delhi: Department of AYUSH, Ministry of Health and Family Welfare; 2003

[6] Anonymous. Pharmcopoeial Standards of Ayurvedic Formulations. Revised ed. New Delhi: CCRAS, Government of India, Ministry of Health and Family Welfare, Department of Health; 1987. pp. 1-20

[7] Lal UR, Triptathi SM, Jachak SM, Bhutani KK, Singh IP. HPLC analysis and standardization of Arjunarishta—An ayurvedic cardioprotective formulation. Scientia Pharmaceutica. 2009;77:605-616

[8] Lal UR, Triptathi SM, Jachak SM, Bhutani KK, Singh IP. Chemical changes during fermentation in Abhayarishta and its standardization by HPLC-DAD. Natural Product Communications. 2010;**5**(4):575-579

[9] Lal UR, Triptathi SM, Jachak SM, Bhutani KK, Singh IP. RP-HPLC-DAD analysis of Jirakadyarishta and chemical changes during fermentation. Natural Product Communications. 2010;**5**(11):1767-1770

[10] Hyun-Sun L, Yoon-Chang K, Hyung Joo S, Kyung-Yong K, Kwang-Won L. Preventive effects of chebulic acid isolated from *Terminalia chebula* on advanced glycation endproduct-induced endothelial cell dysfunction. Journal of Ethnopharmacology. 2010;**131**(3):567-574. DOI: 10.1016/j.jep.2010.07.039

[11] Mi-Hyun N, Won-rak S, Sung-Yong Y, Young-Seok L, Kwang-Won L. Chebulic acid inhibits advanced glycation end products-mediated vascular dysfunction by suppressing ROS via the ERK/Nrf2 pathway. Journal of Functional Foods. 2017;**36**:150-161. DOI: 10.1016/j.jff.2017.06.058

[12] Lin TC, Nonaka GI, Nishioka I, Ho FC. Tannins and related compounds, structure of terchebulin, an ellagitannin having novel tetraphenylcarboxylic acid (terchebulic acid) moiety and biogenetically related tannins from *T. chebula*. Chemical & Pharmaceutical Bulletin. 1990;**38**:3004-3008

[13] Tanaka T, Zhang H, Jiang ZH, Kouno I. Relationship between hydrophobicity and structure of hydrolysable tannins and association of tannin with crude drug constituents in aqueous solutions. Chemical & Pharmaceutical Bulletin. 1997;**45**:1891-1897

[14] Subramanian AP, Jaganathan SK, Mandal M, Supriyanto E, Muhamad II. Gallic acid induced apoptotic events in HCT-15 colon cancer cells. World Journal of Gastroenterology. 2016;**22**(15):3952-3961. DOI: 10.3748/wjg.v22.i15.3952

[15] Lal UR, Singh S, Banerjee S, Singh IP. Nutraceuticals and functional foods—An Indian prespective. In:

Recent Progress in Medicinal Plants Vol-42, Nutraceuticals and Functional Foods. Houston, Texas, U.S.A: Studium Press, LLC; 2016. ISBN-1626990794 EAN- 9781626990791

[16] Piwowarski JP, Granica S, Zwierzyńska M, Stefańska J, Matthias PS, Melzig F, et al. Role of human gut microbiota metabolism in the anti-inflammatory effect of traditionally used ellagitannin-rich plant materials. Journal of Ethnopharmacology. 2014;**155**(1):801-809. DOI: 10.1016/j.jep.2014.06.032

[17] Giménez-Bastida JA, Larrosa M, González-Sarrías A, Tomás-Barberán F, Espín JC, García-Conesa MT. Associated molecular markers in human colon fibroblasts. Journal of Agricultural and Food Chemistry. 2012;**60**:8866-8876. DOI: 10.1021/jf300290f

[18] Kasote DM, Jayaprakasha GK, Patil BS. Chapter 13: Encapsulation of polyphenols: An effective way to enhance their bioavailability for gut health. In: Jayaprakasha GK, Patil BS, Gattuso G. editors. Advances in Plant Phenolics: From Chemistry to Human Health. ACS Division of Agricultural and Food Chemistry Inc. Vol. 1286. Washington, D.C.: ACS Symposium Series, American Chemical Society; 2018. pp. 239-259. DOI: 10.1021/bk-2018-1286. ch013

[19] Millqvist-Fureby A. Approaches to Encapsulation of Active Food Ingredients in Spray-Drying. In: Huang Q , Given P, Qian M, editors. Micro/Nanoencapsulation of Active Food Ingredients. ACS Division of Agricultural and Food Chemistry Inc. Vol. 1007. Washington, D.C.: American Chemical Society; 2009. pp. 233-245. DOI: 10.1021/bk-2009-1007.ch015

[20] Harborne JB, Williams CA. Flavonoid patterns in the fruits of the umbelliferae. Phytochemistry. 1972;**11**:1741

[21] Khafagy SM, Sarg TM, Abdel Salam NA, Gabr O. Isolation of two flavone glycosides from the fruits of *Cuminum cyminum* L. grown in Egypt. Die Pharmazie. 1978;**33**:296-297

[22] Harborne JB. The Flavonoids—Advances in Research Since 1986. London: Chapman and Hall; 1996. pp. 448-460

[23] Sachin BS, Sharma SC, Sethi S, Tasduq SA, Tikoo MK, Satti NK, et al. Herbal modulation of drug bioavailability: Enhancement of rifampicin levels in plasma by herbal products and a flavonoid glycoside derived from *Cuminum cyminum*. Phytotherapy Research. 2007;**21**:157-163

[24] Takayanagi T, Ishikawa T, Kitajima J. Sesquiterpene lactone glucosides and alkyl glycosides from the fruit of cumin. Phytochemistry. 2003;**63**:479-484

[25] Ishikawa T, Takayanagi T, Kitajima J. Water-soluble constituents of cumin: Monoterpenoid glucosides. Chemical & Pharmaceutical Bulletin. 2002;**50**:1471-1478

[26] Noda S, Tanabe S, Suzuki T. Differential effects of flavonoids on barrier integrity in human intestinal Caco-2 cells. Journal of Agricultural and Food Chemistry. 2012;**60**:4628-4633

[27] Selma MV, Espín JC, Tomás-Barberán FA. Interaction between phenolics and gut microbiota: Role in human health. Journal of Agricultural and Food Chemistry. 2009;**57**(15):6485-6501

[28] Oteiza PI, Fraga CG, Mills DA, Taft DH. Flavonoids and the gastrointestinal tract: Local and systemic effects. Molecular Aspects of Medicine. 2018;**61**:41-49

[29] Takagaki A, Ohara M, Nishimura S, Ebitani K. A one-pot reaction for biorefinery: Combination of solid acid and base catalysts for direct production of 5-hydroxymethylfurfural from saccharides. Chemical Communications. 2009;**41**:6276-6278

[30] Severin I, Dumont C, Jondeau-Cabaton A, Graillot V, Chagnon MC. Genotoxic activities of the food contaminant 5-hydroxymethylfurfural using different in vitro bioassays. Toxicology Letters. 2009;**192**:189-194

[31] Kitts DD, Chen XM, Jing H. Demonstration of antioxidant and anti-inflammatory bioactivities from sugar–amino acid Maillard reaction products. Journal of Agricultural and Food Chemistry. 2012;**60**:6718-6727

[32] Zhao Q, Ou J, Huang C, Qiu R, Wang Y, Liu F, et al. Absorption of 1-dicysteinethioacetal–5-hydroxymethylfurfural in rats and its effect on oxidative stress and gut microbiota. Journal of Agricultural and Food Chemistry. 2018;**66**:11451-11458

[33] Singh A, Lal UR, Mukhtar HM, Singh PS, Shah G, Dhawan RK. Phytochemical profile of sugarcane and its potential health aspects. Pharmacognosy Reviews. 2015;**9**(17):45-54

[34] Palla G. Isolation and identification of phenolic glycosides in liquid sugar from cane molasses. Journal of Agriculture and Food Chemistry. 1982;**30**:764-766

[35] Smith P, Paton N. Sugarcane flavonoids. Sugar Technological Review. 1985;**12**:117-142

[36] Paton NH. Sugarcane phenolics and first expressed juice colour. International Sugar Journal. 1992;**94**:99-102

[37] Fabiana CV, Renata C. HPLC microfraction of flavonoids and antioxidants activity of *S. officinarum*. Journal of the Brazilian Chemical Society. 2008;**19**:903-908

[38] Joaguim MD, Novoa AV, Linares AV, Lojalo FM. Antioxidant activity of phenolic compounds from sugarcane juice. Plant Foods for Human Nutrition. 2006;**61**:187-192

[39] Colombo R, Yariwake JH, Queroz EF, Nadijoko K. On line identification of minor flavones from sugarcane juice by LC/UV/MS and post column derivatization. Journal of the Brazilian Chemical Society. 2009;**20**(9):1574-1579

Section 3

Role of Chronic Inflammation in Cancer

Chapter 7

Immuno-Oncology, Imaging Biomarkers and Response to Chemotherapy in Cancer Treatment

Alireza Ziaei and Forough Kheiry

Abstract

Immuno-oncology is a young and growing field in cancer therapy. It stimulates immune system to target and attack the tumor or inhibiting the immune response. Recent findings in cancer immunotherapy has revealed that the immune system can control many cancers across various histologies, producing durable responses in a way which not seen with many small molecule drugs. Advances in understanding the role and molecular mechanisms of immunotherapy are revolutionizing clinical practice in cancer treatment. Immunotherapy is being intensively explored with the aim of improving primary response rates or prolonging overall survival. The purpose of this chapter is to review the different aspect of immunotherapy including blockade of immunological checkpoints, immuno-oncology and imaging biomarkers, immune response, therapeutic resistance and combination therapy, while several additional immuno-therapeutic strategies are also highlighted.

Keywords: immune response, immunotherapy, immuno-oncology, cancer

1. Introduction

Cancer plays a serious role in public health bother. Global demographic features increase the predicted incidence of cancer in the coming decades. Annually, cancer is expected to reach 420 million new cases by 2025. Female breast cancer, colorectal, prostate, and lung are often diagnostic cancers in Europe, while lung cancer is the leading explanation for cancer and death worldwide [1]. The increasing information of biology and tumors over the past 15 years has considerably modified the pattern of cancer. Throughout the past decades, immune therapy has been used as a promising approach to the treatment of a broad variety of human cancers. But these methods such as chemotherapy and radiotherapy seem to be effective enough due to the problems including low target property, drug resistance, severe side effects and immuno-therapies induce host immune system to promote a response against tumors [2]. An important feature of Immunotherapy is to kill malignant tumors whereas healthy tissues not damaged. The issue of immunotherapy is to expand strategies that effectively and securely enhance anti-tumor responses. A few current cancer immunotherapy methods tested for their effectiveness include cytokine treatment, cell-receptor cell transfer, cancer vaccines and monoclonal antibodies (mAbs). The most encouraging of these approaches are those that are specific T-cell stimulants that are capable of long-term tumor immunity [3]. The activity and regulation of T-cell is vital for the development of the tumor, since T-cells have the ability to remove cancerous cells [4].

2. Checkpoint blockade in immuno-oncology therapy

Checkpoint inhibitors are immune synapses which decrease the function of T-lymphocyte [5]. They are against autoimmunity and systemic inflammations. These mechanisms help tumor to escape from immune detection [2, 5]. The most frequent useful checkpoint inhibitor is checkpoint inhibitor mAbs, anti-cytotoxic T lymphocyte-associated protein 4 (CTLA-4) and anti-programmed cell death protein 1 (PD-1) [6, 7]. Checkpoint inhibitors invigorate immune system and persuade tumors. However, stimulation of cancerous T-cell proliferation can provide non-Hodgkin lymphoma (NHL) [2, 8]. Complication of checkpoint inhibitors is an autoimmune disease. Due to PD-1 or CTLA-4 illustrates beneficial result on advanced-stage melanoma [2, 9]. So, cytotoxic T lymphocyte antigen-4 and B7.1 are the most frequent targets in Immunotherapy. They can manage the interaction between T-cell and dendritic cells [1, 10].

2.1 PD-1

PD-1 is a receptor which is increased by T-cells during peripheral activation. PD-1 blockade down regulates the activity of intramural T regulatory cells [10]. Tumors can evade from immune system by inhibiting PD-1. Also, PD-1 is expressed by other immune cells such as lymphocyte B, natural killer (NK) cells and dendritic cells [4, 11–13]. PD-L1 has two ligands including PD-L1 (B7-H1) and PD-L2 (B7-H2). These two ligands expressed by inflammation and tumors tissues [4, 14]. Also, these ligands are expressed on antigen presenting cell (APCs). In addition, tumor tissues express these ligands [13]. PD-1 reduces the activity of T-cells later than CTLA-4. So, PD-1 influences on immune response during the chronic inflammation. PD-1 is important for the monitoring of Tregs suppressor performance [4]. CD80 or B7-1 is linked to PD-L1. Bidirectional interactions can inhibit PD-L1 and B7-1. Evading of PD-1 from immune diagnosis is so important [13]. Overall, PD-L1 in cancer is related to poor prognosis and larger tumor size and reduction in cytotoxic activity [4, 15, 16]. But, PD-1 can stop NHL by diminishing the proliferation of cancerous T-cells [15]. PD-L2 only can regulate the responses of Th2. But, PD-L2 is not selected as a target in cancer. PD-L2 does not have strong relation with survival. However, PD-L1 has the most potent influence and anti-tumor Th1 responses [4, 9]. PD-L1 is a useful ligand to manage several cancers like melanoma, non-small cell lung cancer (NSCLC) and kidney cancer [9].

2.2 CTLA-4

Cytotoxic T lymphocyte antigen 4 (CTLA-4) is a glycoprotein that exists on the surface of T cells [1]. When T-cells activation is regulated in its early stage, T-cells in central lymph nodes express CTLA-4. CTLA-4 which is expressed by regulatory T cells (Tregs) can control the activated lymphocyte's proliferation in the lymph nodes. CTLA-4 plays a role in joining to B7·1 and B7·2 and involves with CD28. So, CTLA-4 can discontinue the activation and production of T cells. Anti-CTLA-4 decreases the Tregs cell to promote the proliferation of T cells [2, 10].

2.3 CD73

The investigations on anti-CD73 or anti-adenosine phase 1 found that they could effectively provoke immune response and improve the functions of first generation immune checkpoint inhibitors [17]. CD73 in Triple-negative breast cancer have poor prognosis [18]. Estrogen receptor (ER) negative has poor prognosis as well. CD73 in ER positive has no prognostic value. Stages I–III have good prognosis [19]. CD73 in B-cell acute lymphoblastic leukemia is a marker of minimal residual disease. B-cell chronic lymphocytic leukemia expresses CD73 as a marker of aggressiveness. CD73 is associated with CD38 and ZAP70 expression; two markers of disease progression in B-cell chronic lymphocytic leukemia [18, 20, 21]. CD73 in glioblastoma multiform (GBM) has poor prognosis [17]. CD73 is associated with limited metastatic potential in melanoma [17]. High-grade serous CD73 expression shows poor prognosis in ovarian cancers. However, CD73 expression indicated good prognosis in Epithelial ovarian cancer [17].

3. First group of immunotherapy medication

3.1 Ipilimumab (Yervoy)

Ipilimumab is a fully human immunoglobulin G1 (IgG1) monoclonal. It up regulates T-cell activation by targeting CTLA-4 and is used in phase 2 data for tumor response and safety by logistic regression models. Ipilimumab dosage is about 0.3, 3, and 10 mg/kg every 3 weeks for maximum four doses. About 10 mg/kg doses of Ipilimumab are more effective than 3 mg/kg in metastatic melanoma. However, 10 mg/kg doses of Ipilimumab have more serious side effects [1, 22, 23]. Clinical efficacy of Ipilimumab shows strong improvement on survival. Its response rate is 9–18% in phase III clinical trial in patients with NSCLC. Also, treatment scenario for Ipilimumab is pretreated and its control arm is Docetaxel. Response rate in patient with melanoma in phase 3 trial is p100 10.9 mo vs. 1.5 mo. Treatment scenario for Ipilimumab is pretreated in management of melanoma [1].

3.2 Tremelimumab

Tremelimumab is fully humanized IgG2 antibody and its target cell is T lymphocyte. Tremelimumab affects T lymphocyte by targeting CTL-4 and is an immune checkpoint inhibitor in hepatocellular carcinoma (HCC) clinical trials [1]. The effect of Tremelimumab has recently been studied in combination with Durvalumab on HCC. The response rate of this combination on HCC was approximately 25%. In phase 3 on metastatic melanoma, Tremelimumab can increase overall survival in comparison to chemotherapy [10]. It is given every 3 weeks for the management of melanoma and has 10% response rate [1]. Another study on phase 1 clinical trial has shown that the combination of Tremelimumab and CP-893,870 (a CD40-agonist mAb) provides the 27% objective response rate and 26 months overall survival. Also this combination provides 8% complete response rate [2].

3.3 Pembrolizumab (Keytruda)

Pembrolizumab is a humanized IgG4 monoclonal antibody against PD-1. It has only influence on tumors express programmed death-ligand 1 (PD-L1) [4, 24]. Pembrolizumab is recommended for the management of advance melanoma along with Ipilimumab. The recommended dosage is 2 mg/kg each 3 weeks in phase 1 clinical trial in patient with metastatic melanoma [1, 4, 24]. Also, Pembrolizumab is suggested for the treatment of metastatic NSCLC [4]. This drug has been studied in various cancer including gastric/gastroesophageal junction cancer (phase III), NSCLC (phase III), squamous cell carcinoma of the head and neck (SCCHN) (phase III), urothelial cancer (phase III), colorectal carcinoma (phase II), gastric/ gastroesophageal junction cancer (phase II), GBM Merkel cell carcinoma (phase II), Hodgkin lymphoma (HL) and NHL (phase II). Pembrolizumab is one of the most important immune checkpoint inhibitors in HCC clinical trials. Response rate of Pembrolizumab is about 25 vs. 4% in patients with melanoma in phase II clinical trial. Also its control arm is investigator's choice chemotherapy. Also, using Pembrolizumab, as first line in treatment of melanoma, has 33.7 vs. 11.9% response rate in phase 3 clinical trial [23]. A recent study shows the saturations of Pemberolizumab is reached to 95% by dosage of 1 mg/kg every 3 week. Some studies revealed that reaching to complete achievement of the goal is 64% by 1 mg/kg each 3 week. However, complete achievements ≥2 mg/kg (such as 10 mg/kg) is higher 90% [25]. Later study has found that Pembrolizumab illustrates equivalence in exposure at dosage body weight-based 2-mg/kg each 3 week. But, Nivolumab does not have equality in exposure at indefinite quantity of two hundred mg each 3 weeks [24, 26]. Pembrolizumab clearance decreases about 20% after first injection. But this clearance is not clinically important [24, 27]. Common side effects of Pembrolizumab are fatigue, pruritus, and decreased appetite. Recent study in lung cancer patients shows 50% of tumors cell has PD-L1 receptors. In addition, Pembrolizumab has 45.2% response rate in patients who has PD-L1 receptors. But, objective response rate is 19.4% through all patients with metastatic lung cancer [27].

3.4 Blinatumomab (connecting bi-specific antibodies)

Blinatumomab is approved for CD19+ B-cell malignancies and its pre-clinical finding has strong in-vitro cytolytic activity. Blinatumomab's pharmacokinetics has clear kinetics and can trigger T lymphocytes to reach tumors cell. One of the recent studies on Blinatumomab shows that its clinical efficacy has high response rates, and its safety has moderate to severe toxicity [23].

3.5 Nivolumab (Optivo)

Nivolumab is a human immunoglobulin G4 (IgG4) monoclonal antibody that targets PD-1. Nivolumab target cell is T lymphocyte and is accepted in cancer with expressing PD-L1 and also without expressing PD-L1 [4]. Nivolumab dosage is about 1–10 mg/kg. Also non-clinical data recommends 0.3 mg/kg as initial dose. Low-immunogenic tumor types needed higher Nivolumab dosage. For instance, beneficial dosage for melanoma and renal cell carcinoma (immunogenic tumors) is 1–10 mg/kg (1 mg/kg each 2 week) [26]. However, higher dosage (3 and 10 mg/kg each 2 week) needs for NSCLC. Thus, lower dose level can have longer progression-free survival in immunogenic tumor types. Nivolumab is approved for both PD-L1 expressers [24, 28]. Recent studies indicate that Nivolumab has increased the survival in patients with melanoma [28, 29]. Nivolumab has 25–40% response rate with long lasting response (2 years) in patients with melanoma. Another study in phase III trial has shown Nivolumab has increased survival in comparison with chemotherapy in patients with advance melanoma and advance NSCLC [4]. Nivolumab should be selected 3 mg/kg each 2 week as monotherapy dose for different type of tumors to improve survival [30]. The investigation exhibited that there was a linear relationship between Nivolumab pharmacokinetics and the dose range. For renal cell carcinoma, metastatic melanoma and NSCLC, suggested dosage is

240 mg IV every 2 week depends on population pharmacokinetics analyses and response analyses of dose and exposure [31]. Also, Nivolumab is prescribed for renal cell carcinoma due to second choice. Pharmacometrics has main role in changing body weight based on dosage to flat dosage. The advantages of using a flat dose include removing excess material waste, the convenience of health care providers, and reducing worries about the exact dose in patients with weight fluctuations. Combination of Nivolumab and Ipilimumab are used in the management of melanoma [28]. Nivolumab are investigated in different types of tumors including gastric cancer (phase III), GBM (phase III), acute myeloid leukemia (AML) (phase II), anal canal (phase II), cervical cancer (phase II), colon cancer (phase II), HL, NHL (phase II), nasopharyngeal carcinoma (phase II), pancreatic cancer (phase II) [4]. Nivolumab is one of important Immune checkpoint inhibitors in HCC clinical trials. Nivolumab's pre-clinical findings has moderate effect and its clinical efficacy has a strong influence on improvement of survival. It is used for the first line treatment of melanoma in phase 3 clinical trial. Nivolumab's control arm is Dacarbazine. Melanoma response rate of Nivolumab is approximately 40 vs. 13.9%. Nivolumab is used in treatment of NSCLC as pretreated with response rate about 32 vs. 11% in phase 3 clinical trial and the control arm is investigator's choice chemotherapy [1].

3.6 Atezolizumab

Atezolizumab is a humanized Fc-engineered IgG1 monoclonal and binds to PD-L1. Atezolizumab promote neither activate antibody-dependent cell-mediated cytotoxicity (ADCC) nor complement-dependent cytotoxicity (CDC). Also, Atezolizumab blocks the interaction with PD-1 and B7.1 receptors on tumor cells. Recent study shows that the best dosage for metastatic urothelial carcinoma and metastatic NSCLC is 1200 mg every 3 weeks. Also later study on dose-escalation in phase 1 indicates dosage of Atezolizumab is about 0.01–20 mg/kg based on body weights [32].

3.7 Durvalumab

Durvalumab is a humanized Fc-engineered IgG1 monoclonal and binds to PD-L1. Durvalumab promote neither ADCC nor CDC, and avoids the ability of toxicity caused by it does not have attraction to joining PD-L2. Recommended dosage of Durvalumab is 10 mg/kg each 2 weeks in carcinoma of urothelial. Proposed concentration in metastatic urothelial carcinoma is about 50 μg/mL. Recommended fixed dosage regimen of Durvalumab is 1500 mg every 4 week or 750 mg every 2 week. This regimen indicates similar overall pharmacokinetic exposure based on body weight [33].

3.8 Avelumab

Avelumab is a fully human IgG1 monoclonal antibody and has short half-life for about 3.9–4.1 days compare to Nivolumab which is about 12–20 days, Pembrolizumab with half-life of 14–22 days, and Atezolizumab with half-life of 21 days. Avelumab shows the reduction in clearance similar to Nivolumab and Pembrolizumab during long treatments. The investigation of avelumab on metastatic Merkel cell carcinoma after 1 year of follow up has shown that avelumab can be effective in treating advance Merkel cell carcinoma due to 33.0% overall response rate (ORR) and 11.4% to complete response rate. The dosage is used in that study was 10 mg/kg every 2 weeks. Also, studies in phase 1 have shown that this drug can also be effective in patients with platinum-refractory metastatic urothelial carcinoma cancer due to 17.3% ORR [24, 34–38].

4. Second group of immunotherapy medication

Next-generation of novel therapeutic target include VISTA, LAG-3, TIGIT, and TIM-3 inhibitors. Also, another potential checkpoint is p-selectin glycoprotein ligand-1 (PSGL-1) which regulates T-cell responses in tumor microenvironment (TME). CTLA-4 and PD-1 are co-target receptors which they are responsible for supporting overall immune self-tolerance. However, TIGIT, LAG-3, and TIM-3 receptors influence on NK and CD8+ T-cell. Treg cell suppressive influence and improving CD8+ and NK cell activity inside malignancy tissues is revoked by synergizing their corresponding blockade. Thus, synergizing of first- and second generation inhibitors provoke immune system to have beneficial response against malignancies [2, 39–41].

4.1 T-cell immunoglobulin-3 (Tim-3)

Tim-3 is expressed on IFNγ producing CD4+ T helper 1 (Th1) and CD8+ T cytotoxic 1 (Tc1) T-cells. Also, Tim-3 is expressed on Treg cells and on innate immune cells (DC, NK cells, and monocytes). Co-inhibition of Tim-3 and PD-1 is more beneficial than PD-1 alone inhibition in anti-tumor effector functions. Tim-3 shows the dysfunction of CD8+ T-cells in cancers. Co-inhibition in Tim-3 and PD-1 has greater effects in managing melanoma, NSCLC, and NHL [37].

4.2 T-cell immunoglobulin and ITIM domain (TIGIT)

T-cell immunoglobulin and ITIM domain (TIGIT) Ligand (CD155 and CD112) are expressed in tumors cells. Negative TIGIT up regulate anti-tumors activities. Dysfunctional phenotype among CD8+ TILs is produced by co-expression of CD8 plus TIGIT+ TILs with PD-1, Tim-3, and Lag3. Co-inhibition of TIGIT with PD-1 increased proliferation, cytokine production, and degranulation In CD8+ TILs from melanoma patients [37]. Moreover, TIGIT synergies with Tim-3 to improve anti-tumor responses. So, both co-inhibition of TIGIT with PD-1 or TIGIT with Tim-3 induce anti-tumor effects. In addition, TIGIT are expressed on tumor infiltrating Treg. Restrictive phenotype of Treg cell is provided by the TIGIT+ Treg in tissues with malignancy cells. Notably, CD8+ T-cell function (direct suppression) and promotion of Treg function (indirect suppression) can suppress anti-tumor immunity by TIGIT [37].

4.3 B-cell and T-cell lymphocyte attenuator (BLTA)

B-cell and T-cell lymphocyte attenuator (BTLA) is an immunoglobulin-like molecule expressed on different cells such as on B-cells, T-cells, NK cells, and APCs. BLTA is a section of CD28 family. BLTA plays a major role in early T-cell regulation and provides early T-cell response gene. Combination of BLTA and herpes virus entry mediator (HVEM) induces reduction of T-cell proliferation and cytokine production. Melanoma cells are expressed HVEM. The combination of BTLA and HVEM inhibits the expansion and IFNγ production. Also, BLTA is related to restricted T-cell expansion. Inhibition of BTLA, PD-1, and TIM3 together increase IL-2. Inhibition of BTLA, PD-1, and TIM3 can restore T-cell dysfunctions. After the BTLA and HVEM interconnections, T-cell activation and level of IFNγ decreases [13].

4.4 V-domain Ig suppressor of T-cell activation (VISTA)

V-domain Ig suppressor of T-cell activation (VISTA) is a powerful suppressor of T-cell [13] which is expressed by hematopoietic tissues and infiltrating leukocytes.

VISTA is predominantly found on leukocytes inside tumors and myeloid hematopoietic section 140. Like PD-L1, it promotes suppression of CD4 and CD8. VISTA also has long-lasting kinetics which can induce the reduction of cytokine production such as IL-10, TNF-alpha, and IFNγ. VISTA inhibition increase the frequency of tumor-infiltrating effector T-cells by combining to a specific antibody. Thus this combination inhibit tumor growth. VISTA can increase overall survival by combining to an agonistic CD40 antibody, TLR agonists, and tumor antigen peptides [13].

4.5 CD160

CD160 is a glycosyl-phosphatidyl-inositol (GPI) which is expressed on CD8þ T-cells, NK cells, and NK-T cells. CD160 inhibition induces T-cell proliferation and cytokine production 147. Also, CD160 is a ligand for HVEM. The combination of CD160 and HVEM promote the suppression of T-cells. So, CD160 is an inhibitory checkpoint for T-cells [13].

4.6 CD244

CD244 is a immunoglobulin which can regulate and activates the lymphocytes. In addition, CD244 can stimulate both T-cell and NK cells. NK cytotoxicity is inhibited opposed the expression of CD48 by CD244. CD244 can provide both suppression and activation of T-cell by cross linking, related to CD244 level of expression and adaptation of intracellular molecule. Recent study shows that CD244, LAG-3, and PD-1 is reduced in tumor-infiltrating antigen-specific CD8þ T-cells by herpes virus glycoprotein (GD) adjutant vaccine [13].

5. Passive immuno-therapy

With the exception of immuno-suppressants, many other important therapies are developing immunization that can be divided into active or inactive Immunotherapy with respect to host immunity when detecting anti-tumor responses. Active immuno-therapies have correlation with capacity of anti-tumor attack of T-cell. However, passive Immunotherapy includes inherent anti-tumor properties of adaptive T-cell therapy [1, 41].

5.1 Tumor-targeting monoclonal antibodies (mAbs)

MAbs have different effects on immune cells. First, mAbs can change the receptor's signaling role which malignant cells expressed them. Second, they neutralize the signals which malignant cells or stromal components or neoplastic lesion provided them. MAbs identify cancer cells due to tumor associated antigen (TAA) expression which expressed by transformed cells [39, 42]. Another anti-cancer immuno-therapies against activatory checkpoint receptors include anti CD137 or anti-CD40 which are being tested in clinical trials [1]. MAbs Cetuximab blocks signaling pathways which determine neoplastic cells' survival or progression. Also Cetuximab is approved for the treatment of head and neck cancer. In addition, it is used in managing colorectal carcinoma [9, 39, 43, 44]. Naked mAbs such as Tigatuzumab activates murderous receptors of malignant cells. Gemtuzumab ozogamicin is an anti-CD33 Calicheamicin. Gemtuzumab ozogamicin binds to a TAA-specific mAbs. It use for acute myeloid leukemia patients [38]. CD20-specific mAb Rituximab is complement-dependent cytotoxicity. Rituximab is activated by TAA-specifics mAbs. Also, naked TAA-specific mAbs activates ADCC and antibody-dependent cellular phagocytosis [39, 45, 46]. A recent study shows that Rituximab has beneficial influence on chronic lymphocytic leukemia, and NHL [39, 46, 47]. Blinatumomab is a CD19- and CD3 bispecific T-cell engagers (BiTE) which is chimeric proteins includes of two single-chain changeable fragments from mAbs. BiTE has two fragments, one of them target a TAA and another target T-cell surface antigen. Blinatumomab is approved for treatment of B-cell acute lymphoblastic leukemia. MAbs and BiTE should be considered active immuno-therapeutic or passive immun0-therapeutics. This implying depends on host immune responses. For example, Cituximab can block epidermal growth factor receptor (EGFR) signaling and also can induce ADCC. In addition, Cituximab can mediate the effects of immuno-stimulatory [39, 48]. Bevacizumab is approved for management of glioblastoma multiform, cervical carcinoma, renal cell carcinoma, and lung cancer due to anti-angiogenesis effects. But, Bevacizumab induces tumor infiltration via lymphocyte B and lymphocyte T. In addition, Bevacizumab blocks CD4+ CD25+ FOXP3+ regulatory T-cells [39, 48, 49].

5.2 Summary of anti mAbs indications

Alemtuzumab's indication is chronic lymphocytic leukemia. Bevacizumab's indications are colorectal carcinoma, lung carcinoma, renal cell carcinoma. Brentuximab vedotin indications are anaplastic large cell lymphoma and HL. Blinatumomab indication is acute lymphoblastic leukemia. Catumaxomab indications are malignant ascites in patients with epithelial cell adhesion molecule (EPCAM) + cancer. Cetuximab indications are head and neck cancer and colorectal carcinoma. Denosumab indications are breast carcinoma, prostate carcinoma, and bone giant cell tumors. Gemtuzumab ozogamicin indication is acute myeloid leukemia. Ibritumomab tiuxetan indication is NHL. Panitumumab indication is colorectal carcinoma. Pertuzumab indication is breast carcinoma. [38]. Obinutuzumab indication is chronic lymphocytic leukemia. Ofatumumab indication is chronic lymphocytic leukemia. Ramucirumab indications are gastric or gastroesophageal junction adenocarcinoma. Rituximab indications are chronic lymphocytic leukemia and NHL. Siltuximab indication is Multicentric Castleman's disease. Tositumomab indication is NHL, and Trastuzumab indications are breast carcinoma, gastric or gastroesophageal and junction adenocarcinoma [38].

5.3 Oncolytic viruses

Oncolytic viruses have potential anti-neoplastic effects and can inherent cytopathic effects. Productive viral infection up regulates the mortal overcharge of cellular metabolism. Oncolytic viruses are lethal for host cells due to endogenous or exogenous gene products, and are approved by US food and drug administration (FDA) [39, 50].

5.4 Oncorine H101

Oncorine H101 is oncolytic viruses. Oncorine indication is head and neck cancer. The mechanism of action is selective lysis of malignant cells [38].

6. Immune oncology biomarker and immune response

Biomarkers have different purpose and are seen as a pre-existing anti-tumor in certain developing tumors. Also, response to immune treatments can provide specific biomarkers [48]. When blockade of the PD-1/PD-L1 checkpoint response increase, PD-L1 expression can be seen in the TME. The high level expression of PD-L1 is related with a higher response rate and its expression increases survival [48]. Immunotherapy can exacerbate tumor lymphocytes (TILs), which illustrates antitumor immune response [48]. CD8 T-cells are associated with tumor regression after stopping of PD-1/L1 in melanoma metastasis. Increased immunogenicity of a tumor shows an increasing of tumor mutational load and neoantigen [49]. High mutational burdens increase survival than low load. Mutational load and neoantigens have been shown in many type of advance tumors including melanoma, NSCLC, and colorectal carcinoma. The investigations on colorectal carcinoma illustrate higher tumor-infiltrating lymphocytes and smokers response which is better than nonsmokers (adenocarcinomas) [1]. Immuno-stimulatory or immune inhibitory cytokines existence in the microscopic environment of the tumor forecast susceptibility or resistance. There are several methods for research in the microscopic environment of the tumor including immuno-histochemistry, immuno-fluorescence, whole-exome sequencing, transciptome analysis, proteomics, flow cytometry and others [48]. Type I interferon-based transcriptomic signatures has beneficial effect in metastatic melanoma. However, it may originally be used for other types of tumors [1]. Several investigations on PD-1/PD-L1 checkpoints indicate that TME PD-L1 (TME cell types express PD-L1) expression is significantly related with response [29]. Tumors with negative PD-L1 are resistance to therapy since tumor or immune cell must have PD-L1 for immune checkpoint therapy [29]. Alone PD-L1 (B7-H1) expression cannot adequately predict the Immunotherapy response. So, adding PD-L1 with another parameters (CD8+ T-cells or an IFNγ gene signature) improves predictive value [48].

6.1 Imaging biomarker

There are two main approaches for imaging in clinical oncology including anatomic and functional imaging. Anatomic change fluorescence and bioluminescence are the most useful imaging techniques. In addition, magnetic resonance imaging (MRI) improves contrast and increase resolution of anatomic images. Also, MRI can improve range of functional measure. Dynamic contrast-enhanced MRI can indicate tumor perfusion and permeability of cell membrane. Diffusion-weighted MRI demonstrates the access of drug by parameters such as rate and distance of water molecule. Recent study evaluates immunotherapy by using cells labeled with either super paramagnetic iron oxide particles or perfluorocarbon nanoemulsions in MRI-based cell follow [51, 52]. Detecting biochemical markers in tumors is possible by single-photon emission computed tomography (SPECT) and PET. These two mature imaging techniques has beneficial effects such as high-resolution images, the potential to quantify metabolic activity for corrects attraction of therapeutic influences [52]. The investigations on lymphoma and solid tumors shows that 18F-FDG-PET imaging which is oncologic nuclear imaging is very useful for disease response evaluations. But, there are few important problem with 18F-FDG-PET such as the distinction between neoplasm and infectious or inflammatory processes. SPECT provide high resolution similar to PET. However, beneficial advantage of SPECT in comparison with PET is ubiquity of SPECT cameras, reduced cost structure, increased logistics for imaging caused by longer half-lives of the radionuclides, and a greater number of radionuclides available for labeling. 99mTc-methyldiphosphonate (99mTc-MDP) is the most useful SPECT agents in imaging of advance osteoblastic bone cancer. Real metastases are not detected by bone scan, while the reaction of the skeleton to metastases can be found [52, 53]. Also, another SPECT agents which they are useful for different cancers including using 123I-metaiodobenzylguanidine (123I-MIBG) in neuroblastoma, using 111In-pentreotide in patients with neuro-endocrine tumors, and 123I-sodium iodide (NaI) for thyroid distinction between expected post immuno-therapeutic results. The most frequent use of PET agent is 18F-fluorothymidine (18F-FLT) which is a marker for proliferation of the cells. 18F-fluorothymidine (18F-FLT) improves the differentiation between tumors and false positive rate associated to infections and inflammations [52]. 18F-FLT has some limitations in comparison with 18F-FDG-PET such as reduction in signal to background ration. Also, 18F-FLT shows background structures such as bone marrow, which cannot show the activity of the tumors and reduces the identification of tumors. Furthermore, 18F-FlT gathers in area of infection and inflammation lesser than 18F-FDG [54].

7. Immune response

Genomic factors play an important role in responding to Immunotherapy. Across several mechanisms, viral proteins have influence on intercommunication alongside T-cells and malignancy. For example anti-tumor cytotoxic activity of the NK cells is increased by hidden cytomegalovirus [55]. In addition, PD-L1 expression is provoked by EBV in NHL and other EBV+ cancers [53]. one of the most responsive cancer to checkpoints inhibitor is HL. Also, HL has high level of PD-L1 expression. PD-L1 expression is reduced in HPV+ tumors; But, T-cell infiltration is increased in HPV+ tumors. Therefore, an important biological biomarkers for Immunotherapy is the presence of viral proteins [56]. Recent study shows that Merkel-cell polyomavirus positive tumors have higher PD-L1 expression (71 vs. 25%). Response rate in virus positive tumor is about 65 vs. 44% higher than virus negatives tumors [48].

8. Combination therapy

Combination therapy can increase response rate, efficacy and improve multiple components of T-cell anti-tumor responses. It has been reported that, Nivolumab + Ipilimumab are beneficial against melanoma. But, this combinations may have many serious side effects such as hepatitis, colitis, pneumonia. Bevacizumab combine with interferon-alpha to manage renal cancer. The combination of Elotuzumab and Dexamethasone and Lenalidomide is useful to control multiple myeloma [7, 59]. Combination of Nivolumab and Pembrolizumab is prescribed for managing squamous and non-squamous NSCLC [4, 33].

8.1 Binary checkpoint inhibition

Combination of Nivolumab (anti-PD-1) and Ipilimumab (anti-CTLA-4) provide total two-year survival in 79% of cases in metastatic melanoma. Also this combination has 53% objective response rate in metastatic melanoma. Recent study shows combinations of Nivolumab and Ipilimumab has 61% objective response rate. However, Ipilimumab alone has 11% objective response rate. Totally, recent study shows 22% remission [2]. Also, later investigations shows that the combination of anti-PD-1 and CTLA-4 stimulate T-cell more than anti-CTLA-4 alone. In combination of PD-1, CTLA-4 and VISTA blockade checkpoint is demonstrated the stimulation of T-cell [2].

8.2 Checkpoint inhibitor and mAbs

Combination of Tremelimumab (anti-PD-1) and a CD40-agonist mAb has 27% objective response rate, 26 months overall survival. T-cell antigen 4-1BB is targeted by mAb's, and improves T-cell stimulation [57]. Combination of 4-1BB agonists with PD-1 blockade has notable results in rejection in murine model with colon adenocarcinoma. This combination therapy led to increase the level of IFNγ-producing CD8+ and CD4+ T-cells in comparison with monotherapies. Efficacy of OX40 agonist is decreased by PD-1 inhibitions. Also, PD-1 blockade causes reduction of CD4+ and CD8+ lymphocyte infiltration and causes 30% breast tumors remissions [58].

8.3 Epigenome regulator

Epigenome regulator is coupled with checkpoint inhibitor, and includes an inhibitor of histone deacetylases (HDAC) or DNA methyl-transferase (DNMT). HADC typically associated with the cancer process [59]. Immune checkpoint management mechanisms contain covalent modifications, microRNAs (miRNAs), and long noncoding RNAs (lncRNAs), and histone modifications. DNA methylation and histone acetylation have the most effects in management of growth and activation of T lymphocyte. Inhibition of HDAC promotes tumor death. Inhibition of HDAC provokes tumor death by different pathway such as reactive oxygen species (ROS) and apoptosis. HDAC inhibitor is prescribed for different type of malignancies including leukemia, gastric carcinoma, NSCLC. HDAC inhibitors have several complications including lymphopenia, leukopenia, neutropenia, and thrombocytopenia. Combination therapy of HDAC and DNMT inhibitors with other immunological agents is used for more efficacy. For example, Entinostat is combined with Nivolumab and Ipilimumab for managing metastatic breast cancer. Also, Entinostat with Pembrolizumab is used for solid tumors, metastatic uveal melanoma and NSCLC. Mocetinostat and Durvalumab are used for managing solid tumors [60–62].

8.4 Selective therapy with checkpoint inhibitor

Checkpoint blockers coupled with receptor and non-receptor tyrosine kinases (TK) play major roles in tumorigenesis. The angiogenesis provides growth factor VEGF and restricts T-cell infiltration through the tumor endothelium. In addition, angiogenesis promotes myeloid-derived suppressor cells (MDSCs) and Treg cells inside tumors. Combination of Bevacizumab (a VEGF inhibitor) with Ipilimumab can control 67% in metastatic melanoma. In addition, this combination can induce T-cell activation inside tumors with approving toleration level. It is currently attempting to coordinate anti-PD-1/PD-L1 MABs with VEGF inhibitor for even greater effectiveness [60]. Imatinib (TKI) with an anti-CTLA-4 mAb decrease Treg cell. Tumor volume is decreased 50% by CTLA-4 and Indoleamine 2,3-dioxygenase (IDO) blockade combination during 80 days [60]. Tumor volume is decreased 50% by CTLA-4 and IDO blockade combination during 80 days [60]. Combination of PD-1 and IDO blockades has favorable effects on advanced melanoma [2].

8.5 Adaptive T-cell therapy (ACT) with checkpoint inhibitor

Adaptive T-cell therapy induces anti-tumor stimulation. CD19-specifics chimeric antigen receptor (CAR) T-cell therapies provide 90% revocation of which 67% of them have response following 6 months in acute lymphoblastic leukemia patients. In addition, more than 53% complete response rate has shown in B-cell lymphoma [61].

8.6 Nanoscale coordination polymer (NCP) with checkpoint inhibitor

Combination of anti-PD-l1 (Pembrolizumab) and nanoscale coordination polymer (NCP) combination increase CD8+ T-cells in tumors. Survival rate is increased by antiPD-1 checkpoint inhibitors and agonistic anti-OX40 antibodies. Anti-OX40 antibodies encourage the stimulation of elevated T-cell due to increased release of IFNγ and increased CD8+/Treg cell ratio [59]. It has recently been shown that presentation of antigen is increased by synthetic polymeric nanoparticle PC7A. Also, flexible nanovaccin platform carry antigens to lymph nodes. The combination of PD-L1 inhibitor and laser light and gold nanostars, which they are called photodermal nanotherapy, can manage advance metastatic bladder malignancy [2].

9. Conclusion

Immunology has changed the way of cancer treatments and control. Primitive immunotherapy with checkpoint inhibitors provides beneficial results. However, the combination of checkpoint inhibitor with other immune target agents provide new generation of immune-oncology treatments. Knowledge about immunological checkpoints, immuno-oncology biomarkers, immune response, therapeutic resistance and combination therapy helps us in the process of cancer diagnosis/follow-up, and imaging during immunotherapy helps to better understand the patients' immune response.

Author details

Alireza Ziaei[1,2]* and Forough Kheiry

1 Brigham and Women's Hospital, Harvard Medical School, Boston, MA, USA

2 Boston Children's Hospital, Harvard Medical School, Boston, MA, USA

*Address all correspondence to: alireza.ziaei@childrens.harvard.edu

References

[1] Zugazagoitia J, Guedes C, Ponce S, Ferrer I, Molina-Pinelo S, Paz-Ares L. Current challenges in cancer treatment. Clinical Therapeutics. 2016;**38**(7):1551-1566

[2] Marshall HT, Djamgoz MB. Immuno-oncology: Emerging targets and combination therapies. Frontiers in Oncology. 2018;**8**:1-29

[3] Robinson TO, Schluns KS. The potential and promise of IL-15 in immuno-oncogenic therapies. Immunology Letters. 2017;**190**:159-168

[4] Medina PJ, Adams VR. PD-1 pathway inhibitors: Immuno-oncology agents for restoring antitumor immune responses. Pharmacotherapy. 2016;**36**(3):317-334

[5] Baumeister SH, Freeman GJ, Dranoff G, Sharpe AH. Coinhibitory pathways in immunotherapy for cancer. Annual Review of Immunology. 2016;**34**(1):539-573

[6] Mahoney KM, Rennert PD, Freeman GJ. Combination cancer immunotherapy and new immunomodulatory targets. Nature Reviews Drug Discovery. 2016;**131**(20):1796-1803

[7] Azoury CS, Straughan MD, Shukla V. Immune checkpoint inhibitors for cancer therapy: Clinical efficacy and safety. Current Cancer Drug Targets. 2015;**15**(6):452-462

[8] Ludin A, Zon LI, Tchekmedyian N, Gray JE, Creelan BC, Chiappori AA, et al. Propelling immunotherapy combinations into the clinic. Oncology. 2015;**29**:990-1002

[9] Topalian SL, Drake CG, Pardoll DM. Immune checkpoint blockade: A common denominator approach to cancer therapy. Cancer Cell. 2015;**27**(4):451-461

[10] Russi AE, Brown MA. The meninges: New therapeutic targets for multiple sclerosis. Translational Research. 2015;**165**(2):255-269

[11] Pardoll DM. The blockade of immune checkpoints in cancer immunotherapy. Nature Reviews. Cancer. 2012;**12**:252-264

[12] Taube JM, Taube JM, Klein AP, Brahmer JR, et al. Association of PD-1, PD-1 ligands, and other features of the tumor immune microenvironment with response to anti-PD-1 therapy. Clinical Cancer Research. 2014;**20**:5064-5074

[13] Baksh K, Weber J. Immune checkpoint protein inhibition for cancer: Preclinical justification for CTLA-4 and PD-1 blockade and new combinations. Seminars in Oncology. 2015;**42**(3):363-377

[14] Rozali EN, Hato SV, Robinson BW, Lake RA, Lesterhuis WJ. Programmed death ligand 2 in cancer-induced immune suppression. Clinical & Developmental Immunology. 2012;**2012**:656340

[15] Couzin-Frankel J. Autoimmune diseases surface after cancer treatment. Science. 2017;**358**(6365):852-852

[16] Peng W, Liu C, Xu C, Lou Y, Chen J, Yang Y, et al. PD-1 blockade enhances T-cell migration to tumors by elevating IFN-γ inducible chemokines. Cancer Research. 2012;**72**(20):5209-5218

[17] Allard D, Allard B, Gaudreau PO, Chrobak P, Stagg J. CD73–adenosine: A next-generation target in immuno-oncology. Immunotherapy. 2016;**8**(2):145-163

[18] Leclerc BG, Charlebois R, Chouinard G, Allard B, Pommey S, Saad F, et al. CD73 expression is an independent prognostic factor

in prostate cancer. Clinical Cancer Research. 2016;**22**(1):158-166

[19] Long JS, Schoonen PM, Graczyk D, O'Prey J, Ryan KM. p73 engages A2B receptor signalling to prime cancer cells to chemotherapy-induced death. Oncogene. 2015;**34**(40):5152-5162

[20] Dent R, Hanna WM, Trudeau M, Rawlinson E, Sun P, Narod SA. Pattern of metastatic spread in triple-negative breast cancer. Breast Cancer Research and Treatment. 2009;**115**(2):423-428

[21] Morgensztern D, Campo MJ, Dahlberg SE, Doebele RC, Garon E, Gerber DE, et al. Molecularly targeted therapies in non-small-cell lung cancer annual update 2014. Journal of Thoracic Oncology. 2015;**10**(1):S1-S63

[22] Kris MG, Johnson BE, Berry LD, Kwiatkowski DJ, Iafrate AJ, Wistuba II, et al. Using multiplexed assays of oncogenic drivers in lung cancers to select targeted drugs. Journal of the American Medical Association. 2014;**311**(19):1998

[23] Diao L, Meibohm B. Pharmacometric applications and challenges in the development of therapeutic antibodies in immuno-oncology. Current Pharmacology Reports. 2018;**4**(4):285-291

[24] Elassaiss-Schaap J, Rossenu S, Lindauer A, Kang S, De Greef R, Sachs J, et al. Using model-based "learn and confirm" to reveal the pharmacokinetics-pharmacodynamics relationship of Pembrolizumab in the KEYNOTE-001 trial. CPT: Pharmacometrics & Systems Pharmacology. 2017;**6**(1):21-28

[25] Freshwater T, Kondic A, Ahamadi M, Li CH, de Greef R, de Alwis D, et al. Evaluation of dosing strategy for pembrolizumab for oncology indications. Journal for Immuno Therapy of Cancer. 2017;**5**(1):1-9

[26] Li H, Yu J, Liu C, Liu J, Subramaniam S, Zhao H, et al. Time dependent pharmacokinetics of pembrolizumab in patients with solid tumor and its correlation with best overall response. Journal of Pharmacokinetics and Pharmacodynamics. 2017;**44**(5): 403-414

[27] Garon EB, Rizvi NA, Hui R, Leighl N, Balmanoukian AS, Eder JP, et al. Pembrolizumab for the treatment of non-small-cell lung cancer. The New England Journal of Medicine. 2015;**372**(21):2018-2028

[28] Morrissey K, Yuraszeck T, Li C-C, Zhang Y, Kasichayanula S. Immunotherapy and novel combinations in oncology: Current landscape, challenges, and opportunities. Clinical and Translational Science. 2016;**9**(2): 89-104

[29] Agrawal S, Feng Y, Roy A, Kollia G, Lestini B. Nivolumab dose selection: Challenges, opportunities, and lessons learned for cancer immunotherapy. Journal for ImmunoTherapy of Cancer. 2016;**4**(1):72

[30] Bajaj G, Wang X, Agrawal S, Gupta M, Roy A, Feng Y. Model-based population pharmacokinetic analysis of Nivolumab in patients with solid tumors. CPT: Pharmacometrics & Systems Pharmacology. 2017;**6**(1):58-66

[31] Zhao X, Suryawanshi S, Hruska M, Feng Y, Wang X, Shen J, et al. Assessment of nivolumab benefit–risk profile of a 240-mg flat dose relative to a 3-mg/kg dosing regimen in patients with advanced tumors. Annals of Oncology. 2017;**28**(8):2002-2008

[32] Stroh M, Winter H, Marchand M, Claret L, Eppler S, Ruppel J, et al. Clinical pharmacokinetics and pharmacodynamics of atezolizumab

in metastatic urothelial carcinoma. Clinical Pharmacology and Therapeutics. 2017;**102**(2):305-312

[33] Baverel P, Dubois V, Jin C, Song X, Jin X, Mukhopadhyay P, et al. Population pharmacokinetics of durvalumab and fixed dosing regimens in patients with advanced solid tumors. Journal of Clinical Oncology. 2017;**35**(15 suppl):2566-2566

[34] Wilkins JJ, Brockhaus B, Dai H, Vugmeyster Y, White JT, Brar S, et al. Time-varying clearance and impact of disease state on the pharmacokinetics of avelumab in Merkel cell carcinoma and urothelial carcinoma. CPT: Pharmacometrics & Systems Pharmacology. 13 Apr 2019

[35] Heery CR, O'Sullivan-Coyne G, Madan RA, Cordes L, Rajan A, Rauckhorst M, et al. Avelumab for metastatic or locally advanced previously treated solid tumours (JAVELIN solid tumor): A phase 1a, multicohort, dose-escalation trial. The Lancet Oncology. 2017;**18**(5):587-598

[36] Anderson AC, Joller N, Kuchroo VK. Lag-3, Tim-3, and TIGIT: Co-inhibitory receptors with specialized functions in immune regulation. Immunity. 2016;**44**(5):989-1004

[37] Anderson AC, Joller N, Kuchroo VK. Lag-3, Tim-3, and TIGIT: Co-inhibitory receptors with specialized functions in immune regulation. Immunity. 2016;**44**(5):989-1004

[38] Galluzzi L, Vacchelli E, Bravo-San Pedro JM, Buqué A, Senovilla L, Baracco EE, et al. Classification of current anticancer immunotherapies. Oncotarget. 2014;**5**(24):12472

[39] Coulie PG, Van den Eynde BJ, van der Bruggen P, Boon T. Tumour antigens recognized by T lymphocytes: At the core of cancer immunotherapy. Nature Reviews Cancer. 2014;**14**(2):135-146

[40] De T, Rouge LM, Galluzzi L, Olaussen KA, Zermati Y, Tasdemir E, et al. A novel epidermal growth factor receptor inhibitor promotes apoptosis in non-small cell lung cancer cells resistant to Erlotinib. Cancer Research. 2007;**67**(13):6253-6262

[41] Lim CM, Stephenson R, Salazar AM, Ferris RL. Tlr3 agonists improve the immunostimulatory potential of cetuximab against egfr+ head and neck cancer cells. Oncoimmunology. 2013;**2**(6):1-10

[42] Forero-Torres A, Infante JR, Waterhouse D, Wong L, Vickers S, Arrowsmith E, et al. Phase 2, multicenter, open-label study of tigatuzumab (CS-1008), a humanized monoclonal antibody targeting death receptor 5, in combination with gemcitabine in chemotherapy-naive patients with unresectable or metastatic pancreatic cancer. Cancer Medicine. 2013;**2**(6):925-932

[43] Battella S, Cox MC, Santoni A, Palmieri G. Natural killer (NK) cells and anti-tumor therapeutic mAb: Unexplored interactions. Journal of Leukocyte Biology. 2016;**99**(1):87-96

[44] van Oers MHJ, Klasa R, Marcus RE, Wolf M, Kimby E, Gascoyne RD, et al. Rituximab maintenance improves clinical outcome of relapsed/resistant follicular non-Hodgkin lymphoma in patients both with and without rituximab during induction: Results of a prospective randomized phase 3 intergroup trial. Blood. 2006;**108**(10):3295-3301

[45] Manzoni M, Rovati B, Ronzoni M, Loupakis F, Mariucci S, Ricci V, et al. Immunological effects of bevacizumab-based treatment in metastatic colorectal cancer. Oncology. 2010;**79**(3-4):187-196

[46] Terme M, Pernot S, Marcheteau E, Sandoval F, Benhamouda N, Colussi O, et al. VEGFA-VEGFR pathway blockade

inhibits tumor-induced regulatory T-cell proliferation in colorectal cancer. Cancer Research. 2013;**73**(2):539-549

[47] Linette GP, Carreno BM. Dendritic cell-based vaccines. Oncoimmunology. 2013;**2**(11):e26512

[48] Janice MM, Monjazeb AM, Beerthuijzen JMT, Collyar D, Rubinstein L, Harris LN. The challenge for development of valuable immuno-oncology biomarkers. 2017:4970-4979

[49] Wilson FH, Johannessen CM, Piccioni F, Tamayo P, Kim JW, Van Allen EM, et al. A functional landscape of resistance to ALK inhibition in lung cancer. Cancer Cell. 2015;**27**(3):397-408

[50] Salgado R, Denkert C, Demaria S, Sirtaine N, Klauschen F, Pruneri G, et al. The evaluation of tumor-infiltrating lymphocytes (TILs) in breast cancer: Recommendations by an international TILs working group 2014. Annals of Oncology. 2015;**26**(2):259-271

[51] Hegde PS, Karanikas V, Evers S. The where, the when, and the how of immune monitoring for cancer immunotherapies in the era of checkpoint inhibition. Clinical Cancer Research. 2016;**22**(8):1865-1874

[52] Juergens RA, Zukotynski KA, Singnurkar A, Snider DP, Valliant JF, Gulenchyn KY. Imaging biomarkers in immunotherapy. Biomarkers in Cancer. 2016;**8s2**(Il):BIC.S31805

[53] Sartor O, Eisenberger M, Kattan MW, Tombal B, Lecouvet F. Unmet needs in the prediction and detection of metastases in prostate cancer. The Oncologist. 2013;**18**(5):549-557

[54] Tan YY, Liang J, Liu DF, Zhu F, Wang GM, Ding XM, et al. 18F-FLT PET/CT imaging in a wister rabbit inflammation model. Experimental and Therapeutic Medicine. 2014;**8**(1):69-72

[55] Bigley AB, Rezvani K, Shah N, Sekine T, Balneger N, Pistillo M, et al. Latent cytomegalovirus infection enhances anti-tumour cytotoxicity through accumulation of NKG2C+ NK cells in healthy humans. Clinical and Experimental Immunology. 2016;**185**(2):239-251

[56] Huehls AM, Coupet TA, Sentman CL. Bispecific T-cell engagers for cancer immunotherapy. Immunology and Cell Biology. 2015;**93**(3):290-296

[57] Gao J, Ward JF, Pettaway CA, Shi LZ, Subudhi SK, Vence LM, et al. VISTA is an inhibitory immune checkpoint that is increased after ipilimumab therapy in patients with prostate cancer. Nature Medicine. 2017;**23**(5):551-555

[58] Messenheimer DJ, Jensen SM, Afentoulis ME, Wegmann KW, Feng Z, Friedman DJ, et al. Cancer therapy: Preclinical timing of PD-1 blockade is critical to effective combination immunotherapy with anti-OX40. Clinical Cancer Research. 2017;**23**(20)

[59] Weintraub K. Take two: Combining immunotherapy with epigenetic drugs to tackle cancer. Nature Medicine. 2016;**22**(1):8-10

[60] Steinsaltz A. What does rabbi Steinsaltz say? There are no final answers. Parabola. 2006;**31**(4):56-58

[61] Kochenderfer JN, Dudley ME, Kassim SH, Somerville RPT, Carpenter RO, Maryalice SS, et al. Chemotherapy-refractory diffuse large B-cell lymphoma and indolent B-cell malignancies can be effectively treated with autologous T cells expressing an anti-CD19 chimeric antigen receptor. Journal of Clinical Oncology. 2015;**33**(6):540-549

[62] Mazzone R, Zwergel C, Mai A, Valente S. Epi-drugs in combination with immunotherapy: A new avenue to improve anticancer efficacy. Clinical Epigenetics. 2017;**9**(1):1-15

Chapter 8

TLR4-Induced Inflammation Is a Key Promoter of Tumor Growth, Vascularization, and Metastasis

Sophia Ran, Nihit Bhattarai, Radhika Patel and Lisa Volk-Draper

Abstract

Toll-like receptor-4 (TLR4) is a powerful pathway best known for inducing inflammation in response to bacteria-produced lipopolysaccharide. TLR4 is also activated by endogenous ligands produced by host-damaged cells and a chemo-drug paclitaxel. Under normal conditions, TLR4 is expressed mainly in macrophages and, at a lower level, in epithelial, endothelial, and stromal cells. Activated TLR4 significantly increases inflammatory cytokines and enhances cell proliferation, migration, invasion, and survival. While these functions in normal cells are essential for host defense and tissue repair, TLR4 overexpression in malignant cells promotes tumor growth and metastasis. This is because pro-oncogenic effects of activated TLR4 in tumor cells are amplified by similar event in TLR4-positive tumor-associated cells including endothelial cells and their mobilized progenitors. The collective activation of multiple cell types within the tumor promotes chemoresistance and metastasis. Here, we summarize the current knowledge of the TLR4 pathway and its functional outcomes in normal and tumor cells. We also discuss its underappreciated role in supporting tumor progression through vascular activation and recruitment of endothelial progenitors. The review considers several open questions regarding the impact of TLR4-mediated pro- and antitumor effects, structural requirements for recognition of the TLR4 complex, and a potential contribution of chemotherapy to tumor spread.

Keywords: Toll-like receptor-4, paclitaxel chemotherapy, tumor growth, tumor blood and lymphatic vessels, metastasis

1. Introduction

Human Toll-like receptor-4 (TLR4) was discovered in 1997 through a bioinformatics approach based on the homology of similar Toll protein found in *Drosophila* [1, 2]. *Drosophila* Toll protein-mediated protection against fungus infection was the first clue suggesting the role of mammalian TLR4 in activation of the immune system. The complex of TLR4 and its co-receptors is the primary sensor and responder to lipopolysaccharides (LPS), the major constituents of membranes of Gram-negative bacteria [3]. Based on exquisite sensitivity to LPS and high level of TLR4 expression in macrophages, it was initially thought that the main function of this protein is restricted to an inflammatory response aimed at eradication of microbial pathogens.

Subsequent studies, however, discovered intricate interactions of TLR4 with multitude of other molecules besides LPS suggesting a much broader role in homeostasis, tissue repair, and longevity in addition to the immune defense. These functions of TLR4 directly relate to cancer initiation, progression, and response to therapy.

2. Basic structure of TLR4 gene and protein

Human TLR4 gene contains four exons, and it is located in the long arm of chromosome 9 [4]. TLR4 is Type-1 transmembrane protein belonging to the family of Toll-like receptors consisting of 10 members in humans and 12 proteins in mice [5]. TLR4 protein is composed of an extracellular domain, a C-terminal leucine-rich repeat (LRR) domain, and a single transmembrane sequence connected to an intracellular Toll/IL-1 receptor (TIR) region that conveys signaling [5]. LRR and TIR domains are responsible for ligand recognition and signal transduction, respectively [6].

3. TLR4 expression in normal organs

The main cell types that express TLR4 under normal conditions are cells of innate immunity including monocytes [7], macrophages [8], neutrophils [9], and dendritic cells [10]. In addition, TLR4 is also found in T cells [11] and B lymphocytes [12] albeit at lower level. Osteoclasts, macrophage-like cells in the bone marrow, also express TLR4 [13]. Embryonic stem cells [14] as well as adult hematopoietic-myeloid [15], lymphoid [15], mesenchymal [16], blood vascular endothelial [17], and lymphatic endothelial [18] progenitors all express TLR4 and signaling components of this pathway. Among non-hematopoietic cells, TLR4 is expressed in blood vascular [19] and lymphatic [20] endothelia as well as at low concentration in fibroblasts [21], keratinocytes [22], and epithelial cells of most normal organs including the colon [23], intestine [24], ovary [25], kidney [26], and lungs [27]. Professional phagocytes and their myeloid precursors express the greatest amount of TLR4 and exhibit the most pronounced response to its ligands [28]. The level and composition of TLR4 signal-transducing molecules vary among different cell types, particularly between myeloid and epithelial cells [29]. However, all positive cells share the basic traits of this pathway such as responsiveness to LPS reflected by activation of transcription factors of the NF-κB family and production of inflammatory cytokines. During inflammation, TLR4-expressing normal cells significantly increase secretion of inflammatory mediators [25, 30] due to co-upregulated TLR4 [31], its intracellular adapters [32], and co-receptors [10] which enhances cooperation among the pathway's components. Likewise, malignant TLR4-positive cells express much higher levels of inflammatory proteins as compared with their normal counterparts [33, 34].

4. Physiological functions of TLR4 in normal organs

In order to understand the full impact of TLR4 on cancer progression, it is useful to be familiar with its physiological role in normal organs. The main function of TLR4 in normal cells is restoration of tissue homeostasis perturbed by either pathogens or sterile injury. Response to pathogens is dictated by its ability to recognize and respond to LPS [3] and other microbial [35] and non-bacterial [36] lipids. The bacterial lipid-containing products are collectively called pattern-associated molecular patterns (PAMPs). Recognition of PAMPs triggers upregulation of inflammatory proteins that mediate proliferation [37], chemotactic migration [38], and survival

[39] of innate immunity cells, all of which is necessary for their division, mobilization to infected tissue, and cytoprotection against bacterial toxins and stresses of inflamed environment. LPS also induces differentiation of myeloid progenitors resulting in rapid maturation of dendritic cells and their superior antigen presentation to T lymphocytes necessary for eradication of invading pathogens [40].

Another broad panel of TLR4-activating molecules are called damage-associated molecular patterns or DAMPs. These molecules are produced by severely damaged or dying cells [41, 42]. The TLR4 responsiveness to this class of activators creates regenerative environment that helps to repair the injured tissue by replacing its lost or damaged components. This function of TLR4 is equally critical for long-term survival of the entire organism as the ability to generate pathogen-destroying cells. Therefore, in this situation TLR4 activates local and bone marrow (BM)-derived myeloid (BMDM) progenitors wired to differentiate the required cell types that replenish the damaged tissue. Not surprisingly, TLR4-expressing macrophages derived from BMDM progenitors dominate the late stages of wound healing acting to restore post-injury homeostasis, including rebuilding of functional vasculature [43]. In parallel to systemic effect, local epithelial and stromal cells activated by TLR4 produce copious amounts of chemotactic factors to recruit these progenitors while also being induced to divide, migrate, and re-populate the wounded area.

Given the TLR4 role in homeostasis, it is not surprising that it activates and induces differentiation of BM-derived progenitors from myeloid and lymphoid lineages [15], mesenchymal stem cells [16], blood vascular endothelial progenitors [17], lymphatic endothelial progenitors [18], and local tissue epithelial stem cells [14]. Chemokines recruiting these progenitors are produced by local stroma and epithelium as demonstrated by TLR4-dependent upregulation of a variety of cytokines in inflamed fibroblasts [42], hepatic stellate cells [44], as well as intestinal [45], alveolar [27], ovarian [25], and renal [26] epithelial cells. In addition to production of chemokines, TLR4 activation of epithelial cells increases their division [46] and survival [47] similarly to its effects on immune and hematopoietic cells described above. Tissue infiltration by immune cells and BM progenitors is facilitated by increased vascular permeability [48, 49] and upregulation of cell adhesion proteins that facilitate leukocyte-endothelial interactions [50]. These two major events permitting recruitment of BM-regenerating cells are induced by TLR4 activation of blood vascular endothelium [51] and vessel-supporting pericytes [52]. Lastly, TLR4 activation of lymphatic endothelial cells [20, 53] is essential for collection of tissue-mobilized macrophages from the inflamed tissue followed by their transportation to locoregional lymph nodes. Lymphatic-mediated removal of macrophages and dendritic cells from the affected site helps in resolving the inflammation and mounting the adaptive immune response through antigen presentation to T cells in the local nodes. Simultaneous activation of TLR4 in epithelium, stroma, endothelium, BM, and immune organs ensures tissue recovery in a coordinated and timely manner. TLR4 plays a central role in this process by coordinating epithelial cytokine release and activation, production of new cells in the BM, their recruitment to injured tissue, and resolution of residual inflammation that collectively promote tissue repair [54, 47]. While all these processes are essential for homeostasis, similar TLR4 activities in the context of cancer result in devastating outcomes including protection of tumor cells against anticancer drugs and their improved ability to generate and invade newly formed vessels.

5. TLR4 expression in malignant tumors

Although TLR4 expression was initially thought to be restricted to hematopoietic cells, subsequent studies discovered functional TLR4 in a variety of normal epithelial

Tumor type	No. patients	Detection method	Comments	P-value	Ref
Various solid tumors	1,294	Meta analysis	Data from 15 independent studies show high correlation between TLR4 expression and poor disease-free and overall survival	0.001 and 0.05	[81]
Breast	665	RT-PCR	Significantly shorter survival of patients with TLR4 polymorphisms	0.006	[82]
Breast	50	IHC	High TLR4 expression in tumor cells significantly correlated with lymph node metastasis	0.022	[76]
Breast	74	IHC	High TLR4 expression in infiltrating mononuclear cells highly correlated with lymphatic metastasis and recurrence	0.0001	[79]
Breast	120	IHC	Elevated TLR4 expression was strongly associated with tumor size and lymphatic metastasis	0.05	[83]
Prostate	133	ELISA	High TLR4 expression correlated with elevated PSA after ablation, an event defined as biochemical recurrence	0.05	[84]
Ovarian	109	RT-PCR and IHC	High expression of TLR4 significantly correlated with worse of overall and disease-free survival	0.01	[85]
Non-small cell lung cancer	126	IHC	Elevated TLR4 expression was strongly associated with TNM stage and lymphatic metastasis	0.001	[86]
Ovarian	57	IHC	TLR4 was detected in 46.3% of cases. Co-expression of TLR4 and its adaptor MyD88 was highly associated with advanced tumor stage	0.05	[87]
Colorectal	108	IHC	High expression of TLR4 strongly correlated with shorter overall survival	0.0001	[77]
Colon	53	IHC	High expression of TLR4 strongly correlated with disease progression	0.05	[73]
Hepatic	106	IHC	TLR4 was expressed in 86% of tumor specimens and significantly correlated with tumor size	0.01	[64]
Pancreatic	30	RT-PCR and IHC	TLR4 was expressed in 69.2% of tumor specimens and significantly correlated with tumor size, vascular invasion and lymphatic metastasis	0.001	[72]
Esophageal	87	RT-PCR and IHC	TLR4 expression in mononuclear cells was detected in 48.3% of specimens and significantly correlated with lymphatic metastasis	0.05	[88]

Tumor type	No. patients	Detection method	Comments	P-value	Ref
Melanoma	35	IHC	TLR4 expression in mononuclear cells significantly correlated with shorter relapse-free survival	0.001	[80]

Table 1.
Correlation of TLR4 expression with tumor growth, metastasis and poor patient survival in clinical human cancers.

cells [25, 26]. Malignant transformation amplifies TLR4 expression while typically preserving its functionality [55]. In fact, constitutive expression of epithelial TLR4 might contribute to development of cancer if persistently activated by pathogenic and environmental ligands which leads to vicious cycles of self-propagating inflammation. For instance, TLR4 interaction with *H. pylori* products in normal gastric epithelium might lead to chronic gastritis and progression into gastric intestinal metaplasia [56]. Analysis of cell lines from other organs also consistently showed substantial upregulation of TLR4 in tumor cells compared with their normal counterparts. Protein, mRNA, and functional activity of the TLR4 pathway have been demonstrated in tumor lines derived from many human epithelial lines including breast [33, 57], ovarian [58, 59], lung [60], prostate [61, 62], head and neck [63], hepatic [64], gastric [65], and pancreatic [66] cancers. It is also expressed in melanoma [67], glioblastoma [68], and various lines derived from hematopoietic malignancies [69]. Mouse tumor cell lines from a variety of tissues replicate these findings [70, 71].

TLR4 expression is not only limited to cultured tumor cell lines but is also detected in malignant cells in clinical human cancers. Moreover, the majority of clinical studies showed that TLR4 expression strongly correlates with poor prognosis due to increased tumor size [72], stage [73], loss of differentiation [74], chemoresistance [73, 75], venous invasion [72], lymph node metastasis [72, 75–78], recurrence [79], and shorter patient survival [77, 80] (**Table 1**). A recently published meta-analysis examining data from 15 independent encompassing analyses of different tumors from 1294 patients found strong associations (P-values 0.001–0.05) between TLR4 expression and reduced overall and disease-free survival [81]. Collectively, these studies demonstrate high expression of TLR4 in a variety of human solid tumors suggesting it plays a prominent role in inflammation-fueled cancer progression and metastasis.

6. Signal transduction and intracellular pathways induced by TLR4

Given the emerging evidence for the TLR4 pro-tumorigenic role (**Table 1**), it is important to understand the basic steps in this pathway, its positive and negative molecular regulators, as well as biochemical requirements for intracellular signal transduction in both normal myeloid and malignant epithelial cells. The best understanding of this pathway is derived from the studies of macrophages activated by LPS. Initiation of a signal cascade is mediated through recruitment of adapters interacting with the TIR domain of TLR4. Upon ligand-induced oligomerization of TLR4, the TIR domain recruits myeloid differentiation factor-88 (MyD88) that forms heterodimers with Mal (MyD88 adapter-like) partner, a protein specific for TLR4 pathway [89]. Upon binding to TIR, MyD88-Mal complex recruits members of the IL-1R associated kinase (IRAK) family, IRAK1 and IRAK4 [90]. Once phosphorylated, IRAK1/4 dissociates from the complex and recruits TNF receptor associate factor-6 (TRAF6), an E3 ubiquitin ligase and a critical mediator of

TLR2 and TLR4 signaling [91]. Polyubiquitination mediated by TRAF6 activates MAP3 kinases and TGF-beta associated kinase (TAK1) [92]. MAP3K activation leads to stimulation of p38/JNK pathways, whereas TAK1 together with TAB1/2 kinases phosphorylates the inhibitor of cytosolic NF-κB complex leading to release and nuclear translocation of NF-κB p65/p50 heterodimers [92]. This initiates the canonical NF-κB cascade resulting in transcription of a broad panel of inflammatory and pro-survival genes. This is amplified by genes transcribed by AP-1, CREB, and Sp1, factors activated through the parallel p38/JNK cascade.

Independently of MyD88 pathway, viruses and some TLR4 ligands also activate TIR domain-containing adapter inducing interferon-beta protein (TRIF) that is associated with TRIF-related adapter molecule (TRAM). TRIF also activates NF-κB; however, the expression level and the composition of the downstream transcribed genes are distinct from the MyD88-dependent activation. For instance, TRIF specifically activates IRF3 factor that induces robust transcription of antiviral interferons necessary to fight viral infections as opposed to classic MyD88-NF-κB targets such as TNFα and IL-6 that are predominantly upregulated after exposure to bacterial LPS.

7. Role of co-receptors in activation of TLR4

One persistent misconception in the cancer research literature is that TLR4 directly binds LPS and other activating ligands. However, it has been firmly established that TLR4, as a single protein, has very low affinity to LPS. Triggering the TLR4 pathway by LPS in monocytes and macrophages requires at least four co-receptors: myeloid differentiation protein-2 (MD2), CD14, and CD11b bound to CD18 (a complex of integrins known as Mac-1). Secreted MD2 binds to and stabilizes extracellular portion of TLR4 which creates a highly specific site for LPS recognition [93]. Intracellular MD2 also aids cytosolic trafficking of TLR4 from Golgi to the plasma membrane [94]. Physical interaction among MD2, LPS, and TLR4 has been shown in multiple elegant studies employing a combination of high-resolution structural analyses, phenotype comparison in genetically modified mice, and other rigorous approaches [95] that show a critical role of MD2 in LPS recognition by TLR4 in either mouse or human cells.

Likewise, the essential role of CD14 has been shown by physical binding of CD14 to lipid A portion of LPS using crystal structure analyses [35] and resonance energy transfer [96] as well as by hypo-responsiveness to LPS in mice lacking CD14 [97] or in the presence of CD14-blocking antibodies [7]. The function of CD14 is to accept a monomer of LPS from a blood-circulating LPS-binding protein and transfer it to a pre-made pocket in the MD2/TLR4 complex [98]. The absence of CD14 from TLR4-/MD2-positive cells results in a 1000-fold reduced sensitivity to LPS compared with cells expressing this protein [99]. The involvement of CD11b/CD18 in reactivity to LPS is somewhat less certain although some studies using a point mutation identified a specific LPS-binding site in CD18 integrin [100]. Additional studies showed lack of cytokine production in Mac-1-deficient mice [101] and other deficiencies in TLR4 signaling upon treatment with anti-CD11b or anti-CD18 antibodies in vivo [9]. While some studies suggested that optimal signaling requires LPS engagement with TLR4/MD2 complex and Mac-1, others found lesser requirements for CD11b/CD18 [102]. This issue, therefore, remains unresolved as well as the mechanisms of TLR4 signal transduction induced by various endogenous ligands dissimilar from LPS. Importantly, very few structural studies were performed in TLR4-expressing normal or tumor epithelial cells that might have entirely different requirements for TLR4 co-receptors and signal transduction than macrophages. Tumor epithelial cells are unlikely to express myeloid-specific CD14 and CD11b and might not uniformly express MyD88, MD2, and other TLR4 pathway essential proteins. How exactly TLR4 transmits the multitude of functional effects in the epithelial cell context is largely unknown.

8. LPS is the most rigorously confirmed TLR4 agonist

The best-studied ligands of TLR4 are various LPS molecules expressed in Gram-negative bacteria. The basic structure of LPS includes a lipid A component with 4–6 fatty acyl chains, an oligosaccharide core, and covalently attached O-antigen polysaccharide side chain [103]. The presence of phosphates in the lipid A and oligosaccharides confers the highly negative charge to LPS enabling its reactivity with cationic bactericidal host molecules such as beta-defensins [104]. CD14 binds the lipid A portion of LPS leaving acyl chains exposed to an LPS-binding site on the TLR4/MD2 complex. The presence of six acyl chains (as opposed to five or four) confers the best potency in activating TLR4 [105], presumably because the four acyl chains perfectly fit the hydrophobic cavity in MD2 [106] and the other two chains support the complex and promote its oligomerization [107]. This structural requirement illustrates the exquisite specificity of the binding site in the TLR4/MD2 complex to LPS raising reservations about the potential suitability of this complex for binding alternative ligands [95]. A functional and some structural evidence exists demonstrating TLR4-dependent cell activation triggered by lipid-like molecules (e.g., lipoteichoic acid [108], minimally oxidized LDL [109], and free saturated fatty acid palmitate [110]) whose binding might be supported by a hydrophobic site on CD14. Among other proposed TLR4-activating ligands, some structural evidence exists for a chemotherapeutic drug paclitaxel (PXL) [95, 101] and endogenous ligands HMGB1 [111] and S100A8 [112]. At the present, mechanisms by which other functional TLR4 ligands induce signal transduction are largely unknown.

9. Chemotherapeutic drug paclitaxel as a TLR4 ligand and a promoter of tumor growth and metastasis

For cancer researchers, a TLR4 stimulating effect of PXL is of special significance. This is because PXL and the entire class of its derivatives known as taxanes are widely used as anticancer cytotoxic drugs against a variety of human malignancies [113]. Resistance, however, occurs frequently [114], and the underlying mechanisms are poorly understood. PXL, the active component of all taxanes, exerts its cytotoxic action via binding to microtubules leading to their over-stabilization which results in apoptotic death of dividing cells [115]. The pro-survival effects of activated TLR4 pathway can explain many attributes associated with PXL chemoresistance including activation of NF-κB [116], phosphorylation of Bcl-2 and Bcl-XL [117], and resultant evasion of apoptosis [33, 58] in spite of continuous therapy.

Despite somewhat limited direct evidence confirming physical interactions of PXL with the TLR4 complex, there is overwhelming functional evidence for PXL activation of the TLR4 pathway in malignant human and mouse cells (**Table 2**). The early studies demonstrated that wild-type (WT) mice with functional TLR4 injected with PXL upregulated nearly an identical panel of inflammatory cytokines as those injected with LPS [3]. That was in sharp contrast to myeloid cells from TLR4-deficient mice that failed to respond to either molecule [118]. Mice lacking MyD88, the major intracellular adapter of TLR4, also did not respond to LPS

Tumor type	Specie	Study type	Taxane-mediated effects	Ref
Breast and ovarian	Human	In vitro	PXL induced degradation of IkappaB alpha followed by activation of NF-κB and MAPK	[126]
Renal	Human	In vitro	PXL activated ERK1/2 and induced Bcl-2 and EGFR	[127]
Breast	Human	In vitro	Only PXL-responsive tumor lines showed marked increase in AP-1 and NF-κB binding to IL-8 promoter	[128]
Breast	Human	In vitro & In vivo	Curcumin, an inhibitor of NF-κB, blocked PXL-dependent upregulation of pro-survival, proliferative and angiogenic proteins including MMP9 & VEGF-A	[129]
Prostate	Human	In vitro	Docetaxel increased tumor cell survival by activating PI3K/AKT pathway and TLR4 silencing reduced this effect	[61]
Breast	Human	Tumor xenografts in mice	PXL therapy induced NF-κB, Bcl-2, and VEGF-A, and anti-VEGF-A antibody blocked this effect	[130]
Various	Human	In vitro	In a cell-based screening of 1,280 compounds, PXL was identified as one of the most potent inducers of invasion	[131]
Non-small cell lung carcinoma	Human	Clinical study	Pre-operative taxane therapy increased COX2, PGE2 and microvessel density in patients	[132]
Breast	Human	In vitro & models in vivo	PXL upregulated cytokines mainly in TLR4-positive tumor lines; an anti-TLR4 antibody blocked this effect	[33]
Breast	Human	Clinical study	Taxane chemotherapy increased circulating angiogenic factors and endothelial cell progenitors in patients	[133]
Breast	Human & Mouse	Tumor models in mice	Taxane chemotherapy increased circulating CSF1 and tumor homing of BM pro-vascular myeloid cells	[134]
Breast	Human	Clinical study	Neoadjuvant taxane therapy increased angiogenesis in patients, possibly through VEGF-A and Notch pathways	[135]
Breast	Human	Tumor xenografts in mice	TLR4-positive tumors responded to PXL by increasing cytokines, homing of myeloid pro-vascular cells, lymphangiogenesis, and metastasis to lymph nodes	[136]
Breast	Human & Mouse	In vitro	PXL induced differentiation of lymphatic endothelial progenitors in TLR4-positive BM myeloid precursors	[18]
Breast	Human & Mouse	Tumor models in vivo	Docetaxel increased tumor lymphatic formation and metastasis to lymph nodes	[137]

Table 2.
Pro-oncogenic Effects of Paclitaxel and Docetaxel (selected list)

or PXL [119]. Treatment with PXL faithfully reproduced all known events in the LPS-inducing cascade including dual activation of MyD88 and TRIF pathways [58, 119–121]; phosphorylation of IRAK1 and IRAK4 [58, 122]; NF-κB activation

[33, 118, 122]; signaling through PI3K/pAKT [61, 121, 123] and activation of MAP kinases [119], p38 [124], JNK [123], ERK1/2 [33, 125], AP-1, and STAT3 [116]; and transcription of inflammatory genes and pro-survival factors [33, 118].

PXL-induced upregulation of inflammatory, promitotic, and pro-survival genes is evidenced by transcriptional analyses of drug-treated human cancer lines from breast [33, 122, 136], ovarian [58, 121], prostate [61], lung [116, 138], and melanoma [139] origins. Upregulation of these genes is evidenced as early as 6 hours posttreatment [138] which eliminates the possibility that this is a secondary effect resulting from cell death. Inhibition of IRAK1, an intracellular kinase whose phosphorylation is required for TLR4-dependent activation of NF-κB [90], in breast cancer lines suppressed an inflammatory response to PXL concomitant with decreased chemoresistance in vivo [122]. Correlation with chemoresistance was also recorded in an independent study that employed two different models of isogenic TLR4-negative and TLR4-positive lines [33, 136]. Mediation of PXL signaling through TLR4 is also suggested by studies with TAK-242 (also known as CLI-095), a TLR4-specific inhibitor that blocks interactions between the TIR domain and intracellular adapters [140]. Breast carcinoma cells pre-treated with TAK-242 reduced PXL-induced expression of inflammatory cytokines by nearly 90% [33]. Multiple studies showed that PXL effects on tumor epithelial or immune cells are largely TLR4-dependent since silencing TLR4 by siRNAs or blocking its actions by specific antibodies or sequence-based peptide inhibitors significantly reduced both NF-κB activation and subsequent molecular (e.g., cytokine upregulation) and cellular (e.g., division and migration) activities [33, 61, 121].

While the notion of PXL sharing the TLR4 pathway with LPS is generally accepted, the molecular basis for physical TLR4 recognition by PXL is still a matter of debate, particularly in the context of nonmyeloid cells. CD14 was reported to play a minimal role in transmission of PXL signals [141], and it is typically absent in normal and tumor epithelial cells. PXL was reported to bind to CD18 [101], but the partner for the Mac-1 complex, CD11b, is typically absent from non-hematopoietic cells such as tumor cells from epithelial malignancies. The requirement for MD2 turned out to be particularly contentious as several studies reported an exclusive specificity of mouse but not human MD2 in supporting PXL-induced signaling [142, 143]. The implication would be that PXL affects only cells from the mouse specie, but this contradicts extensive evidence demonstrating functional LPS-mimetic effects of PXL on human tumor cells (**Table 2**) and normal monocytes [18]. One group found that PXL does bind to human TLR4/MD2 complex but acts as an antagonist [143]. However, this is inconsistent with increased migration, invasion, and other activities of human tumor cells [62, 144] as well as with direct stimulating effects on multiple signaling pathways [122]. It should be noted that two studies that identified PXL as an inhibitor of TLR4 were performed in HEK-293 cells, a human embryonic kidney line immortalized by adenovirus A5 which caused substantial deviations from the epithelial phenotype including expression of neuron-specific genes [145]. HEK-293 cell line was very useful for identification of structural components of the TLR4 complex but might not necessarily reflect the biology of human tumor cells due to differences in organ origin (many responders are derived from tissues other than kidney), stemness status (embryonic vs. adult), and unique genetic changes caused by virus. The latter could lead to significant differences in expression of TLR4 co-receptors and other regulatory proteins. In general, the majority of structural studies with PXL have been performed with either HEK-293 or macrophages. It therefore remains to be established whether the same mechanisms control PXL interactions with the TLR4 complex in human epithelial neoplastic cells.

10. Endogenous ligands of TLR4 released from damaged and necrotic cells

The class of endogenous ligands comprises more than 30 molecules that share no structural resemblance within the members of the group and either LPS or PXL. The list of proposed endogenous TLR4 ligands includes a variety of structurally dissimilar molecules ranging from high-mobility group box-1 (HMBG1) [146] to S100A8 [27, 147] and fibronectin [148]. Alternative names for endogenous ligands are DAMPs mentioned above [41], danger factors [42], and alarmins [149]. The current concept suggests that DAMPs normally segregated into cytosol or intracellular compartments are secreted upon exposure to inflammatory cytokines [146] or passively released from damaged or necrotic cells [71]. Soluble DAMPs then activate receptors of innate immunity such as TLR2, TLR4, and RAGE that are charged not only with protection against pathogens but also with restoration of homeostasis [41]. This is an appealing concept that fits well with well-established activation of TLR4 during sterile injury [150] and remodeling of wounded tissue or tumor [151]. It might also explain activation of TLR4 in cancers developed at sterile anatomic sites and, particularly, during cytotoxic therapy that produces massive cell death.

DAMP-mediated activation of the TLR4 pathway in tumor cells has been shown by numerous independent studies using genetically modified mice with absent or mutated TLR4 [152], blocking anti-TLR4 antibodies [153], specific inhibitors [152], and gain- of-function or loss-of-function approaches [153]. For instance, anti-TLR4 antibody reduced HMGB1-induced proliferation of mouse lung carcinoma cells [154]. HMGB1-dependent recruitment of c-Kit+ progenitors [155], angiogenesis [156], and lymphangiogenesis [157] was significantly reduced in TLR4 −/− non-tumor-bearing mice suggesting similar outcomes in the presence of tumor. HMGB1-induced angiogenesis was also shown in study with UV-damaged keratinocytes in which the released factor increased inflammation, cell proliferation, and migration of melanoma cell toward the endothelial monolayer [144]. All effects were reduced in TLR4- and MyD88-deficient mice as well as in the presence of TAK-242, a specific peptide inhibitor of TLR4 signal transduction [144]. Consistent with this finding, HMGB1 released from necrotic skin cells enhanced inflammation and recruitment of BM myeloid cells and promoted tumor formation, all of which were reduced in TLR4 null mice [158]. Overexpression of HMGB1 in hepatic carcinoma correlated with tumor invasion, and knockdown of this protein suppressed metastasis [159]. Chemotherapy that produces massive necrosis and hence release of HMGB1 and other pro-inflammatory intracellular factors was shown to enhance tumor relapse and metastasis in a model of colon cancer [71]. A variety of tumor- and metastasis-promoting effects have also been reported for other endogenous TLR4 ligands including S100A8/A9 [152], SAA3 [147], hyaluronic acid [153], heat-shock proteins [68, 160], and peroxiredoxin-1 [161].

While the existing functional evidence strongly supports DAMP activation of the TLR4 pathway, the question remains whether these factors are truly ligands for TLR4 or ancillary molecules that stabilize its membrane complex or potentiate intracellular signaling. This uncertainty stems from structural dissimilarity between LPS and many TLR4-activating molecules; a potential risk by LPS contamination of recombinant factors produced in Gram-negative bacteria [162]; and lack of clear structural evidence for physical interaction with TLR4 or MD2 proteins for some ligands [95]. That said, binding of mammalian cell-produced, endotoxin-free SAA3 and S100A8 to TLR4/MD2 complex was shown by surface plasmon resonance [163], and binding of HMGB1 to the same complex was demonstrated by a point mutation in Cys106 that severely reduced the HMGB1 capacity to activate TLR4 [111]. Determination of other ligands as binding partners, amplifiers [164], or assistants might need to be resolved in the future studies.

11. Cellular and molecular consequences of TLR4 activation in the context of cancer

TLR4 is a powerful pathway that simultaneously enhances several key cell functions including differentiation, proliferation, migration, invasion, and survival. On molecular level, the hallmark of TLR4 stimulation is strong upregulation of inflammatory cytokines that act as autocrine and paracrine activators of the first cell responders to TLR4 ligands and nearby stroma, respectively, as well as systemic alert signals for immune organs. In tumors, parallel TLR4 activation of neoplastic and immune cells often results in "double-edge sword" effects [165] due to conflicting functional implications for each cell type. An antitumor effect of TLR4 activation of dendritic cells (DC) is evident by enhanced maturation [166], migration [167], improved antigen presentation [168], better activation of cytotoxic T cells [168], and increased tumor cell death [169]. However, induction of similar pro-mitotic, survival, and migratory functions in malignant and tumor-associated cells has a pro-tumorigenic effect. TLR4 agonists are often proposed to be used clinically for enhancing antitumor therapy [170]; however, it is worth considering both local and systemic consequences of TLR4 activation. The effects on host immune and hematopoietic cells are not straightforward as improved DC functions are counterbalanced by increased generation of myeloid-derived suppressor cells [171] that inhibit antitumor responses. TLR4 activation of BM immature myeloid cells leads to generation of provascular progenitors [17, 18] that increase tumor vessel formation and metastasis [136, 172]. Lung recruitment of the host BM-derived myeloid cells by TLR4 ligands SAA3 in combination with S100A8/A9 has been shown to create a pulmonary pre-metastatic niche, thus ensuring successful establishment of tumor lesions in distant organs [147]. Likewise, TLR4 activation of T cells may enhance their immunosuppressive effects [173] rather than anticancer activities. In our studies performed in tumor-bearing immunocompetent and immunodeficient mice, we often observe a transiently reduced growth upon injection of TLR4-differentiated myeloid progenitors. However, tumor growth resumes at later stages along with substantial increase in lymph node metastasis which correlates with injection of myeloid-derived progenitors [18]. These studies suggest that development of either TLR4-suppressing or TLR4-activating therapeutic strategies should take into account the impact of modulators on all TLR4-positive cells at both tumor and systemic organs.

12. Direct functional effects of TLR4 on tumor cells

Most solid tumors that originated from epithelial, neuronal, and skin cells do not exhibit the same level of responsiveness to LPS as myeloid cells. Nevertheless, functionally, TLR4 activation of tumor cells largely reproduces the known effects in cells of innate immunity. On molecular level, this includes MyD88-dependent activation of NF-κB [33, 71, 174], MAPK [75], PI3K/AKT [61, 175], ERK1/2 [176], c-Jun [69], p38 [75, 176, 177], and other pathways that collectively upregulate inflammatory cytokines [174, 178], metalloproteases [179], and pro-survival factors [59, 180]. Among multiple LPS-induced cytokines in cancer cells are particularly important angiogenic factor VEGF-A [55, 60, 181], immunosuppressive TGF-beta [60, 182], and a variety of chemokines recruiting BM-derived myeloid cells [34, 178] that promote tumor progression through their own mechanisms. On a cellular level, TLR4 activation increases tumor cell proliferation [69, 177, 183], migration [64, 175], invasion [159], and survival [58, 176, 184] that collectively results in resistance to therapy [58, 61, 69, 136, 183]. Some studies also reported increased stemness due to expansion of cancer stem cells [153, 183]. Additional effects include induction of epithelial-mesenchymal transition (EMT) [66, 180] and evasion of immunosurveillance [183], both of which might reflect TLR4-activated macrophage properties enabling tissue repair and resilience against pathogen-produced toxins. Undoubtedly, combination of these effects profoundly impacts tumor growth, chemoresistance, and metastasis.

While it is not possible to discuss all relevant reports due to very extensive literature on the subject, it is worthwhile to highlight several general points. First, the majority of reports showed a significant increase in oncogenic and metastatic potential of tumor cells treated with TLR4 ligands, whereas a minority described an opposite effect [185]. This suggests that in most situations, although both pro- and antitumor effects are induced by TLR4 signaling, the former might be prevailing over the latter. Second, the pro-oncogenic effects have been observed across the entire tumor source spectrum including breast [136, 174, 175], ovarian [58, 121], prostate [61, 62, 184], lung [55, 70], pancreatic [186], colon [176, 180], colorectal [75, 78], and hepatocellular [159, 177] carcinoma lines as well as glioma [183], myeloma [69], and melanoma [144] cells. This indicates a widespread role of TLR4 signaling in human solid cancers which should be considered by clinical therapeutic strategies. Third, TLR4 pathway activated by PXL [33, 58, 62], LPS [175, 184], or other ligands [154] equally affects mouse [178] and human [33, 58] cancer cells. This point is important not only because of the widespread use of mice for modeling human cancers but also because of a lingering debate whether PXL-dependent activation is restricted to mouse cells [142, 187]. Evidence from multiple studies demonstrating PXL-dependent activation of human tumor cells (**Table 2**; reviewed in [188]) indicates that this is not a case. Lastly, mediation through the TLR4 protein by PXL and endogenous ligands has been shown by many approaches including RNA interference [61, 62], anti-TLR4 blocking antibodies [33, 189], TLR4-specific inhibitors [33, 144], as well as use of TLR4−/− mice [30, 144, 158] and isogenic tumor lines with differential TLR4 expression [33]. Although the studies of alternative TLR4 ligands would still benefit from stronger structural evidence for direct recognition of the TLR4 complex, the combined functional evidence derived from multiple independent studies cannot be dismissed. The currently available data show mainly a pro-tumorigenic impact of TLR4 expressed in human and mouse cancer cells resulting from exposure to LPS or TLR4 alternative ligands.

13. Importance of TLR4-induced autocrine loops in normal myeloid cell physiology and tumor pathology

One important function of the TLR4 pathway in macrophages during pathogenic invasion is to amplify the signaling to hasten proliferation and survival of resident macrophages as well as recruitment of BM-derived myeloid cells to the septic site. Macrophages effectively achieve this goal by establishing autocrine loops through coincided upregulation of secreted cytokines and corresponding membrane-inserted receptors. This positive reinforcement ensures sustained expression of downstream targets necessary for prolonged survival, resilience, and heightened activities of immune cells. For instance, LPS-upregulated IL-1 and IL-18 are co-expressed with their receptors that signal through the MyD88 pathway in addition to TLR4 [190] which doubles the outcomes of the combined signaling [191]. LPS-induced co-expression of IL-8, TNF alpha, and other cytokines with their receptors was reported to amplify macrophage functions by enhancing activation of NF-κB [39] and STAT1 [192]. This pattern is mimicked by TLR4-positive tumor cells activated by either LPS [178] or PXL [33]. In our study with TLR4-expressing breast carcinoma lines, we observed that PXL-induced transcription of multiple cytokines was coordinated with upregulation of matching receptors evident by parallel elevation of CXCL2/CXCR2, CCL20/CCR6, and CSF1/CSF1R pairs [33]. Similarly to positive reinforcement in activated macrophages, signaling through these additional pathways in tumor cells significantly increased expression of pro-survival proteins such as pAKT and ERK1/2 [33]. These findings highlight a cytoprotective program naturally induced by TLR4 in macrophages and reproduced by tumor cells that might represent a key mechanism underlying tumor evasion of apoptosis and resistance to therapy.

14. Indirect pro-oncogenic effects of TLR4 mediated by cells in the tumor microenvironment (TME)

TME has profound effects on tumor progression [193, 194]. Some of the pro-oncogenic and pro-metastatic effects of TLR4 are mediated by TME cells such as macrophages, fibroblasts, smooth muscle cells, and pericytes as well as endothelium lining blood and lymphatic vessels. Macrophages are natural responders to TLR4 ligands having the highest expression of this receptor. Under inflammatory conditions, TLR4 is further upregulated by LPS [31] and cytokines [195] through positive feedback loops. Tumor-associated macrophages (TAMs) are well-known promoters of metastasis through secretion of growth-promoting cytokines, proteases [196], and immunosuppressive factors [197]. TAMs are also significant source for lymphangiogenic factors that increase lymphatic density and metastasis [198]. Importantly, TAMs from TLR4-deficient mice have a significantly reduced capacity to activate NF-κB leading to deficient production of angiogenic and inflammatory factors that promote tumor growth [55].

Cancer-associated fibroblasts (CAFs) are another cell type found in most solid tumors but particularly pronounced in pancreatic [199], colorectal [200], and breast [201] cancers. Inflamed human and mouse fibroblasts express TLR4/MD2 complex and respond to TLR4 ligands [202]. Deletion of TLR4 prevents fibrosis in vivo [202] suggesting that CAF-expressed TLR4 might play a non-redundant role in tumor pathology. This is, indeed, supported by several studies. TLR4 expression in CAFs in human colorectal cancer was associated with high recurrence rate and poor patient survival [200]. CAFs associated with breast cancer were identified as a main source of HMGB1 that activated neighboring TLR4-positive tumor cells [203]. Functional TLR4 was also found to be expressed in another TME component, tumor-recruited mesenchymal stem cells (MSC), which was evidenced by LPS-activated NF-κB, PI3K and IRF1, and upregulation of downstream cytokines [204]. High level of TLR4 was also detected in human pericytes that are ontogenically related to MSC [52]. When activated by either LPS or HMGB1, pericytes upregulated classic NF-κB genes including cytokines and cell adhesion molecules (CAMs) such as VCAM-1 and ICAM-1. The latter greatly increase leukocyte adhesion to pericyte monolayer [52] which might play a key role in transmigration of blood-circulating immune cells and hematopoietic progenitors through the vascular barrier and infiltration of the tumor interstitium. Tumor-recruited cells harbor BM-derived myeloid-suppressive cells that promote immuno-evasion [205] as well as provascular progenitors that expand tumor vasculature [206, 207]. Both of these TME populations are known to advance tumor progression. Collectively, these studies illustrate a prominent role of TLR4 signaling in cross-talk of various TME compartments that propagate circuits supporting tumor-associated and malignant cells.

15. Role of TLR4 in tumor angiogenesis and lymphangiogenesis

Although majority of studies have been focused on myeloid cells, it is difficult to overstate the functional impact of the TLR4 pathway on vasculature. Blood vessels are the first responders to circulating septic molecules, and lymphatic vessels, among other functions, help mounting the adaptive immune response by collecting pathogenic antigens from the infected tissue and delivering them to regional lymph nodes. Blood vascular endothelial cells (BEC) and lymphatic endothelial cells (LEC) from human [19, 208] and mouse [50] origins express TLR4 and are naturally equipped to sense and respond to TLR4 ligands [49, 209]. Endothelial cells (EC) from both large [208] and microvessels [19] express TLR4 and accessory molecules for ligand recognition [32] and intracellular signaling [49, 209, 210]. The TLR4 specificity of endothelial response to LPS and other ligands has been documented using mice with deleted receptor [50], ectopic overexpression of nonfunctional protein [19], siRNA [211], and anti-TLR4 monoclonal antibodies [19].

Similarly to myeloid cells, activation of endothelial TLR4 results in NF-κB-mediated upregulation of inflammatory cytokines [19] that includes prominent expression of angiogenic factors VEGF-A and PDGF-BB [212]. Along with this shared pattern, EC also display a distinct response to TLR4 activation such as high upregulation of transcription factor FOXC2 and induction of DLL4-Notch signaling [210] regulating vascular sprouting [213]. Likewise, CAM upregulation, which is detected in all TLR4-activated cells, is particularly pronounced in endothelium [212]. TRAF6, the key regulator of the TLR4 pathway, also mediates endothelial-specific responses, e.g., disruption of the vascular barrier [48, 49]. The resultant increase in vascular permeability combined with CAM upregulation strongly promotes recruitment of blood-circulating cells [50, 155] many of which (e.g., BM-derived immature myeloid cells) have potent independent effects on generation of tumor vessels [206]. Indeed, microvessel density in clinical human pancreatic cancers was found to be strongly associated with TLR4 expression [211]. A putative endogenous ligand of TLR4, peroxiredoxin-1, was shown to increase tumor growth by promoting tumor vasculature [161]. These studies support the concept that TLR4 activation of tumor endothelium promotes vascular formation through direct induction of angiogenic factors and sprouting and, indirectly, by facilitating transmigration of blood-circulating tumor-promoting immune cells.

Whereas tumor angiogenesis is indispensable for expansion of tumor mass, it might be less relevant to metastasis than lymphatic vessels that have invasion-prone discontinuous basement membrane [214] and are naturally equipped to transport cells to regional lymph nodes [215]. Hematogenous metastasis typically occurs later from the blood vessels in the lymphatic lesions as has recently been shown in several mouse models [216, 217]. Cell trafficking to lymph nodes is mediated exclusively by tumor-associated lymphatic vessels, and increase in density of these vessels is directly associated with metastasis in breast [218] and many other human cancers [188]. Functional TLR4 is highly expressed in LEC as evidenced by substantial upregulation of NF-κB-dependent chemokines that recruit macrophages from inflamed tissue to the lymphatic vessels leading to the draining nodes [20]. The absence of TLR4 significantly reduces lymphatic vessel formation resulting in increased edema and decreased transport through the lymphatic channels [53]. Paclitaxel, a potent mimetic of LPS, promotes lymphangiogenesis in breast cancer models concomitant with highly elevated lymphatic metastasis and, subsequently, increased recurrence [136]. Collectively, these studies present strong evidence for TLR4-dependent promotion of metastasis through activation of both blood and lymphatic endothelia in the tumor.

16. Indirect provascular effects of TLR4 through differentiation of BM-derived endothelial progenitors and their recruitment to tumors

One often overlooked aspect of systemic TLR4 signaling is its tremendous impact on differentiation and recruitment of BM-derived provascular progenitors. Angiogenesis and lymphangiogenesis are tightly regulated in adult organism and, with few exceptions (e.g., wound healing and a female reproductive cycle), are induced only during sustained unresolved inflammation or cancer. The latter are one and the same because all solid tumors have a persistent inflammatory component. Physiologically, any increase in tissue mass or remodeling is accompanied by expansion of blood and lymphatic vessels necessary to serve the new vascular bed. TLR4 responds to this host default program not only by activating local endothelium but also by inducing differentiation of provascular progenitors from early BM precursors.

In all vertebrates, embryonic stem cells derived from hemogenic endothelium express TLR4-NF-κB pathway that is necessary and sufficient to create hematopoietic stem/progenitor cells [15]. The latter give rise to both immune and vascular endothelial cells [219, 220]. Adult mesenchymal [16, 204] and hematopoietic stem cells express functional TLR4 as evidenced by LPS-induced self-renewal and their differentiation into appropriate lineages. Both blood vascular [17, 221] and lymphatic endothelial [18] progenitors vigorously respond to LPS [17] and other TLR4 ligands [221] by increasing proliferation, migration, and expression of transcription factors that control their differentiation into endothelial-like cells. When ligands are present systemically (e.g., released from necrotic tumors and during bolus PXL chemotherapy), TLR4-induced differentiation of BM progenitors occurs in parallel with upregulation of TLR4-dependent CCL2, CCL20, and other chemokines that recruit these progenitors to tumor [136, 174, 178, 222]. In experimental models, mobilization of genetically traceable BM-derived provascular progenitors increased tumor angiogenesis [172], whereas recruitment of myeloid-derived lymphatic endothelial progenitors (M-LECP) substantially increased tumor lymphangiogenesis [136] and lymphatic metastasis [18]. Taken together, these studies demonstrate how TLR4-induced differentiation of BM endothelial precursors and upregulation of tumor chemokines act in concert to increase blood and lymphatic networks that ultimately promote metastasis.

While both LPS and PXL can expand provascular progenitors, the latter is more pertinent to oncology due to widespread use of taxanes in clinical practice. PXL is an active component of all taxanes including widely clinically used docetaxel and nab-paclitaxel. Although counterintuitive, the new concept of chemotherapy-driven metastasis mediated by the TLR4-PXL axis [188, 223, 224] is substantiated by ample evidence from clinical studies. A single dose of PXL to breast cancer (BC) patients doubles the blood level of inflammatory cytokines [225]. An independent study of BC patients before and after PXL therapy confirmed these data and further demonstrated in mice that PXL significantly increases tumor recruitment of BM-derived progenitors [226]. An additional study in BC patients found that PXL increased mobilization of myeloid-derived progenitors by >300% [227]. A separate analysis conducted before and after taxane therapy in BC patients showed a > five-fold increase in tumor-infiltrating myeloid cells and subsequent metastasis [228] Similar extent of tumor enrichment by $CD11b^{+}/CD14^{+}$ myeloid cells concomitant with enhanced metastasis was shown in a large study of patients (N = 699) treated by taxanes [134]. Tumor recruitment of these cells was strongly associated with lymphatic metastasis that doubled in taxane-treated compared with untreated patients [134]. In experimental models, PXL treatment increased angiogenesis and metastatic properties in tumor cells [229]. We recently showed that PXL

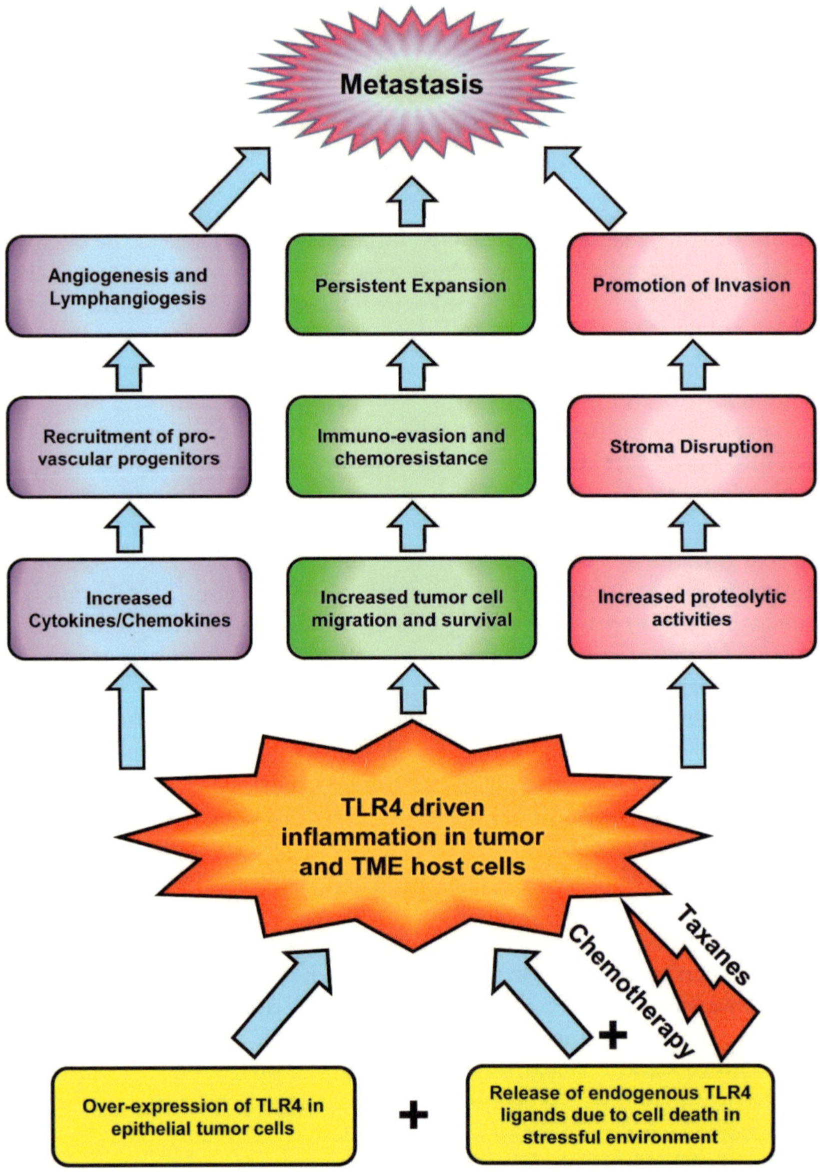

Figure 1.
Activation of TLR4 in tumor cells and tumor microenvironment. TLR4 is overexpressed in malignant cells and in a variety of host cells within the tumor mass including endothelial cells, fibroblasts, pericytes, immune cells, and various progenitors recruited by TLR4-dependent chemokines to tumor inflammatory environment. TLR4 is activated mainly by endogenous ligands released from all expressing cells due to necrotic death induced by pathological surroundings as well as by taxane chemotherapy due to direct activation of the receptor and, indirectly, through increase of endogenous ligands from dead and damaged cells. Following, TLR4 signaling leads to upregulation of inflammatory cytokines, pro-survival and migratory factors, and proteases that disrupt extracellular matrix. This collectively increases not only tumor growth but also its metastatic potential due to enhanced vascular invasion and resistance to cytotoxic therapies. Metastasis is also enhanced because of direct activating effects on tumor endothelium as well as recruitment of provascular progenitors that aid in generation of new vessels.

chemotherapy increased differentiation of BM hematopoietic-myeloid precursors into lymphatic progenitors [18], tumor mobilization of these progenitors, intratumoral lymphangiogenesis, and enhanced metastasis to lymph nodes [18, 136]. Broader recognition of this emerging concept should help in developing novel approaches to combat metastasis such as targeting TLR4-dependent BM differentiation and tumor recruitment of provascular myeloid cells.

17. Summary of TLR4-dependent mechanisms that specifically promote metastasis

Among multitude of pro-oncogenic effects of TLR4, those that specifically affect metastasis relate first and foremost to acquisition of traits normally restricted to inflamed macrophages, that is, enhanced migration, invasion, proliferation, and survival (**Figure 1**). However, this is strongly supplemented by effects on TLR4-expressing cells in the tumor environment from which most relevant are BEC and LEC. Undoubtedly, expansion of angiogenesis and lymphangiogenesis confers direct enhancement of tumor spread through these channels which may occur independently of TLR4 expression in tumor cells. Additionally, the ability to expand BM provascular and stromal progenitors and recruit them to tumor by chemokines—a specific property of inflamed macrophages—substantially supports new vessel and stroma formation. Importantly, the newly acquired properties enabled by the TLR4 signaling are further enhanced by endogenous factors released due to spontaneous necrotic death and chemotherapeutic treatments. Under these conditions, PXL, as an activator of TLR4, takes a special place because of its pro-inflammatory effects through release of endogenous ligands due to tumor cell kill as well through direct action on the TLR4 complex. Ultimately, these processes occur in parallel at tumor and systemic, mainly immune organs, sites. TLR4-positive tumor cells have a pro-metastatic advantage by coordinating generation of new transporting channels and enhanced migratory/invasive potential as well as the enhanced capacity to survive in the circulation and at new sites (**Figure 1**). TLR4-negative tumor cells might have a reduced metastatic potential due to the absence of direct stimulating effects, but they are still benefited from the regenerative tumor environment that is strongly supported by inflammation orchestrated by TLR4. Taking into account a comprehensive systemic view on tumor and chemotherapy effects on TLR4-mediated activities should facilitate the rational development of new anti-metastatic strategies.

Acknowledgements

Preparation of this manuscript was supported by grants from the National Institute of Health (1R01-CA199649), the Team Science Grant (TSG) from the Simmons Cancer Institute at Southern Illinois University, and Illinois William E. McElroy Foundation awarded to Sophia Ran.

Conflict of interest

The authors have no conflicts of interest.

Acronyms and abbreviations

BEC	blood vascular endothelial cell(s)
BM	bone marrow
BMDM	bone marrow-derived myeloid cells
CAFs	cancer-associated fibroblasts
DAMPs	damage-associated molecular patterns
ECP	endothelial cell progenitor(s)
LN(s)	lymph node(s)

LEC	lymphatic endothelial cell(s)
LPS	lipopolysaccharide
LVD	lymphatic vessel density
M-LECP	myeloid-derived lymphatic endothelial cell progenitor(s)
MMP	matrix metalloproteinase(s)
NF-κB	nuclear factor-kappa B
PAMPs	pathogen-associated molecular patterns
PXL	paclitaxel
TAM(s)	tumor-associated macrophage(s)
TME	tumor microenvironment
VEGF-A	vascular endothelial growth factor-A

Author details

Sophia Ran*, Nihit Bhattarai, Radhika Patel and Lisa Volk-Draper
Department of Medical Microbiology, Immunology and Cell Biology, Southern Illinois University School of Medicine, Springfield, IL, USA

*Address all correspondence to: sran@siumed.edu

References

[1] Medzhitov R, Preston-Hurlburt P, Janeway CA Jr. A human homologue of the Drosophila Toll protein signals activation of adaptive immunity. Nature. 1997;**388**:394-397. DOI: 10.1038/41131

[2] Kawai T, Akira S. Toll-like receptor downstream signaling. Arthritis Research and Therapy. 2005;7:12-19. DOI: 10.1186/ar1469

[3] Poltorak A, He X, Smirnova I, Liu MY, Van HC, Du X, et al. Defective LPS signaling in C3H/HeJ and C57BL/10ScCr mice: Mutations in Tlr4 gene. Science. 1998;**282**:2085-2088

[4] Rock FL, Hardiman G, Timans JC, Kastelein RA, Bazan JF. A family of human receptors structurally related to Drosophila Toll. Proceedings of the National Academy of Sciences of the United States of America. 1998;**95**:588-593

[5] Kawai T, Akira S. The role of pattern-recognition receptors in innate immunity: Update on Toll-like receptors. Nature Immunology. 2010;**11**:373-384. DOI: 10.1038/ni.1863

[6] Kaisho T, Akira S. Toll-like receptor function and signaling. Journal of Allergy and Clinical Immunology. 2006;**117**:979-987. DOI: 10.1016/j.jaci.2006.02.023

[7] Kim D, Kim JY. Anti-CD14 antibody reduces LPS responsiveness via TLR4 internalization in human monocytes. Molecular Immunology. 2014;**57**:210-215. DOI: 10.1016/j.molimm.2013.09.009

[8] Akashi S, Shimazu R, Ogata H, Nagai Y, Takeda K, Kimoto M, et al. Cutting edge: Cell surface expression and lipopolysaccharide signaling via the Toll-like receptor 4-MD-2 complex on mouse peritoneal macrophages. Journal of Immunology. 2000;**164**:3471-3475. pii: ji_v164n7p3471

[9] Zhou X, Gao XP, Fan J, Liu Q, Anwar KN, Frey RS, et al. LPS activation of Toll-like receptor 4 signals CD11b/CD18 expression in neutrophils. American Journal of Physiology. Lung Cellular and Molecular Physiology. 2005;**288**:L655-L662. DOI: 10.1152/ajplung.00327.2004

[10] Zanoni I, Ostuni R, Capuano G, Collini M, Caccia M, Ronchi AE, et al. CD14 regulates the dendritic cell life cycle after LPS exposure through NFAT activation. Nature. 2009;**460**:264-268. DOI: 10.1038/nature08118

[11] Komai-Koma M, Gilchrist DS, Xu D. Direct recognition of LPS by human but not murine CD8+ T cells via TLR4 complex. European Journal of Immunology. 2009;**39**:1564-1572. DOI: 10.1002/eji.200838866

[12] Schweighoffer E, Nys J, Vanes L, Smithers N, Tybulewicz VLJ. TLR4 signals in B lymphocytes are transduced via the B cell antigen receptor and SYK. Journal of Experimental Medicine. 2017;**214**:1269-1280. DOI: 10.1084/jem.20161117

[13] Chang EJ, Kim HJ, Ha J, Kim H, Ryu J, Park KH, et al. Hyaluronan inhibits osteoclast differentiation via Toll-like receptor 4. Journal of Cell Science. 2007;**120**:166-176. DOI: 10.1242/jcs.03310

[14] Lee SH, Hong B, Sharabi A, Huang XF, Chen SY. Embryonic stem cells and mammary luminal progenitors directly sense and respond to microbial products. Stem Cells. 2009;**27**:1604-1615. DOI: 10.1002/stem.75

[15] He Q, Zhang C, Wang L, Zhang P, Ma D, Lv J, et al. Inflammatory signaling regulates hematopoietic stem and progenitor cell emergence in

vertebrates. Blood. 2015;**125**:1098-1106. DOI: 10.1182/blood-2014-09-601542

[16] He X, Wang H, Jin T, Xu Y, Mei L, Yang J. TLR4 activation promotes bone marrow MSC proliferation and osteogenic differentiation via Wnt3a and Wnt5a signaling. PLoS One. 2016;**11**:e0149876. DOI: 10.1371/journal.pone.0149876

[17] He J, Xiao Z, Chen X, Chen M, Fang L, Yang M, et al. The expression of functional Toll-like receptor 4 is associated with proliferation and maintenance of stem cell phenotype in endothelial progenitor cells (EPCs). Journal of Cellular Biochemistry. 2010;**111**:179-186. DOI: 10.1002/jcb.22686

[18] Volk-Draper LD, Hall KL, Wilber AC, Ran S. Lymphatic endothelial progenitors originate from plastic myeloid cells activated by Toll-like receptor-4. PLoS One. 2017;**12**:e0179257. DOI: 10.1371/journal.pone.0179257

[19] Faure E, Equils O, Sieling PA, Thomas L, Zhang FX, Kirschning CJ, et al. Bacterial lipopolysaccharide activates NF-kappaB through Toll-like receptor 4 (TLR-4) in cultured human dermal endothelial cells. Differential expression of TLR-4 and TLR-2 in endothelial cells. The Journal of Biological Chemistry. 2000;**275**:11058-11063

[20] Kang S, Lee SP, Kim KE, Kim HZ, Memet S, Koh GY. Toll-like receptor 4 in lymphatic endothelial cells contributes to LPS-induced lymphangiogenesis by chemotactic recruitment of macrophages. Blood. 2009;**113**:2605-2613. DOI: 10.1182/blood-2008-07-166934

[21] Vink A, Schoneveld AH, van der Meer JJ, van Middelaar BJ, Sluijter JP, Smeets MB, et al. In vivo evidence for a role of Toll-like receptor 4 in the development of intimal lesions. Circulation. 2002;**106**:1985-1990

[22] Miller LS, Modlin RL. Human keratinocyte Toll-like receptors promote distinct immune responses. The Journal of Investigative Dermatology. 2007;**127**:262-263. DOI: 10.1038/sj.jid.5700559

[23] Ohkawara T, Takeda H, Miyashita K, Nishiwaki M, Nakayama T, Taniguchi M, et al. Regulation of Toll-like receptor 4 expression in mouse colon by macrophage migration inhibitory factor. Histochemistry and Cell Biology. 2006;**125**:575-582. DOI: 10.1007/s00418-005-0092-y

[24] Ungaro R, Fukata M, Hsu D, Hernandez Y, Breglio K, Chen A, et al. A novel Toll-like receptor 4 antagonist antibody ameliorates inflammation but impairs mucosal healing in murine colitis. American Journal of Physiology. Gastrointestinal and Liver Physiology. 2009;**296**:G1167-G1179. DOI: 10.1152/ajpgi.90496.2008

[25] Zhou M, Farland-Mancini MM, Funk HM, Husseinzadeh N, Mounajjed T, Drew AF. Toll-like receptor expression in normal ovary and ovarian tumors. Cancer Immunology, Immunotherapy. 2009;**58**:1375-1385. DOI: 10.1007/s00262-008-0650-y

[26] Wolfs TG, Buurman WA, van Schadewijk A, de Vries B, Daemen MA, Hiemstra PS, et al. In vivo expression of Toll-like receptor 2 and 4 by renal epithelial cells: IFN-gamma and TNF-alpha mediated up-regulation during inflammation. Journal of Immunology. 2002;**168**:1286-1293

[27] Chakraborty D, Zenker S, Rossaint J, Holscher A, Pohlen M, Zarbock A, et al. Alarmin S100A8 activates alveolar epithelial cells in the context of acute lung injury in a TLR4-dependent manner. Frontiers in Immunology. 2017;**8**:1493. DOI: 10.3389/fimmu.2017.01493

[28] Zarember KA, Godowski PJ. Tissue expression of human Toll-like receptors

and differential regulation of Toll-like receptor mRNAs in leukocytes in response to microbes, their products, and cytokines. Journal of Immunology. 2002;**168**:554-561

[29] Palha De SC, Blum CM, Sgroe EP, Crespo AM, Kurt RA. Murine mammary carcinoma cells and CD11c(+) dendritic cells elicit distinct responses to lipopolysaccharide and exhibit differential expression of genes required for TLR4 signaling. Cellular Immunology. 2010;**266**:67-75. DOI: 10.1016/j.cellimm.2010.08.015

[30] Fukata M, Chen A, Vamadevan AS, Cohen J, Breglio K, Krishnareddy S, et al. Toll-like receptor-4 promotes the development of colitis-associated colorectal tumors. Gastroenterology. 2007;**133**:1869-1881. DOI: 10.1053/j.gastro.2007.09.008

[31] Liu YH, Huang D, Li ZJ, Li XH, Wang X, Yang HP, et al. Toll-like receptor-4-dependence of the lipopolysaccharide-mediated inhibition of osteoblast differentiation. Genetics and Molecular Research. 2016;**15**:1-11. DOI: 10.4238/gmr.15027191

[32] Wang W, Deng M, Liu X, Ai W, Tang Q, Hu J. TLR4 activation induces nontolerant inflammatory response in endothelial cells. Inflammation. 2011;**34**:509-518. DOI: 10.1007/s10753-010-9258-4

[33] Rajput S, Volk-Draper LD, Ran S. TLR4 is a novel determinant of the response to paclitaxel in breast cancer. Molecular Cancer Therapeutics. 2013;**12**:1676-1687. DOI: 10.1158/1535-7163.MCT-12-1019

[34] Son DS, Parl AK, Rice VM, Khabele D. Keratinocyte chemoattractant (KC)/human growth-regulated oncogene (GRO) chemokines and pro-inflammatory chemokine networks in mouse and human ovarian epithelial cancer cells. Cancer Biology and Therapy. 2007;**6**:1302-1312

[35] Kim JI, Lee CJ, Jin MS, Lee CH, Paik SG, Lee H, et al. Crystal structure of CD14 and its implications for lipopolysaccharide signaling. The Journal of Biological Chemistry. 2005;**280**:11347-11351. DOI: 10.1074/jbc.M414607200

[36] Zhou ZB, Yang B, Li X, Liu H, Lei G. Lysophosphatidic acid promotes expression and activation of matrix metalloproteinase 9 (MMP9) in THP-1 cells via Toll-like receptor 4/nuclear factor-kappaB (TLR4/NF-kappaB) signaling pathway. Medical Science Monitor. 2018;**24**:4861-4868. DOI: 10.12659/MSM.906450

[37] Finnin M, Hamilton JA, Moss ST. Characterization of a CSF-induced proliferating subpopulation of human peripheral blood monocytes by surface marker expression and cytokine production. Journal of Leukocyte Biology. 1999;**66**:953-960

[38] Fan J, Malik AB. Toll-like receptor-4 (TLR4) signaling augments chemokine-induced neutrophil migration by modulating cell surface expression of chemokine receptors. Nature Medicine. 2003;**9**:315-321. DOI: 10.1038/nm832

[39] Lombardo E, varez-Barrientos A, Maroto B, Bosca L, Knaus UG. TLR4-mediated survival of macrophages is MyD88 dependent and requires TNF-alpha autocrine signalling. Journal of Immunology. 2007;**178**:3731-3739

[40] Kawai T, Akira S. TLR signaling. Cell Death and Differentiation. 2006;**13**:816-825. DOI: 10.1038/sj.cdd.4401850

[41] Sirisinha S. Insight into the mechanisms regulating immune homeostasis in health and disease. Asian Pac. Journal of Allergy and Clinical Immunology. 2011;**29**:1-14

[42] Bhattacharyya S, Varga J. Endogenous ligands of TLR4 promote unresolving tissue fibrosis: Implications for systemic sclerosis and its targeted therapy. Immunology Letters. 2018;**195**:9-17. DOI: 10.1016/j.imlet.2017.09.011

[43] Mantovani A, Biswas SK, Galdiero MR, Sica A, Locati M. Macrophage plasticity and polarization in tissue repair and remodelling. The Journal of Pathology. 2013;**229**:176-185. DOI: 10.1002/path.4133

[44] Ouyang Y, Guo J, Lin C, Lin J, Cao Y, Zhang Y, et al. Transcriptomic analysis of the effects of Toll-like receptor 4 and its ligands on the gene expression network of hepatic stellate cells. Fibrogenesis and Tissue Repair. 2016;**9**. DOI: 2. DOI: 10.1186/s13069-016-0039-z

[45] Takahashi K, Sugi Y, Hosono A, Kaminogawa S. Epigenetic regulation of TLR4 gene expression in intestinal epithelial cells for the maintenance of intestinal homeostasis. Journal of Immunology. 2009;**183**:6522-6529. DOI: 10.4049/jimmunol.0901271

[46] Yokota S, Okabayashi T, Rehli M, Fujii N, Amano K. *Helicobacter pylori* lipopolysaccharides upregulate Toll-like receptor 4 expression and proliferation of gastric epithelial cells via the MEK1/2-ERK1/2 mitogen-activated protein kinase pathway. Infection and Immunity. 2010;**78**:468-476. DOI: 10.1128/IAI.00903-09

[47] Jiang D, Liang J, Li Y, Noble PW. The role of Toll-like receptors in non-infectious lung injury. Cell Research. 2006;**16**:693-701. DOI: 10.1038/sj.cr7310085

[48] Wolfson RK, Chiang ET, Garcia JG. HMGB1 induces human lung endothelial cell cytoskeletal rearrangement and barrier disruption. Microvascular Research. 2011;**81**:189-197. DOI: 10.1016/j.mvr.2010.11.010

[49] Liu A, Gong P, Hyun SW, Wang KZ, Cates EA, Perkins D, et al. TRAF6 protein couples Toll-like receptor 4 signaling to Src family kinase activation and opening of paracellular pathway in human lung microvascular endothelia. The Journal of Biological Chemistry. 2012;**287**:16132-16145. DOI: 10.1074/jbc.M111.310102

[50] Andonegui G, Bonder CS, Green F, Mullaly SC, Zbytnuik L, Raharjo E, et al. Endothelium-derived Toll-like receptor-4 is the key molecule in LPS-induced neutrophil sequestration into lungs. The Journal of Clinical Investigation. 2003;**111**:1011-1020. DOI: 10.1172/JCI16510

[51] Harari OA, Alcaide P, Ahl D, Luscinskas FW, Liao JK. Absence of TRAM restricts Toll-like receptor 4 signaling in vascular endothelial cells to the MyD88 pathway. Circulation Research. 2006;**98**:1134-1140. DOI: 10.1161/01.RES.0000220105.85182.28

[52] Guijarro-Munoz I, Compte M, Alvarez-Cienfuegos A, Alvarez-Vallina L, Sanz L. Lipopolysaccharide activates Toll-like receptor 4 (TLR4)-mediated NF-kappaB signaling pathway and proinflammatory response in human pericytes. The Journal of Biological Chemistry. 2014;**289**:2457-2468. DOI: 10.1074/jbc.M113.521161

[53] Zampell J, Elhadad S, Avraham T, Weitman E, Aschen S, Yan A, et al. Toll-like receptor deficiency worsens inflammation and lymphedema after lymphatic injury. American Journal of Physiology. Cell Physiology. 2011;**4**:709-719. DOI: 10.1152/ajpcell.00284.2011

[54] Chao W. Toll-like receptor signaling: A critical modulator of cell survival and ischemic injury in the heart. American Journal of Physiology. Heart and Circulatory Physiology.

2009;**296**:H1-H12. DOI: 10.1152/ajpheart.00995.2008

[55] Lee CH, Wu CL, Shiau AL. Toll-like receptor 4 signaling promotes tumor growth. Journal of Immunotherapy. 2010;**33**:73-82. DOI: 10.1097/CJI.0b013e3181b7a0a4

[56] Hishida A, Matsuo K, Goto Y, Hamajima N. Genetic predisposition to *Helicobacter pylori*-induced gastric precancerous conditions. World Journal of Gastrointestinal Oncology. 2010;**2**:369-379. DOI: 10.4251/wjgo.v2.i10.369

[57] Zaks-Zilberman M, Zaks TZ, Vogel SN. Induction of proinflammatory and chemokine genes by lipopolysaccharide and paclitaxel (Taxol) in murine and human breast cancer cell lines. Cytokine. 2001;**15**:156-165. DOI: 10.1006/cyto.2001.0935

[58] Szajnik M, Szczepanski MJ, Czystowska M, Elishaev E, Mandapathil M, Nowak-Markwitz E, et al. TLR4 signaling induced by lipopolysaccharide or paclitaxel regulates tumor survival and chemoresistance in ovarian cancer. Oncogene. 2009;**28**:4353-4363. DOI: 10.1038/onc.2009.289

[59] Kelly MG, Alvero AB, Chen R, Silasi DA, Abrahams VM, Chan S, et al. TLR-4 signaling promotes tumor growth and paclitaxel chemoresistance in ovarian cancer. Cancer Research. 2006;**66**:3859-3868. DOI: 10.1158/0008-5472.CAN-05-3948

[60] He W, Liu Q, Wang L, Chen W, Li N, Cao X. TLR4 signaling promotes immune escape of human lung cancer cells by inducing immunosuppressive cytokines and apoptosis resistance. Molecular Immunology. 2007;**44**:2850-2859. DOI: 10.1016/j.molimm.2007.01.022

[61] Zhang Y, Wang Y, Yuan J, Qin W, Liu F, Wang F, et al. Toll-like receptor 4 ligation confers chemoresistance to docetaxel on PC-3 human prostate cancer cells. Cell Biology and Toxicology. 2012;**28**:269-277. DOI: 10.1007/s10565-012-9221-2

[62] Hua D, Liu MY, Cheng ZD, Qin XJ, Zhang HM, Chen Y, et al. Small interfering RNA-directed targeting of Toll-like receptor 4 inhibits human prostate cancer cell invasion, survival, and tumorigenicity. Molecular Immunology. 2009;**46**:2876-2884. DOI: 10.1016/j.molimm.2009.06.016

[63] Shuyi Y, Feng W, Jing T, Hongzhang H, Haiyan W, Pingping M, et al. Human beta-defensin-3 (hBD-3) upregulated by LPS via epidermal growth factor receptor (EGFR) signaling pathways to enhance lymphatic invasion of oral squamous cell carcinoma. Oral Surgery, Oral Medicine, Oral Pathology, Oral Radiology, and Endodontics. 2011;**112**:616-625. DOI: 10.106/j.triplo.2011.02.053

[64] Jing YY, Han ZP, Sun K, Zhang SS, Hou J, Liu Y, et al. Toll-like receptor 4 signaling promotes epithelial-mesenchymal transition in human hepatocellular carcinoma induced by lipopolysaccharide. BMC Medicine. 2012;**10**. DOI: 98. DOI: 10.1186/1741-7015-10-98

[65] Basu S, Pathak SK, Chatterjee G, Pathak S, Basu J, Kundu M. *Helicobacter pylori* protein HP0175 Transactivates epidermal growth factor receptor through TLR4 in gastric epithelial cells. The Journal of Biological Chemistry. 2008;**283**:32369-32376. DOI: 10.1074/jbc.M805053200

[66] Liu CY, Xu JY, Shi XY, Huang W, Ruan TY, Xie P, et al. M2-polarized tumor-associated macrophages promoted epithelial-mesenchymal transition in pancreatic cancer cells, partially through TLR4/IL-10 signaling pathway. Laboratory Investigation. 2013;**93**:844-854. DOI: 10.1038/labinvest.2013.69

[67] Molteni M, Marabella D, Orlandi C, Rossetti C. Melanoma cell lines are responsive in vitro to lipopolysaccharide and express TLR-4. Cancer Letters. 2006;**235**:75-83. DOI: 10.1016/j.canlet.2005.04.006

[68] Thuringer D, Hammann A, Benikhlef N, Fourmaux E, Bouchot A, Wettstein G, et al. Transactivation of the epidermal growth factor receptor by heat shock protein 90 via Toll-like receptor 4 contributes to the migration of glioblastoma cells. The Journal of Biological Chemistry. 2011;**286**:3418-3428. DOI: 10.1074/jbc.M110.154823

[69] Bao H, Lu P, Li Y, Wang L, Li H, He D, et al. Triggering of Toll-like receptor-4 in human multiple myeloma cells promotes proliferation and alters cell responses to immune and chemotherapy drug attack. Cancer Biology and Therapy. 2011;**11**:58-67. DOI: 10.4161/cbt.11.1.13878

[70] Ieguchi K, Omori T, Komatsu A, Tomita T, Deguchi A, Maru Y. Ephrin-A1 expression induced by S100A8 is mediated by the Toll-like receptor 4. Biochemical and Biophysical Research Communications. 2013;**440**:623-629. DOI: 10.1016/j.bbrc.2013.09.119

[71] Luo Y, Chihara Y, Fujimoto K, Sasahira T, Kuwada M, Fujiwara R, et al. High mobility group box 1 released from necrotic cells enhances regrowth and metastasis of cancer cells that have survived chemotherapy. European Journal of Cancer. 2013;**49**:741-751. DOI: 10.1016/j.ejca.2012.09.016

[72] Zhang JJ, Wu HS, Wang L, Tian Y, Zhang JH, Wu HL. Expression and significance of TLR4 and HIF-1alpha in pancreatic ductal adenocarcinoma. World Journal of Gastroenterology. 2010;**16**:2881-2888

[73] Cammarota R, Bertolini V, Pennesi G, Bucci EO, Gottardi O, Garlanda C, et al. The tumor microenvironment of colorectal cancer: Stromal TLR-4 expression as a potential prognostic marker. Journal of Translational Medicine. 2010;**8**:112. DOI: 10.1186/1479-5876-8-112

[74] Hasimu A, Ge L, Li QZ, Zhang RP, Guo X. Expressions of Toll-like receptors 3, 4, 7, and 9 in cervical lesions and their correlation with HPV16 infection in Uighur women. Chinese Journal of Cancer. 2011;**30**:344-350

[75] Hsu RY, Chan CH, Spicer JD, Rousseau MC, Giannias B, Rousseau S, et al. LPS-induced TLR4 signaling in human colorectal cancer cells increases beta1 integrin-mediated cell adhesion and liver metastasis. Cancer Research. 2011;**71**:1989-1998. DOI: 10.1158/0008-5472.CAN.2833

[76] Ehsan N, Murad S, Ashiq T, Mansoor MU, Gul S, Khalid S, et al. Significant correlation of TLR4 expression with the clinicopathological features of invasive ductal carcinoma of the breast. Tumour Biology. 2013;**34**:1053-1059. DOI: 10.1007/s13277-013-0645-y

[77] Wang EL, Qian ZR, Nakasono M, Tanahashi T, Yoshimoto K, Bando Y, et al. High expression of Toll-like receptor 4/myeloid differentiation factor 88 signals correlates with poor prognosis in colorectal cancer. British Journal of Cancer. 2010;**102**:908-915. DOI: 10.1038/sj.bjc.6605558

[78] Xu H, Wu Q, Dang S, Jin M, Xu J, Cheng Y, et al. Alteration of CXCR7 expression mediated by TLR4 promotes tumor cell proliferation and migration in human colorectal carcinoma. PLoS One. 2011;**6**:e27399. DOI: 10.1371/journal.pone.0027399

[79] Gonzalez-Reyes S, Marin L, Gonzalez L, Gonzalez LO, Del Casar JM, Lamelas ML, et al. Study of TLR3, TLR4 and TLR9 in breast carcinomas

and their association with metastasis. BMC Cancer. 2010;**10**. DOI: 665. DOI: 10.1186/1471-2407-10-665

[80] Eiro N, Ovies C, Fernandez-Garcia B, Alvarez-Cuesta CC, Gonzalez L, Gonzalez LO, et al. Expression of TLR3, 4, 7 and 9 in cutaneous malignant melanoma: Relationship with clinicopathological characteristics and prognosis. Archives of Dermatological Research. 2013;**305**:59-67. DOI: 10.1007/s00403-012-1300-y

[81] Hao B, Chen Z, Bi B, Yu M, Yao S, Feng Y, et al. Role of TLR4 as a prognostic factor for survival in various cancers: A meta-analysis. Oncotarget. 2018;**9**:13088-13099. DOI: 10.18632/oncotarget.24178

[82] Yang CX, Li CY, Feng W. Toll-like receptor 4 genetic variants and prognosis of breast cancer. Tissue Antigens. 2013;**81**:221-226.10. DOI: 10.1111/tan.12096

[83] Wang X, Yu X, Wang Q, Lu Y, Chen H. Expression and clinical significance of SATB1 and TLR4 in breast cancer. Oncology Letters. 2017;**14**:3611-3615. DOI: 10.3892/ol.2017.6571

[84] Gonzalez-Reyes S, Fernandez JM, Gonzalez LO, Aguirre A, Suarez A, Gonzalez JM, et al. Study of TLR3, TLR4, and TLR9 in prostate carcinomas and their association with biochemical recurrence. Cancer Immunology, Immunotherapy. 2010;**60**:217-226. DOI: 10.1007/s00262-010-0931-0

[85] Zhu Y, Huang JM, Zhang GN, Zha X, Deng BF. Prognostic significance of MyD88 expression by human epithelial ovarian carcinoma cells. Journal of Translational Medicine. 2012;**10**. DOI: 77. DOI: 10.1186/1479-5876-10-77

[86] Wang K, Wang J, Wei F, Zhao N, Yang F, Ren X. Expression of TLR4 in non-small cell lung cancer is associated with PD-L1 and poor prognosis in patients receiving Pulmonectomy. Frontiers in Immunology. 2017;**8**:456. DOI: 10.3389/fimmu.2017.00456

[87] Kim KH, Jo MS, Suh DS, Yoon MS, Shin DH, Lee JH, et al. Expression and significance of the TLR4/MyD88 signaling pathway in ovarian epithelial cancers. World Journal of Surgical Oncology. 2012;**10**:193. DOI: 10.1186/1477-7819-10-193

[88] Sheyhidin I, Nabi G, Hasim A, Zhang RP, Ainiwaer J, Ma H, et al. Overexpression of TLR3, TLR4, TLR7 and TLR9 in esophageal squamous cell carcinoma. World Journal of Gastroenterology. 2011;**17**:3745-3751. DOI: 10.3748/wjg.v17.i32.3745

[89] Fitzgerald KA, Palsson-McDermott EM, Bowie AG, Jefferies CA, Mansell AS, Brady G, et al. Mal (MyD88-adapter-like) is required for Toll-like receptor-4 signal transduction. Nature. 2001;**413**:78-83. DOI: 10.1038/35092578

[90] Cheng Z, Taylor B, Ourthiague DR, Hoffmann A. Distinct single-cell signaling characteristics are conferred by the MyD88 and TRIF pathways during TLR4 activation. Science Signaling. 2015;**8**. DOI: ra69. DOI: 10.1126/scisignal.aaa5208

[91] Verstak B, Nagpal K, Bottomley SP, Golenbock DT, Hertzog PJ, Mansell A. MyD88 adapter-like (Mal)/TIRAP interaction with TRAF6 is critical for. The Journal of Biological Chemistry. 2009;**284**:24192-24203. DOI: 10.1074/jbc.M109.023044

[92] Hamidi A, von B, V, Hamidi R, Winssinger N, Barluenga S, Heldin CH, Landstrom M. Polyubiquitination of transforming growth factor beta (TGFbeta)-associated kinase 1 mediates nuclear factor-kappaB activation in response to different inflammatory stimuli. The Journal of Biological Chemistry 2012; 287: 123-133. DOI: 10.1074/jbc.M111.285122

[93] Shimazu R, Akashi S, Ogata H, Nagai Y, Fukudome K, Miyake K, et al. MD-2, a molecule that confers lipopolysaccharide responsiveness on Toll-like receptor 4. Journal of Experimental Medicine. 1999;**189**:1777-1782

[94] Latz E, Visintin A, Lien E, Fitzgerald KA, Monks BG, Kurt-Jones EA, et al. Lipopolysaccharide rapidly traffics to and from the Golgi apparatus with the Toll-like receptor 4-MD-2-CD14 complex in a process that is distinct from the initiation of signal transduction. The Journal of Biological Chemistry. 2002;**277**:47834-47843. DOI: 10.1074/jbc.M207873200

[95] Mancek-Keber M, Jerala R. Postulates for validating TLR4 agonists. European Journal of Immunology. 2015;**45**:356-370. DOI: 10.1002/eji.201444462

[96] Jiang Q, Akashi S, Miyake K, Petty HR. Lipopolysaccharide induces physical proximity between CD14 and Toll-like receptor 4 (TLR4) prior to nuclear translocation of NF-kappa B. Journal of Immunology. 2000;**165**:3541-3544

[97] Moore KJ, Andersson LP, Ingalls RR, Monks BG, Li R, Arnaout MA, et al. Divergent response to LPS and bacteria in CD14-deficient murine macrophages. Journal of Immunology. 2000;**165**:4272-4280

[98] Hailman E, Lichenstein HS, Wurfel MM, Miller DS, Johnson DA, Kelley M, et al. Lipopolysaccharide (LPS)-binding protein accelerates the binding of LPS to CD14. Journal of Experimental Medicine. 1994;**179**:269-277

[99] Golenbock DT, Liu Y, Millham FH, Freeman MW, Zoeller RA. Surface expression of human CD14 in Chinese hamster ovary fibroblasts imparts macrophage-like responsiveness to bacterial endotoxin. The Journal of Biological Chemistry. 1993;**268**:22055-22059

[100] Wong KF, Luk JM, Cheng RH, Klickstein LB, Fan ST. Characterization of two novel LPS-binding sites in leukocyte integrin betaA domain. The FASEB Journal. 2007;**21**:3231-3239. DOI: 10.1096/fj.06-7579com

[101] Bhat N, Perera PY, Carboni JM, Blanco J, Golenbock DT, Mayadas TN, et al. Use of a photoactivatable taxol analogue to identify unique cellular targets in murine macrophages: Identification of murine CD18 as a major taxol-binding protein and a role for Mac-1 in taxol-induced gene expression. Journal of Immunology. 1999;**162**:7335-7342

[102] Han C, Jin J, Xu S, Liu H, Li N, Cao X. Integrin CD11b negatively regulates TLR-triggered inflammatory responses by activating Syk and promoting degradation of MyD88 and TRIF via Cbl-b. Nature Immunology. 2010;**11**:734-742. DOI: 10.1038/ni.1908

[103] Dixon DR, Darveau RP. Lipopolysaccharide heterogeneity: Innate host responses to bacterial modification of lipid a structure. Journal of Dental Research. 2005;**84**:584-595. DOI: 10.1777/154405910508400702

[104] Fruitwala S, El-Naccache DW, Chang TL. Multifaceted immune functions of human defensins and underlying mechanisms. Seminars in Cell and Developmental Biology. 2018;**88**:163-172. DOI: 10.1016/j.semcdb.2018.02.023

[105] Teghanemt A, Zhang D, Levis EN, Weiss JP, Gioannini TL. Molecular basis of reduced potency of underacylated endotoxins. Journal of Immunology. 2005;**175**:4669-4676

[106] Ohto U, Fukase K, Miyake K, Satow Y. Crystal structures of human MD-2 and its complex with antiendotoxic lipid

IVa. Science. 2007;**316**:1632-1634. DOI: 10.1126/science.1139111

[107] Saitoh S, Akashi S, Yamada T, Tanimura N, Matsumoto F, Fukase K, et al. Ligand-dependent Toll-like receptor 4 (TLR4)-oligomerization is directly linked with TLR4-signaling. Journal of Endotoxin Research. 2004;**10**:257-260. DOI: 10.1179/096805104225005904

[108] Cleveland MG, Gorham JD, Murphy TL, Tuomanen E, Murphy KM. Lipoteichoic acid preparations of gram-positive bacteria induce interleukin-12 through a CD14-dependent pathway. Infection and Immunity. 1996;**64**:1906-1912

[109] Miller YI, Choi SH, Wiesner P, Bae YS. The SYK side of TLR4: Signalling mechanisms in response to LPS and minimally oxidized LDL. British Journal of Pharmacology. 2012;**167**:990-999. DOI: 10.1111/j.1476-5381.2012.02097.x

[110] Kochumon S, Wilson A, Chandy B, Shenouda S, Tuomilehto J, Sindhu S, et al. Palmitate activates CCL4 expression in human monocytic cells via TLR4/MyD88 dependent activation of NF-kappaB/MAPK/PI3K signaling systems. Cellular Physiology and Biochemistry. 2018;**46**:953-964. DOI: 10.1159/000488824

[111] Yang H, Hreggvidsdottir HS, Palmblad K, Wang H, Ochani M, Li J, et al. A critical cysteine is required for HMGB1 binding to Toll-like receptor 4 and activation of macrophage cytokine release. Proceedings of the National Academy of Sciences of the United States of America. 2010;**107**:11942-11947. DOI: 10.1073/pnas.1003893107

[112] Vogl T, Tenbrock K, Ludwig S, Leukert N, Ehrhardt C, van Zoelen MA, et al. Mrp8 and Mrp14 are endogenous activators of Toll-like receptor 4, promoting lethal, endotoxin-induced shock. Nature Medicine. 2007;**13**:1042-1049. DOI: 10.1038/nm1638

[113] Schutz FA, Buzaid AC, Sartor O. Taxanes in the management of metastatic castration-resistant prostate cancer: Efficacy and management of toxicity. Critical Reviews in Oncology/Hematology. 2014;**91**:248-256. DOI: 10.1016/j.critrevonc.2014.02.003

[114] McGrogan BT, Gilmartin B, Carney DN, McCann A. Taxanes, microtubules and chemoresistant breast cancer. Biochimica et Biophysica Acta. 2008;**1785**:96-132. DOI: 10.106/j.bbcan.2007.10.004

[115] Torres K, Horwitz SB. Mechanisms of Taxol-induced cell death are concentration dependent. Cancer Research. 1998;**58**:3620-3626

[116] Collins TS, Lee LF, Ting JP. Paclitaxel up-regulates interleukin-8 synthesis in human lung carcinoma through an NF-kappaB- and AP-1-dependent mechanism. Cancer Immunology, Immunotherapy. 2000;**49**:78-84

[117] Poruchynsky MS, Wang EE, Rudin CM, Blagosklonny MV, Fojo T. Bcl-xL is phosphorylated in malignant cells following microtubule disruption. Cancer Research. 1998;**58**:3331-3338

[118] Perera PY, Qureshi N, Vogel SN. Paclitaxel (Taxol)-induced NF-kappaB translocation in murine macrophages. Infection and Immunity. 1996;**64**:878-884

[119] Byrd-Leifer CA, Block EF, Takeda K, Akira S, Ding A. The role of MyD88 and TLR4 in the LPS-mimetic activity of Taxol. European Journal of Immunology. 2001;**31**:2448-2457. DOI. 10.1002/1521-4141(200108)31:8<2448::AID-IMMU2448qt:3.0CO;2-N

[120] Silasi DA, Alvero AB, Illuzzi J, Kelly M, Chen R, Fu HH, et al. MyD88

predicts chemoresistance to paclitaxel in epithelial ovarian cancer. The Yale Journal of Biology and Medicine. 2006;**79**:153-163

[121] Wang AC, Su QB, Wu FX, Zhang XL, Liu PS. Role of TLR4 for paclitaxel chemotherapy in human epithelial ovarian cancer cells. European Journal of Clinical Investigation. 2009;**39**:157-164. DOI: 10.1111/j.1365-2362.2008.02070.x

[122] Wee ZN, Yatim SM, Kohlbauer VK, Feng M, Goh JY, Bao Y, et al. IRAK1 is a therapeutic target that drives breast cancer metastasis and resistance to paclitaxel. Nature Communications. 2015;**6**:8746. DOI: 10.1038/ncomms9746

[123] Le XF, Hittelman WN, Liu J, McWatters A, Li C, Mills GB, et al. Paclitaxel induces inactivation of p70 S6 kinase and phosphorylation of Thr421 and Ser424 via multiple signaling pathways in mitosis. Oncogene. 2003;**22**:484-497. DOI: 10.1038/sj.onc.1206175

[124] Subbaramaiah K, Hart JC, Norton L, Dannenberg AJ. Microtubule-interfering agents stimulate the transcription of cyclooxygenase-2. Evidence for involvement of ERK1/2 AND p38 mitogen-activated protein kinase pathways. Journal of Biological Chemistry. 2000;**275**:14838-14845. pii: 275/20/14838

[125] Wang Y, Qu Y, Niu XL, Sun WJ, Zhang XL, Li LZ. Autocrine production of interleukin-8 confers cisplatin and paclitaxel resistance in ovarian cancer cells. Cytokine. 2011;**56**:365-375. DOI: 10.1016/j.cyto.2011.06.005

[126] Huang Y, Fan W. IkappaB kinase activation is involved in regulation of paclitaxel-induced apoptosis in human tumor cell lines. Molecular Pharmacology. 2002;**61**:105-113

[127] Sumitomo M, Asano T, Asakuma J, Asano T, Horiguchi A, Hayakawa M. ZD1839 modulates paclitaxel response in renal cancer by blocking paclitaxel-induced activation of the epidermal growth factor receptor-extracellular signal-regulated kinase pathway. Clinical Cancer Research. 2004;**10**:794-801

[128] Lee LF, Haskill JS, Mukaida N, Matsushima K, Ting JP. Identification of tumor-specific paclitaxel (Taxol)-responsive regulatory elements in the interleukin-8 promoter. Molecular and Cellular Biology. 1997;**17**:5097-5105

[129] Kang HJ, Lee SH, Price JE, Kim LS. Curcumin suppresses the paclitaxel-induced nuclear factor-kappaB in breast cancer cells and potentiates the growth inhibitory effect of paclitaxel in a breast cancer nude mice model. The Breast Journal. 2009;**15**:223-229. DOI: 10.1111/j.1524-4741.2009.00709.x

[130] Volk LD, Flister MJ, Chihade D, Desai N, Trieu V, Ran S. Synergy of nab-paclitaxel and bevacizumab in eradicating large orthotopic breast tumors and preexisting metastases. Neoplasia. 2011;**13**:327-338

[131] Quintavalle M, Elia L, Price JH, Heynen-Genel S, Courtneidge SA. A cell-based high-content screening assay reveals activators and inhibitors of cancer cell invasion. Science Signaling. 2011;**4**:ra49. DOI: 10.1126/scisignal.2002032

[132] Altorki NK, Port JL, Zhang F, Golijanin D, Thaler HT, Duffield-Lillico AJ, et al. Chemotherapy induces the expression of cyclooxygenase-2 in non-small cell lung cancer. Clinical Cancer Research. 2005;**11**:4191-4197. DOI: 10.1158/1078-0432.CCR-05-0108

[133] Furstenberger G, von Moos R, Lucas R, Thurlimann B, Senn HJ, Hamacher J, et al. Circulating endothelial cells and angiogenic

serum factors during neoadjuvant chemotherapy of primary breast cancer. British Journal of Cancer. 2006;**94**:524-531. DOI: 10.1038/sj.bjc.6602952

[134] DeNardo DG, Brennan DJ, Rexhepaj E, Ruffell B, Shiao SL, Madden SF, et al. Leukocyte complexity predicts breast cancer survival and functionally regulates response to chemotherapy. Cancer Discovery. 2011;**1**:54-67. DOI: 10.1158/2159-8274.CD-10-0028

[135] Zhang P, He D, Chen Z, Pan Q, Du F, Zang X, et al. Chemotherapy enhances tumor vascularization via notch signaling-mediated formation of tumor-derived endothelium in breast cancer. Biochemical Pharmacology. 2016;**118**:18-30. DOI: 10.1016/j.bcp.2016.08.008

[136] Volk-Draper L, Hall K, Griggs C, Rajput S, Kohio P, DeNardo D, et al. Paclitaxel therapy promotes breast cancer metastasis in a TLR4-dependent manner. Cancer Research. 2014;**74**:5421-5434. DOI: 10.1158/0008-5472.CAN-14-0067

[137] Harris AR, Perez MJ, Munson JM. Docetaxel facilitates lymphatic-tumor crosstalk to promote lymphangiogenesis and cancer progression. BMC Cancer. 2018;**18**:718. DOI: 10.1186/s12885-018-4619-8

[138] Taxman DJ, MacKeigan JP, Clements C, Bergstralh DT, Ting JP. Transcriptional profiling of targets for combination therapy of lung carcinoma with paclitaxel and mitogen-activated protein/extracellular signal-regulated kinase kinase inhibitor. Cancer Research. 2003;**63**:5095-5104

[139] Wu J, Guan M, Wong PF, Yu H, Dong J, Xu J. Icariside II potentiates paclitaxel-induced apoptosis in human melanoma A375 cells by inhibiting TLR4 signaling pathway. Food and Chemical Toxicology. 2012;**50**:3019-3024. DOI: 10.1016/j.fct.2012.06.027

[140] Matsunaga N, Tsuchimori N, Matsumoto T, Ii M. TAK-242 (resatorvid), a small-molecule inhibitor of Toll-like receptor (TLR) 4 signaling, binds selectively to TLR4 and interferes with interactions between TLR4 and its adaptor molecules. Molecular Pharmacology. 2011;**79**:34-41. DOI: 10.1124/mol.110.068064

[141] Kirikae F, Kirikae T, Qureshi N, Takayama K, Morrison DC, Nakano M. CD14 is not involved in Rhodobacter sphaeroides diphosphoryl lipid a inhibition of tumor necrosis factor alpha and nitric oxide induction by taxol in murine macrophages. Infection and Immunity. 1995;**63**:486-497

[142] Kawasaki K, Akashi S, Shimazu R, Yoshida T, Miyake K, Nishijima M. Involvement of TLR4/MD-2 complex in species-specific lipopolysaccharide-mimetic signal transduction by Taxol. Journal of Endotoxin Research. 2001;7:232-236

[143] Resman N, Gradisar H, Vasl J, Keber MM, Pristovsek P, Jerala R. Taxanes inhibit human TLR4 signaling by binding to MD-2. FEBS Letters. 2008;**582**:3929-3934. DOI: 10.106/j.febslet.2008.10.037

[144] Bald T, Quast T, Landsberg J, Rogava M, Glodde N, Lopez-Ramos D, et al. Ultraviolet-radiation-induced inflammation promotes angiotropism and metastasis in melanoma. Nature. 2014;**507**:109-113. DOI: 10.1038/nature13111

[145] Shaw G, Morse S, Ararat M, Graham FL. Preferential transformation of human neuronal cells by human adenoviruses and the origin of HEK 293 cells. The FASEB Journal. 2002;**16**:869-871. DOI: 10.1096/fj.01-0995fje

[146] Sims GP, Rowe DC, Rietdijk ST, Herbst R, Coyle AJ. HMGB1 and RAGE in inflammation and Cancer. Annual Review of Immunology.

2010;**28**:367-388. DOI: 10.1146/annurev.immunol.021908.132603

[147] Hiratsuka S, Watanabe A, Sakurai Y, kashi-Takamura S, Ishibashi S, Miyake K, et al. The S100A8-serum amyloid A3-TLR4 paracrine cascade establishes a pre-metastatic phase. Nature Cell Biology. 2008;**10**:1349-1355. DOI: 10.1038/ncb1794

[148] Okamura Y, Watari M, Jerud ES, Young DW, Ishizaka ST, Rose J, et al. The extra domain A of fibronectin activates Toll-like receptor 4. The Journal of Biological Chemistry. 2001;**276**:10229-10233. DOI: 10.1074/jbc.M100099200

[149] Wei F, Yang D, Tewary P, Li Y, Li S, Chen X, et al. The alarmin HMGN1 contributes to anti-tumor immunity and is a potent immunoadjuvant. Cancer Research. 2014;**74**:5989-5998. DOI: 10.1158/0008-5472.CAN-13-2042

[150] Cohen MJ, Brohi K, Calfee CS, Rahn P, Chesebro BB, Christiaans SC, et al. Early release of high mobility group box nuclear protein 1 after severe trauma in humans: Role of injury severity and tissue hypoperfusion. Critical Care. 2009;**13**:R174. DOI: 10.1186/cc8152

[151] Kelsh RM, McKeown-Longo PJ. Topographical changes in extracellular matrix: Activation of TLR4 signaling and solid tumor progression. Trends in Cancer Research. 2013;**9**:1-13

[152] Kallberg E, Vogl T, Liberg D, Olsson A, Bjork P, Wikstrom P, et al. S100A9 interaction with TLR4 promotes tumor growth. PLoS One. 2012;**7**:e34207. DOI: 10.1371/journal.pone.0034207

[153] Ferrandez E, Gutierrez O, Segundo DS, Fernandez-Luna JL. NFkappaB activation in differentiating glioblastoma stem-like cells is promoted by hyaluronic acid signaling through TLR4. Scientific Reports. 2018;**8**:6341. DOI: 10.1038/s41598-018-24444-6

[154] Xu X, Zhu H, Wang T, Sun Y, Ni P, Liu Y, et al. Exogenous high-mobility group box 1 inhibits apoptosis and promotes the proliferation of Lewis cells via RAGE/TLR4-dependent signal pathways. Scandinavian Journal of Immunology. 2014;**79**:386-394. DOI: 10.1111/sji.12174

[155] Furlani D, Donndorf P, Westien I, Ugurlucan M, Pittermann E, Wang W, et al. HMGB-1 induces c-kit+ cell microvascular rolling and adhesion via both Toll-like receptor-2 and Toll-like receptor-4 of endothelial cells. Journal of Cellular and Molecular Medicine. 2012;**16**:1094-1105. DOI: 10.1111/j.1582-4934.2011.01381.x

[156] Lin Q, Yang XP, Fang D, Ren X, Zhou H, Fang J, et al. High-mobility group box-1 mediates Toll-like receptor 4-dependent angiogenesis. Arteriosclerosis, Thrombosis, and Vascular Biology. 2011;**31**:1024-1032. DOI: 10.1161/ATVBAHA.111.224048

[157] Han L, Zhang M, Wang M, Jia J, Zhao M, Fan Y, et al. High mobility group Box-1 promotes inflammation-induced lymphangiogenesis via Toll-like receptor 4-dependent signalling pathway. PLoS One. 2016;**11**:e0154187. DOI: 10.1371/journal.pone.0154187

[158] Mittal D, Saccheri F, Venereau E, Pusterla T, Bianchi ME, Rescigno M. TLR4-mediated skin carcinogenesis is dependent on immune and radioresistant cells. The EMBO Journal. 2010;**29**:2242-2252. DOI: 10.1038/emboj.2010.94

[159] Yan W, Chang Y, Liang X, Cardinal JS, Huang H, Thorne SH, et al. High-mobility group box 1 activates caspase-1 and promotes hepatocellular carcinoma invasiveness and metastases. Hepatology. 2012;**55**:1863-1875. DOI: 10.1002/hep.25572

[160] Galluzzi L, Buque A, Kepp O, Zitvogel L, Kroemer G. Immunogenic cell death in cancer and infectious disease. Nature Reviews. Immunology. 2017;**17**:97-111. DOI: 10.1038/nri.2016.107

[161] Riddell JR, Bshara W, Moser MT, Spernyak JA, Foster BA, Gollnick SO. Peroxiredoxin 1 controls prostate cancer growth through Toll-like receptor 4-dependent regulation of tumor vasculature. Cancer Research. 2011;**71**:1637-1646. DOI: 10.1158/0008-5472.CAN-10-3674

[162] Tsan MF, Gao B. Endogenous ligands of Toll-like receptors. Journal of Leukocyte Biology. 2004;**76**:514-519. DOI: 10.1189/jlb.0304127

[163] Maru Y, Tomita T, Deguchi A, Ieguchi K, Takita M, Tsukahara F, et al. Drug targeting based on a new concept-targeting against TLR4 as an example. Endocrine, Metabolic & Immune Disorders—Drug Targets. 2015;**15**:83-87

[164] Ehrchen JM, Sunderkotter C, Foell D, Vogl T, Roth J. The endogenous Toll-like receptor 4 agonist S100A8/S100A9 (calprotectin) as innate amplifier of infection, autoimmunity, and cancer. Journal of Leukocyte Biology. 2009;**86**:557-566. DOI: 10.1189/jlb.1008647

[165] Basith S, Manavalan B, Yoo TH, Kim SG, Choi S. Roles of Toll-like receptors in cancer: A double-edged sword for defense and offense. Archives of Pharmacal Research. 2012;**35**:1297-1316.1. DOI: 10.1007/s12272-012-0802-7

[166] Kim JY, Kim YJ, Kim JS, Ryu HS, Lee HK, Kang JS, et al. Adjuvant effect of a natural TLR4 ligand on dendritic cell-based cancer immunotherapy. Cancer Letters. 2011;**313**:226-234. DOI: 10.1016/j.canlet.2011.09.009

[167] Grobner S, Lukowski R, Autenrieth IB, Ruth P. Lipopolysaccharide induces cell volume increase and migration of dendritic cells. Microbiology and Immunology. 2013;**8**:61-67. DOI: 10.1111/1348-0421.12116

[168] Apetoh L, Ghiringhelli F, Tesniere A, Obeid M, Ortiz C, Criollo A, et al. Toll-like receptor 4-dependent contribution of the immune system to anticancer chemotherapy and radiotherapy. Nature Medicine. 2007;**13**:1050-1059. DOI: 10.1038/nm1622

[169] Matsuzawa A, Saegusa K, Noguchi T, Sadamitsu C, Nishitoh H, Nagai S, et al. ROS-dependent activation of the TRAF6-ASK1-p38 pathway is selectively required for TLR4-mediated innate immunity. Nature Immunology. 2005;**6**:587-592. DOI: 10.1038/ni1200

[170] Wolska A, Lech-Maranda E, Robak T. Toll-like receptors and their role in carcinogenesis and anti-tumor treatment. Cellular and Molecular Biology Letters. 2009;**14**:248-272. DOI: 10.2478/s11658-008-0048-z

[171] Chen J, Sun B, Zhao X, Liang D, Liu J, Huang Y, et al. Monophosphoryl lipid a induces bone marrow precursor cells to differentiate into myeloid-derived suppressor cells. Molecular Medicine Reports. 2013;**8**:1074-1078. DOI: 10.3892/mmr.2013.1653

[172] Roodhart JM, He H, Daenen LG, Monvoisin A, Barber CL, van AM, et al. Notch1 regulates angio-supportive bone marrow-derived cells in mice: Relevance to chemoresistance. Blood. 2013;**122**:143-153. DOI: 10.1182/blood-2012-11-459347

[173] Zhu XM, Yao YM, Liang HP, Xu CT, Dong N, Yu Y, et al. High mobility group box-1 protein regulate immunosuppression of regulatory T cells through Toll-like receptor 4. Cytokine. 2011;**54**:296-304. DOI: 10.1016/j.cyto.2011.02.017

[174] Egunsola AT, Zawislak CL, Akuffo AA, Chalmers SA, Ewer JC, Vail CM, et al. Growth, metastasis, and expression of CCL2 and CCL5 by murine mammary carcinomas are dependent upon Myd88. Cellular Immunology. 2012;**272**:220-229. DOI: 10.1016/j.cellimm.2011.10.008

[175] Li J, Yin J, Shen W, Gao R, Liu Y, Chen Y, et al. TLR4 promotes breast Cancer metastasis via Akt/GSK3beta/beta-catenin pathway upon LPS stimulation. The Anatomical Record (Hoboken.). 2017;**300**:1219-1229. DOI: 10.1002/ar.23590

[176] Tang X, Zhu Y. TLR4 signaling promotes immune escape of human colon cancer cells by inducing immunosuppressive cytokines and apoptosis resistance. Oncology Research. 2012;**20**:15-24

[177] Wang L, Zhu R, Huang Z, Li H, Zhu H. Lipopolysaccharide-induced Toll-like receptor 4 signaling in cancer cells promotes cell survival and proliferation in hepatocellular carcinoma. Digestive Diseases and Sciences. 2013;**58**:2223-2236. DOI: 10.1007/s10620-013-2745-3

[178] Wang L, Liu Q, Sun Q, Zhang C, Chen T, Cao X. TLR4 signaling in cancer cells promotes chemoattraction of immature dendritic cells via autocrine CCL20. Biochemical and Biophysical Research Communications. 2008;**366**:852-856. DOI: 10.1016/j.bbrc.2007.12.030

[179] Yang H, Wang B, Wang T, Xu L, He C, Wen H, et al. Toll-like receptor 4 prompts human breast cancer cells invasiveness via lipopolysaccharide stimulation and is overexpressed in patients with lymph node metastasis. PLoS One. 2014;**9**:e109980. DOI: 10.1371/journal.pone.0109980

[180] Chung YH, Kim D. Enhanced TLR4 expression on colon cancer cells after chemotherapy promotes cell survival and epithelial-Mesenchymal transition through phosphorylation of GSK3beta. Anticancer Research. 2016;**36**:3383-3394

[181] Pei Z, Li H, Guo Y, Jin Y, Lin D. Sodium selenite inhibits the expression of VEGF, TGFbeta(1) and IL-6 induced by LPS in human PC3 cells via TLR4-NF-(K)B signaling blockage. International Immunopharmacology. 2010;**10**:50-56. DOI: 10.1016/j.intimp.2009.09.020

[182] Li C, Li H, Jiang K, Li J, Gai X. TLR4 signaling pathway in mouse Lewis lung cancer cells promotes the expression of TGF-beta1 and IL-10 and tumor cells migration. Biomedical Materials and Engineering. 2014;**24**:869-875. DOI: 10.3233/BME-130879

[183] Che F, Yin J, Quan Y, Xie X, Heng X, Du Y, et al. TLR4 interaction with LPS in glioma CD133+ cancer stem cells induces cell proliferation, resistance to chemotherapy and evasion from cytotoxic T lymphocyte-induced cytolysis. Oncotarget. 2017;**8**:53495-53507. DOI: 10.18632/oncotarget.18586

[184] Jain S, Suklabaidya S, Das B, Raghav SK, Batra SK, Senapati S. TLR4 activation by lipopolysaccharide confers survival advantage to growth factor deprived prostate cancer cells. The Prostate. 2015;**75**:1020-1033. DOI: 10.1002/pros.22983

[185] Andreani V, Gatti G, Simonella L, Rivero V, Maccioni M. Activation of Toll-like receptor 4 on tumor cells in vitro inhibits subsequent tumor growth in vivo. Cancer Research. 2007;**67**:10519-10527. DOI: 10.1158/0008-5472.CAN-07-0079

[186] Liu J, Xu D, Wang Q, Zheng D, Jiang X, Xu L. LPS induced miR-181a promotes pancreatic cancer cell migration via targeting PTEN and MAP2K4. Digestive Diseases and

Sciences. 2014;**59**:1452-1460. DOI: 10.1007/s10620-014-3049-y

[187] Zimmer SM, Liu J, Clayton JL, Stephens DS, Snyder JP. Paclitaxel binding to human and murine MD-2. The Journal of Biological Chemistry. 2008;**283**:27916-27926. DOI: 10.1074/jbc.M802826200

[188] Ran S. The role of TLR4 in chemotherapy-driven metastasis. Cancer Research. 2015;**75**:2405-2410. DOI: 10.1158/0008-5472.CAN-14-3525

[189] Yang H, Zhou H, Feng P, Zhou X, Wen H, Xie X, et al. Reduced expression of Toll-like receptor 4 inhibits human breast cancer cells proliferation and inflammatory cytokines secretion. Journal of Experimental and Clinical Cancer Research. 2010;**29**:92. DOI: 10.1186/1756-9966-29-92

[190] Ohnishi H, Tochio H, Kato Z, Kawamoto N, Kimura T, Kubota K, et al. TRAM is involved in IL-18 signaling and functions as a sorting adaptor for MyD88. PLoS One. 2012;**7**:e38423. DOI: 10.1371/journal.pone.0038423

[191] Desbien AL, Dubois CN, Reed SJ, Bailor HR, Liang H, Carter D, et al. IL-18 and subcapsular lymph node macrophages are essential for enhanced B cell responses with TLR4 agonist adjuvants. Journal of Immunology. 2016;**197**:4351-4359. DOI: 10.4049/jimmunol.1600993

[192] Luu K, Greenhill CJ, Majoros A, Decker T, Jenkins BJ, Mansell A. STAT1 plays a role in TLR signal transduction and inflammatory responses. Immunology and Cell Biology. 2014;**92**:761-769. DOI: 10.1038/icb.2014.51

[193] Pietras K, Ostman A. Hallmarks of cancer: Interactions with the tumor stroma. Experimental Cell Research. 2010;**316**:1324-1331. DOI: 10.1016/j.yexcr.2010.02.045

[194] Quail DF, Joyce JA. Microenvironmental regulation of tumor progression and metastasis. Nature Medicine. 2013;**19**:1423-1437. DOI: 10.1038/nm.3394

[195] Guzzo C, Ayer A, Basta S, Banfield BW, Gee K. IL-27 enhances LPS-induced proinflammatory cytokine production via upregulation of TLR4 expression and signaling in human monocytes. Journal of Immunology. 2012;**188**:864-873. DOI: 10.4049/jimmunol.1101912

[196] Liguori M, Solinas G, Germano G, Mantovani A, Allavena P. Tumor-associated macrophages as incessant builders and destroyers of the cancer stroma. Cancers (Basel). 2011;**3**:3740-3761. DOI: 10.3390/cancers3043740

[197] Chanmee T, Ontong P, Konno K, Itano N. Tumor-associated macrophages as major players in the tumor microenvironment. Cancers (Basel). 2014;**6**:1670-1690. DOI: 10.3390/cancers6031670

[198] Schoppmann SF, Fenzl A, Nagy K, Unger S, Bayer G, Geleff S, et al. VEGF-C expressing tumor-associated macrophages in lymph node positive breast cancer: Impact on lymphangiogenesis and survival. Surgery. 2006;**139**:839-846. DOI: 10.1016/j.surg.2005.12.008

[199] Ijichi H, Chytil A, Gorska AE, Aakre ME, Bierie B, Tada M, et al. Inhibiting Cxcr2 disrupts tumor-stromal interactions and improves survival in a mouse model of pancreatic ductal adenocarcinoma. The Journal of Clinical Investigation. 2011;**121**:4106-4117. DOI: 10.1172/JCI42754

[200] Eiro N, Gonzalez L, Gonzalez LO, Fernandez-Garcia B, Andicoechea A, Barbon E, et al. Toll-like receptor-4 expression by stromal fibroblasts is associated with poor prognosis in colorectal cancer. Journal of

Immunotherapy. 2013;**36**:342-349. DOI: 10.1097/CJI.0b013e31829d85e6

[201] Radisky ES, Radisky DC. Stromal induction of breast cancer: Inflammation and invasion. Reviews in Endocrine and Metabolic Disorders. 2007;**8**:279-287. DOI: 10.1007/s11154-007-9037-1

[202] Bhattacharyya S, Wang W, Qin W, Cheng K, Coulup S, Chavez S, et al. TLR4-dependent fibroblast activation drives persistent organ fibrosis in skin and lung. JCI Insight. 2018;**3**:1-17. DOI: 10.1172/jci.insight.98850

[203] Zhao XL, Lin Y, Jiang J, Tang Z, Yang S, Lu L, et al. HMGB1 released by autophagic cancer-associated fibroblasts maintains the stemness of luminal breast cancer cells. The Journal of Pathology. 2017;**243**:376-389. DOI: 10.1002/path.4958

[204] Kim SH, Das A, Chai JC, Binas B, Choi MR, Park KS, et al. Transcriptome sequencing wide functional analysis of human mesenchymal stem cells in response to TLR4 ligand. Scientific Reports. 2016;**6**:30311. DOI: 10.1038/srep30311

[205] Eruslanov E, Stoffs T, Kim WJ, Daurkin I, Gilbert SM, Su LM, et al. Expansion of CCR8(+) inflammatory myeloid cells in cancer patients with urothelial and renal carcinomas. Clinical Cancer Research. 2013;**19**: 1670-1680. DOI: 10.1158/1078-0432.CCR-12-2091

[206] Ahn GO, Brown JM. Role of endothelial progenitors and other bone marrow-derived cells in the development of the tumor vasculature. Angiogenesis. 2009;**12**:159-164. DOI: 10.1007/s10456-009-9135-7

[207] Ran S, Wilber A. Novel role of immature myeloid cells in formation of new lymphatic vessels associated with inflammation and tumors. Journal of Leukocyte Biology. 2017;**102**:253-263. DOI: 10.1189/jlb.1MR1016-434RR

[208] Hijiya N, Miyake K, Akashi S, Matsuura K, Higuchi Y, Yamamoto S. Possible involvement of Toll-like receptor 4 in endothelial cell activation of larger vessels in response to lipopolysaccharide. Pathobiology. 2002;**70**:18-25. DOI: 10.1159/000066000

[209] Zabini D, Crnkovic S, Xu H, Tscherner M, Ghanim B, Klepetko W, et al. High-mobility group box-1 induces vascular remodelling processes via c-Jun activation. Journal of Cellular and Molecular Medicine. 2015;**19**:1151-1161. DOI: 10.1111/jcmm.12519

[210] Xia S, Menden HL, Korfhagen TR, Kume T, Sampath V. Endothelial immune activation programmes cell-fate decisions and angiogenesis by inducing angiogenesis regulator DLL4 through TLR4-ERK-FOXC2 signalling. The Journal of Physiology. 2018;**596**:1397-1417. DOI: 10.1113/JP275453

[211] Sun Y, Wu C, Ma J, Yang Y, Man X, Wu H, et al. Toll-like receptor 4 promotes angiogenesis in pancreatic cancer via PI3K/AKT signaling. Experimental Cell Research. 2016;**347**:274-282. DOI: 10.1016/j.yexcr.2016.07.009

[212] Ma B, Dohle E, Li M, Kirkpatrick CJ. TLR4 stimulation by LPS enhances angiogenesis in a co-culture system consisting of primary human osteoblasts and outgrowth endothelial cells. Journal of Tissue Engineering and Regenerative Medicine. 2017;**11**: 1779-1791. DOI: 10.1002/term.2075

[213] Hellstrom M, Phng LK, Hofmann JJ, Wallgard E, Coultas L, Lindblom P, et al. Dll4 signalling through Notch1 regulates formation of tip cells during angiogenesis. Nature. 2007;**445**:776-780. DOI: 10.1038/nature05571

[214] Zhu Y, Maric J, Nilsson M, Brannstrom M, Janson PO, Sundfeldt K. Formation and barrier function of tight junctions in human ovarian surface epithelium. Biology of Reproduction. 2004;**71**:53-59. DOI: 10.1095/biolreprod.103.022913

[215] Betterman KL, Harvey NL. The lymphatic vasculature: Development and role in shaping immunity. Immunological Reviews. 2016;**271**: 276-292. DOI: 10.1111/imr.12413

[216] Keklikoglou I, Cianciaruso C, Guc E, Squadrito ML, Spring LM, Tazzyman S, et al. Chemotherapy elicits pro-metastatic extracellular vesicles in breast cancer models. Nature Cell Biology. 2018;**21**:190-202. DOI: 10.1038/s41556-018-0256-3

[217] Brown M, Assen FP, Leithner A, Abe J, Schachner H, Asfour G, et al. Lymph node blood vessels provide exit routes for metastatic tumor cell dissemination in mice. Science. 2018;**359**:1408-1411. DOI: 10.1126/science.aal3662

[218] Ran S, Volk L, Hall K, Flister MJ. Lymphangiogenesis and lymphatic metastasis in breast cancer. Pathophysiology. 2009;**17**:229-251. DOI: 10.1016/j.pathophys.2009.11.003

[219] Lee LK, Ghorbanian Y, Wang W, Wang Y, Kim YJ, Weissman IL, et al. LYVE1 marks the divergence of yolk sac definitive hemogenic endothelium from the primitive erythroid lineage. Cell Reports. 2016;**17**:2286-2298. DOI: 10.1016/j.celrep.2016.10.080

[220] Bailey AS, Willenbring H, Jiang S, Anderson DA, Schroeder DA, Wong MH, et al. Myeloid lineage progenitors give rise to vascular endothelium. Proceedings of the National Academy of Sciences of the United States of America. 2006;**103**:13156-13161. DOI: 10.1073/pnas.0604203103

[221] Nakamura Y, Suzuki S, Shimizu T, Miyata M, Shishido T, Ikeda K, et al. High mobility group box 1 promotes angiogenesis from bone marrow-derived endothelial progenitor cells after myocardial infarction. Journal of Atherosclerosis and Thrombosis. 2015;**122**:570-581. DOI: 10.5551/jat.27235

[222] Fukata M, Hernandez Y, Conduah D, Cohen J, Chen A, Breglio K, et al. Innate immune signaling by Toll-like receptor-4 (TLR4) shapes the inflammatory microenvironment in colitis-associated tumors. Inflammatory Bowel Diseases. 2009;**15**:997-1006. DOI: 10.1002/jbd.20880

[223] Voloshin T, Voest EE, Shaked Y. The host immunological response to cancer therapy: An emerging concept in tumor biology. Experimental Cell Research. 2013;**319**:1687-1695. DOI: 10.1016/j.yexcr.2013.03.007

[224] Daenen LG, Houthuijzen JM, Cirkel GA, Roodhart JM, Shaked Y, Voest EE. Treatment-induced host-mediated mechanisms reducing the efficacy of antitumor therapies. Oncogene. 2014;**33**:1341-1347. DOI: 10.1038/onc.2013.94

[225] Pusztai L, Mendoza TR, Reuben JM, Martinez MM, Willey JS, Lara J, et al. Changes in plasma levels of inflammatory cytokines in response to paclitaxel chemotherapy. Cytokine. 2004;**25**:94-102

[226] Liu G, Chen Y, Qi F, Jia L, Lu XA, He T, et al. Specific chemotherapeutic agents induce metastatic behaviour through stromal- and tumour-derived cytokine and angiogenic factor signalling. The Journal of Pathology. 2015;**237**:190-202. DOI: 10.1002/path.4564

[227] Roodhart JM, Langenberg MH, Vermaat JS, Lolkema MP, Baars A, Giles RH, et al. Late release of circulating endothelial cells and endothelial

progenitor cells after chemotherapy predicts response and survival in cancer patients. Neoplasia. 2010;**12**:87-94

[228] Ruffell B, Au A, Rugo HS, Esserman LJ, Hwang ES, Coussens LM. Leukocyte composition of human breast cancer. Proceedings of the National Academy of Sciences of the United States of America. 2012;**109**:2796-2801. DOI: 10.1073/pnas.1104303108

[229] Gingis-Velitski S, Loven D, Benayoun L, Munster M, Bril R, Voloshin T, et al. Host response to short-term, single-agent chemotherapy induces matrix metalloproteinase-9 expression and accelerates metastasis in mice. Cancer Research. 2011;**71**: 6986-6996. DOI: 10.1158/0008-5472. CAN-11-0629

Section 4

Therapeutic Perspectives for Inflammation

Chapter 9

The Potential Contribution of Nanoparticles in the Treatment of Inflammatory Diseases

Mona A. Elsayed, Ayman Norredin

Abstract

The scope of this chapter is to review the significant effect that nanomedicine has had in the treatment of inflammatory diseases. Nanotechnology has been widely studied in the last decade and proved to be an encouraging strategy in the healthcare system and the medical field. This novel technology provides a vast number of nanomaterials and tools that could actually diagnose and treat different inflammatory disorders and conditions. An enormous amount of in vivo and in vitro research was conducted by many groups to validate the positive contribution that nanoparticles have in regard to the treatment of inflammation and its associated illnesses. This contribution is due to the fact that nanoparticles could be modulated to pass through metabolic barriers and specifically targeted to deliver drugs to the required sites without affecting healthy cells and tissues. This makes them a promising therapeutical choice for the treatment of inflammatory diseases in the future.

Keywords: nanoparticles, inflammation, nanomedicine, drug delivery, nanotechnology

1. Introduction

Along with the advances in drug development recently, a new technology has gained a lot of attention in the last decades; this technology is nanotechnology [1]. Pharmaceutical industries have become increasingly interested in nanomedicine, due to the huge advantages this technology provides. Nanomedicine is the application of nanotechnology to diagnose and treat biological systems in health and disease [2]. Nanomedicine has led to the development of powerful tools for biological and medical research; these developments include targeted drug delivery, implantable materials for tissue engineering, and creating nanoscale probes for medical diagnostics and tracking cell movements [3]. At times of infection or injury, inflammation plays a very important role in protecting the injured tissue from further infection by starting the healing process [4]. It does this by increasing blood flow to the damaged tissue, which increases the activity of the cells and makes the tissue appear red, hot, and swelling. So, inflammation is actually the body's own response to any damage occurred in the body, which makes it an important part of the healing process. However, if inflammation occurs by mistake, for example, in autoimmune diseases where the body attacks itself or if the inflammation stays too long, even after the infection or injury had passed, then this could cause an inflammatory disease. Therefore, short periods of inflammation, such as with an allergic reaction or with an infection, are generally fully treatable and leave no long-term problems. On the other hand, if inflammation lasts more than several months or years, then it is particularly severe and may cause lasting damage to the affected area or organ, for example, deformed joints. Although, there are an extensive number of medications that are available for the treatment of acute and chronic inflammation in the market. However, scientists have recently started to guide their research toward nanomedicine treatments for inflammatory diseases. Many researches have been studied in vivo and in vitro regarding the treatment of inflammatory diseases with different kinds of nanoparticles. The results of most of the studies reveal a lot of promising and very successful developments. The focus of this chapter is to provide an overview in nanotechnology contribution in treating inflammatory diseases.

2. Inflammation

When a body is injured or attacked by microbial organisms such as bacteria, viruses, or fungi, the immune system is signaled for invaders by the process of inflammation. Inflammation is simply the body's mechanism of defending itself by responding to stimuli to repair and heal any signs of damaged cells or tissues. That's why inflammation is an important part of the immune system's physiological response, without which, infections and injuries could become fatal. However, if the inflammatory process is not working as it should be, it can turn into a disease. Inflammatory diseases include a massive number of disorders and conditions [4–6]. Examples include allergy, asthma, glomerulonephritis, hepatitis, and inflammatory bowel disease [5]. Chronic inflammation has been linked to certain diseases such as heart disease or stroke and may also lead to autoimmune disorders, such as rheumatoid arthritis or cancer [4].

2.1 Causes of inflammation

An infection or injury affecting the body will most probably trigger a number of physical reactions by the immune system that will eventually cause inflammation [5]. On the other hand, inflammation in any part of the body does not necessarily mean that there is a microbial infection.

The most common causes of inflammation are:

- Pathogens like viruses, bacteria, or fungi
- Injuries like external cuts or wounds
- Chemicals or radiation affecting the lungs or body

Diseases or conditions that can cause inflammation:

- Cystitis: an inflammation of the bladder
- Bronchitis: an inflammation of the bronchi in the lungs
- Otitis media: an inflammation in the middle ear
- Dermatitis: an inflammation of the skin

2.2 Kinds of inflammation

2.2.1 Acute inflammation

Acute inflammation is a short-term response with localized effects that means it works at a specific place where the problem exists. It usually occurs after an injury or wound on the skin, a sprained ankle, or a sore throat due to a bacterial infection. It starts rapidly, and symptoms are usually severe, but they subside in a couple of days or weeks. During an acute inflammation episode, the blood vessels in the area affected dilate, and therefore blood flow increases, and the white blood cells cover the injured area to promote healing. This response is what causes the injured area to turn red and become swollen [5].

2.2.2 Chronic inflammation

Chronic inflammation is a long-term response; it's mostly a persistent, low-level inflammation that can last for months or even a lifetime [7]. Inflammation begins as a defensive process in which the body is ready to protect itself from harmful pathogens or chemicals that were exposed to the body for a long period of time. However, sometimes, this defense mechanism can become uncontrolled, and hence, damage to vital organs, nervous and musculoskeletal systems, and blood vessels could occur. In some diseases the immune system might attack its own normal cells mistaking it for a foreign organism or pathogen, such as in autoimmune disorders, causing harmful inflammatory responses.

Chronic inflammatory diseases include:

- Rheumatoid arthritis, where many joints throughout the entire body are permanently inflamed

- Psoriasis, a chronic skin disease

- Inflammations of the bowel such as ulcerative colitis

- Active hepatitis

2.3 Signs and symptoms of inflammation

Signs and symptoms of inflammation can be uncomfortable, but they show that the body is trying to heal itself. They vary in severity and intensity depending whether the inflammation is acute or chronic. The most important signs that may indicate an acute inflammation are [5, 6]:

- Redness: this occurs because the capillaries in the area are filled with more blood than usual.

- Heat: this occurs because more blood flows to the affected area, and this makes it feel warm to the touch.

- Swelling: this is caused by a buildup of fluid.

- Pain: this is due to the release of chemicals during inflammation that stimulate nerve endings, making the area more sensitive to the touch.

- Immobility: there may be some loss of function in the region of the inflammation.

Not all of the signs must occur simultaneously; some might appear before the others. Some inflammations, however, could occur silently without any symptoms, especially when the inflammation is deep inside the body such as in an internal organ. The loss of function symptom, for example, is when you cannot breathe properly if you have asthma, when an inflamed arm or leg is difficult to move or when the sense of smell is lost during a nasal allergy. Inflammation does not necessarily start exactly when a person has been infected by a virus or bacteria, but it actually begins when the body starts to fight against the harmful stimulus or the infection.

Symptoms of chronic inflammation present in a different way [5, 7]. These can include:

- Constant fatigue
- Mouth sores
- Joint, chest, or abdominal pain
- Rash
- Fever

When people have inflammation, they will feel pain, discomfort, distress, and stiffness in the inflamed area, depending on the severity of the inflammation; the type of pain varies. Although inflammation, in most cases, does indicate that the immune system is working properly, the symptoms are still an unpleasant feeling and usually need treatment to ease the pain.

2.4 Treatments of inflammation

The treatment of inflammatory disorders must rely on targets present in the diseased tissues [8]. To achieve the desired therapeutic effect on inflammatory cells, high drug doses will be required which sometime can induce unwanted effects on healthy tissues. The main anti-inflammatory drugs are either steroidal such as betamethasone, prednisone, and dexamethasone or nonsteroidal anti-inflammatory drugs (NSAIDS) such as aspirin, ibuprofen, and naproxen [4]. NSAIDs are available in low doses over the counter mostly to treat the pain associated with inflammation, while higher doses of NSAIDs and steroidal medication are available as prescription medications [5]. Both are used to treat acute and chronic inflammatory diseases. However, their prolonged use is associated with a lot of side effects. Steroidal drugs can cause adrenal atrophy, fluid retention, thinning of bones which can lead to osteoporosis, and increased risk of infection or injury. NSAIDS can cause peptic ulcers, allergies, high blood pressure, or liver and kidney problems. Thus, the search for new anti-inflammatory agents is getting popular with the objective to obtain greater safety, better efficacy, and a more economical way to treat inflammation [5].

Nanomedicine has grown rapidly due to the need for improved therapies for inflammatory, developmental, infectious, and degenerative nervous system disorders [9]. These disorders are a significant burden due to the increased number of people affected, disease severity, and financial cost. Therefore, the need for an improved diagnosis and treatment is urgent. Nanotechnology has been widely studied in the last decade and proved to be an encouraging strategy in the healthcare system and the medical field. This novel technology provides a vast number of nanomaterials and tools that could actually diagnose and treat different inflammatory disorders and conditions. This chapter focuses on the current and future potential of nanomedicine to positively treat inflammatory disorders.

3. Nanotechnology

The last decade has been a tremendous growth for nanotechnology; it encompasses different scientific disciplines. This field aims at designing materials with new functions and beneficial properties at the nanometer level [10]. The nanomaterials designed are mostly any shape with a size in the range of 1–100 nm [11]. The huge and unique advantages that nanoparticles (NPs) offer made them an important research in the medical field, which created a new field called nanomedicine [12]. They can be used for the prevention, diagnosis, and treatment of many diseases, due to their very small size and large surface area. In addition to their easy preparation, NPs can be used to encapsulate and protect drugs, genes, or proteins in which they are carrying from degradation, thus, enhancing their biodistribution and allowing sustained release [13]. They also improve the bioavailability of hydrophobic molecules and can be modulated for site-specific targeting, hence, decreasing the side effects of drugs. Moreover, their unique ability to pass through the physiological barriers and intercellular spaces through different mechanisms due to their small size is an important property in the treatment of different kinds of diseases such as brain disorders [13]. In many cases nowadays, current treatments are simply inadequate to decrease disease progression or even remove symptoms and signs of inflammation [9]. However, nanoparticles can solve such problems, for example, increasing drug penetration into sites of active microbial infection while decreasing its side effects by working as drug carriers. In recent years, the goal for nanoparticle development was for the treatment, detection, and prevention of inflammatory and infected sites [14–16].

Different types of nanocarriers are available, and they are fabricated and chosen depending on different aspects such as the kind of application, what is carried by the nanoparticles whether it's a drug or gene, way of administration, materials used, and method of fabrication. Types of nanoparticles include, but not limited to, polymeric nanoparticles, solid lipid nanoparticles (SLNs), liposomes, metallic nanoparticles, and dendrimers [1]. Below are the different types of nanoparticles that are mostly used.

3.1 Polymeric nanoparticles

Polymeric nanoparticles are made from natural or artificial biodegradable and biocompatible polymers; they represent a promising formulation for drug delivery [17]. They work as carriers to control drug release and target specific locations. When compared to conventional formulations, polymeric nanoparticles can increase the solubility of the drug, hence, increasing its absorption and reducing the therapeutic dose. Furthermore, these nanoparticles are stable and safe. Polymeric nanoparticles can be fabricated using various methods of synthesis, according to their intended application. They can be designed as nanocapsules or nanospheres and range from 10 to 1000 nm in diameter, differing in their composition and structural organization [1]. A nanocapsule has a polymeric membrane surrounding an oily core in which the active ingredient can be adsorbed to the membrane and/or dissolved in the oily core. Nanospheres, on the other hand, are made only from a polymeric structure, where the active constituent is adsorbed or retained. Polymeric materials that have been used extensively for nanoparticles include poly-lactic-acid (PLA) and poly-lactic-co-glycolic acid (PLGA) [1, 18].

3.2 Solid lipid nanoparticles

Solid lipid nanoparticles (SLNs) are colloidal carrier systems that contain highly purified triglycerides, composed mainly of lipids. These structures are produced from solid lipids and are stabilized by surfactants. They combine the advantages of other colloidal systems such as liposomes and polymeric nanoparticles, in their biodegradability, biocompatibility, and low toxicity [19]. SLNs can be produced on a large scale; they have high physicochemical stability and offer good protection against drug degradation [1, 19]. Their size ranges from 50 to 1000 nm and may be used in the pharmaceutical field for the delivery of drugs using different routes of administration such as oral and parenteral routes [1].

3.3 Liposomes

Liposomes for drug delivery are spherical small-sized vesicles composed of natural or synthetic lipid bilayers, separated by an aqueous medium in their core [1, 2, 17]. Hydrophilic substances are encapsulated inside the aqueous compartment, while lipophilic substances are adsorbed or incorporated in the lipid bilayers. Liposomes are classified according to their surface charge, size, lipid composition, and method of preparation. The surface charge could be anionic, cationic, or neutral. According to the size and number of lamellae, liposomes can be classified as small, large, or giant and oligo-, uni- or multi-lamellar, respectively [1]. Liposomes have helped decrease the side effects of different drugs such as anticancer and antifungal drugs, simultaneously with improving their efficacy [2]. Liposomal drug delivery preparations have also been studied in various chronic inflammatory diseases. This is a promising approach since it limits the side effects of anti-inflammatory drugs on healthy tissues [2].

3.4 Metallic nanoparticles

Metallic nanoparticles comprise a class of materials that are made from metals such as titanium, gold, and platinum. They exhibit remarkable optical and electronic properties, which make them very useful in the medical field [20]. These nanoparticles are ranged in size from 1 to 100 nm, and they can be fabricated and modulated with several functional groups, due to their high surface area to volume ratio that allows them to be conjugated with antibodies, ligands, and vehicles for gene drug delivery and diagnostic imaging [17, 19, 21]. Moreover, metallic nanoparticles have the potential to carry large doses of drugs and increase their circulatory half-life [19]. Examples of metallic nanoparticles used in research nowadays include but are not limited to gold, silver, zinc oxide, and iron nanoparticles.

3.5 Dendrimers

Dendrimers, one of the most interesting classes of nanoparticles, are synthetic polymers with repetitively branched molecules ranging in size from 1 to 100 nm [22]. Dendrimers are radially symmetrical molecules with well-defined and homogeneous structure consisting of treelike branches [23]. A typical dendrimer is composed of different parts; it is composed of a central core surrounded by repeated units that start from the inside and grow outward like branches with multiple peripheral functional groups [24]. The functional groups have a high degree of molecular uniformity and could be adjusted in size, valency, solubility, and biodegradation [17]. The dendrimers have very high stability and huge surface area, which made them gain a lot of interest and have a wide number of applications in the biomedical field.

4. Contribution of nanoparticles in inflammatory diseases

Pharmacists, physicians, and patients have long desired better pharmaceutical formulations to improve drug efficacy, reduce toxicity, and reduce the costs of preparation and treatment [2]. The conventional treatments available for inflammatory diseases involve nontargeted treatment options with extensive adverse effects. However, nanodrug delivery has shown, in many studies over the years, a numerous number of promising approaches for delivery of therapeutic agents, and most of them proved to reduce side effects and toxicity, increase a drug's bioavailability and effectiveness at the site, and reduce cost. The focus of this section is to highlight the contribution of several nanoparticle applications that have made an immediate major impact in the treatment of different inflammatory disorders.

4.1 Rheumatoid arthritis

Rheumatoid arthritis (RA) is the most common inflammatory disease and is the major cause of disability of the joints [13, 17, 25]. This disease is associated with progressive disability, systemic complications, and socioeconomic costs [13, 17]. To deliver drugs to the target site directly is still a major problem nowadays. Thus, bounding drugs to carriers, like nanoparticles, can make cell-specific targeting become more achievable. The drugs available conventionally for the treatment of RA include three main groups; these are disease-modifying antirheumatic drugs (DMARDs), steroids, and anti-inflammatory drugs such as NSAIDS. Discussed below are examples for the contribution of nanoparticles to each group.

In one study scientists explored the use of multifunctional nanoparticles in the treatment of RA that involves small synovial joints. This study used near-infrared (NIR) light technology along with the nanoparticles [25]. In this study methotrexate (MTX), which is a DMARD, was loaded to a PLGA polymer-gold (Au) half shell nanoparticle. Then arginine-glycine-aspartic acid (RGD) peptide was conjugated to the surface of the Au NP forming a multifunctional NP (RGD-MTX-PLGA-Au). The RGD peptide was used as a targeting moiety for inflammation, the Au half shell was used to generate heat, and MTX was used for the treatment of RA. The NPs were injected into collagen-induced arthritic (CIA) mice. They were effectively delivered and accumulated in the inflamed joints due to RGD peptides. After delivery, heat was generated upon NIR exposure due to Au, and the MTX was then rapidly released from PLGA nanoparticles. The application of this multifactorial NP in CIA mice had better therapeutic efficacy with a much smaller dose of MTX, when compared to conventional treatment [25]. These results demonstrate that the targeted NPs treatment is a useful and effective strategy for increasing the therapeutic efficacy and decreasing side effects of drugs used in the treatment of RA.

Steroids have been used for the treatment of chronic inflammatory disorders for decades [26]. Normally, to reach efficacious concentrations in the blood, they are frequently injected in high doses due to their rapid clearance from the body. However, the chronic use of corticosteroids is associated with severe side effects such as osteoporosis, hypertension, and weight gain. Therefore, current corticosteroids should have active targeting, controlled release and retention in the inflamed tissue. This could be done using engineered nanomaterials as delivery vehicles. In one study, glucocorticoids were loaded into liposomes to prolong the drug circulation time and change drug distribution. As a consequence, number of injections and doses were reduced while still achieving similar efficacy to that of free glucocorticoid in rat models of rheumatoid arthritis [26].

Nano-carriers that were also successful in delivering anti-inflammatory drugs were PAMAM dendrimers [17, 26]. In one study, they have been used to deliver indomethacin to reduce inflammation in the rat model of arthritis. The polyethylene glycol (PEG) dendrimers were functionalized with folate as a targeting ligand to target only activated macrophages, since folate receptor is expressed on activated macrophages only and not on resting ones. This folate-PEG-PAMAM dendrimer was loaded with indomethacin to study its anti-inflammatory effect. This conjugation resulted in a 10–20-fold increase in drug loading efficiency and was found to release indomethacin in the joints in a sustained manner [17].

4.2 Dermatitis

Dermatologic therapy is mainly aimed to prevent or decrease inflammation in the skin. Topical corticosteroids are the keystone of dermatologic therapy and have been used for various inflammatory conditions for their treatment or prevention [11]. Corticosteroids are often prescribed, though their use can carry significant side effects, as mentioned earlier.

In several studies, SLN corticosteroid formulations showed increased penetration compared to its traditional counterparts, resulting in penetration beyond the epidermis and into the dermis [11]. Moreover, SLN provide the added benefit of sustained release, which is a desirable feature for controlling concentration of drug in tissue over time; these properties may improve side effect profiles and dosing schedules of drugs.

NSAIDs are another main drug used in the treatment of inflammatory diseases because of their excellent anti-inflammatory and analgesic actions [10]. However, NSAIDs are associated with serious adverse effects. Therefore, whenever possible, drugs are used topically for dealing with local inflammatory diseases. Topical ointments that contain NSAIDs nanoparticles were studied for skin penetration, safety, and anti-inflammatory effects in animal models of acute and chronic inflammation. In one study, two ointments, one with normal NSAIDs and the other containing NSAIDs in nanoform, were compared [10]. Following the application of both, the study revealed that NSAID in the nanoform had increased penetration of the drug into the skin compared with the normal NSAID, suggesting a higher local activity of NSAID nanoform when applied to the skin. In chronic inflammation model, both formulations decreased foot swelling in a time-dependent manner. However, the healing rate at 7 days of post treatment was significantly higher following treatment with NSAID nanoform compared with the normal NSAID [10]. Moreover, the concentration of NSAID nanoform was much lower than those required of the normal NSAID. Hence, the potency of the nanoformulations is much higher than normal treatment [10]. NSAID nanoformulations are expected to be the basis for new dermatological products, due to their effective treatment and low side effects.

Another major dermatological product that is used by many consumers is sunscreen. Sunscreens are important tools for skincare and the first line of choice for the prevention of inflammation caused by ultraviolet (UV) rays. UV filters are crucial for the prevention of sunburn and UV-induced mutations that may lead to skin cancer. Inorganic UV filters such as titanium oxide (TiO_2) and zinc oxide (ZnO) have been used in sunscreen formulations for a long time, and they are effective in protecting against both UVA and UVB rays. Despite that, TiO_2 and ZnO filters leave an opaque white residue on the skin, which limits its use by many customers [11]. However, by reducing TiO_2 and ZnO sizes to the nanoscale, the production of translucent products is possible rather than the white coarse raw material. It has been shown that sunscreens using particles between 40 and 60 nm are capable of providing good transparency without weakening UVA and UVB protection [27]. Although there has been some concern about the use of nanomaterials in sunscreens, there is no indication that the use of TiO_2 or ZnO holds any danger, and studies showed that nanoparticle preparations do not penetrate past the stratum corneum [28]. Therefore, further study is still needed to fully evaluate the safety of these filters and fully prove their safety.

4.3 Asthma

Asthma is a chronic inflammatory condition characterized by narrowing and swelling of the airways with extra production of mucus, which makes it difficult for the person to breathe [29]. Theophylline is a drug that had been used conventionally worldwide for the treatment of allergic asthma for several years [30]. Although it's still widely prescribed, its use has decreased due to the use of inhaled glucocorticoids instead. Moreover, theophylline has severe side effects due to its low therapeutic window, such as nausea, headache, and cardiac arrhythmias, which limits its use. The adsorption of theophylline to chitosan nanoparticles, modified by the addition of thiol groups, was studied in vivo using mouse models of allergic asthma [29].

Chitosan is a polymer derived from chitin that has been used for nanodrug delivery due to its beneficial properties such as biocompatibility, biodegradability, and bio-adhesiveness [31]. The mice were treated intranasally with theophylline alone, chitosan nanoparticles alone, or theophylline adsorbed to chitosan nanoparticles [29]. The effects of theophylline on cellular infiltration, histopathology of lung sections, and apoptosis of lung cells were investigated to determine the effectiveness of theophylline chitosan NPs as a drug-delivery vehicle for theophylline. Intranasal delivery of theophylline conjugated nanoparticles augmented the anti-inflammatory effects of the drug compared to theophylline administered alone [29]. Thus, the clinical effects of theophylline in treating asthma could be enhanced through the use of nanodrug delivery system. Nasal drug delivery is indeed a promising technique because of the large surface area in the nose, high blood flow, avoidance of first-pass metabolism, and the quick onset of pharmacological activity. Furthermore, it is reasonable to point out that the bioavailability, adsorption, and residence time of drugs administered through the nasal route would be increased using drug delivery carriers such as nanoparticles [32].

4.4 Inflammatory bowel disease

Ulcerative colitis (UC) and Crohn's disease (CD) are the two major types of inflammatory bowel disease (IBD). IBD is a chronic but relapsing inflammatory disorder of the gastrointestinal tract [33]. UC is characterized by inflammation that is limited to the colon, while CD involves any part of the gastrointestinal tract. Abdominal pain, diarrhea, and rectal bleeding are frequent symptoms in patients suffering from IBD [33]. For years, the conventional treatment of IBD consisted of anti-inflammatory medications, such as corticosteroids, aminosalicylates, and immune suppressants. However, these drugs have several side effects due to their unspecific targeting upon administration. A promising strategy toward IBD treatment would be to selectively target the inflamed colonic tissue in order to decrease side effects and increase therapeutic efficacy of the drug administered.

In one study they used mesalamine, an anti-inflammatory medication used conventionally to treat UC, in a nanoparticle formulation [34]. Free mesalamine undergoes rapid and almost complete systemic absorption from the intestine, which causes side effects and drug loss, lowering the therapeutic effect of the medication. The drug then undergoes extensive metabolism. Therefore, it is important to deliver mesalamine (5ASA) locally to the colon, in order to reduce the systemic drug absorption and thus slow down the metabolism. The drug was covalently bound to a NP matrix polymer. Experiments in mice with colon inflammation showed a distinct retention of the mesalamine inside the NP matrix, which allowed efficient colonic targeting and slowed down the release of the drug. This approach elevated the selectivity of the drug toward the inflammation site by decreasing the rapid drug release in the proximal intestine after oral administration [34].

Nano-drug delivery represents a promising approach in inflammatory disorders, mostly due to their accumulation in the inflamed regions [33]. In another study, the drug release was triggered by the sensitivity of polymer to pH during gastrointestinal (GI) transit. Scientists combined PLGA nanoparticles with pH-triggered polymer, to provide both specific accumulation in inflamed tissue and selective drug release in the colon [33]. They used curcumin (C) as the drug of choice to treat IBD, which is known for decades for its anti-inflammatory, antioxidant, antimicrobial, anticarcinogenic, and hepato-protective effects. Anti-inflammatory effects of C have been studied in several diseases before, such as Alzheimer's disease, Parkinson's disease, multiple sclerosis, and cerebral injury [35]. However, we must note that raw C is known for its poor solubility and thus low bioavailability. Moreover, it has a high rate of metabolism and rapid elimination. Thus, an IBD-specific delivery system is needed to protect C from fast degradation. This study aimed to evaluate the effects of C loaded in polymeric pH-sensitive nanoparticles in the treatment of IBD. They were also compared to a C suspension to assess the selectivity and specific delivery of C to the colon. The negative charge of the surface of nanoparticles attracted them to positively charged ulcerated tissues [36]. Hence, C-NPs exhibited suitable physicochemical characteristics, due to their small size and opposite surface charge, for colonic delivery. In vitro studies reported that encapsulated C was found to cross through the epithelial barrier better than C suspension [33].

4.5 Alzheimer's disease

AD is a type of chronic low-level inflammation that mainly affects the elderly [37]. It's considered as a progressive and devastating neurodegenerative disorder that is characterized by cognitive deterioration and decline in the quality of the patient's life [38]. An enormous amount of in vivo and in vitro research was conducted by many groups to study the effect of NPs on the treatment of AD. The following are some examples of nanomaterials that are intended to target the brain and treat AD:

Albumin NPs loaded with tacrine, which was an AD medication previously, was synthesized and administered through the intranasal route of sheep to avoid the first-pass metabolism of the drug and deliver it rapidly to the brain. Due to the small size and large surface area of albumin NPs, the delivery of tacrine was improved through the mucosa to the brain. This research was tested on sheep nasal mucosa in permeation cell [39].

Dendrimers, as mentioned earlier, are globular macromolecular structures with a densely packed surface. It was found that dendrimers could block the aggregation of Amyloid β (Aβ), which is one of the causes of AD. This is by binding to the protofibrils and fibrils, therefore preventing the cytotoxic effect of Aβ plaques. In one study it was suggested that conjugated and unconjugated dendrimers had the ability to separate Aβ deposits in vitro [40].

Gold (Au) NPs were designed to dissolve the Aβ aggregates by the use of local thermal energy at a molecular level and preventing further aggregation. When Au NPs attach to Aβ aggregates and a weak microwave field is applied, they produce thermal energy which dissolve the aggregation and prevent them from reforming.

Au NPs are known to have the advantage of large surface area, biocompatibility, and small size which make them very suitable in this application [41].

Polymeric NPs such as PLGA have great biocompatibility and biodegradability properties. They have the ability to encapsulate different kind of drugs and transport them to the brain by surface modification. For example, curcumin has been encapsulated by PLGA in several studies. This formulation was found to be a potential candidate for the treatment of AD due to the great properties of curcumin as mentioned earlier. Curcumin was found to bind to the Aβ plaques and disaggregating them, due to its anti-amyloid property, which makes this C-NP formulation a very promising drug in the treatment of AD [41].

5. Future directions

Anti-inflammatory effects of engineered nanomaterials can be intentionally achieved. This is by modulating the nanoparticle physicochemical properties and by using nanoparticles as carriers for anti-inflammatory agents. However, structure activity relationship (SAR) studies are needed to further improve this area of nanotechnology. Despite the huge amount of benefits that nanoparticle holds as drug carriers, there are still some disadvantages [13]. For example, NPs might generate toxicity due to their small size, which widen the biodistribution of the drug in the body. Hence, increasing the drugs' potency, which although beneficial, also might affect the immune response of the body and trigger toxicity. Moreover, clinical researchers have mentioned some negative factors, such as high cost and the difficulty of scaling-up processes [1]. Therefore, future nanodrug delivery studies are recommended, and these studies should focus on toxicity and on identifying key elements like dose, route of administration, physicochemical properties, and composition that might provoke toxicity. Understanding what makes the same nanoparticle beneficial in one model and toxic in another model is critical. This will aid drug delivery formulation scientists in choosing appropriate nanoparticle carriers and will clearly enhance the rapidly growing field of nanodrug delivery.

6. Conclusion

Most drugs available nowadays are limited by their poor solubility, number of side effects, frequent dosing, and nonspecific delivery. Therefore, scientists have shifted their research to using nanoparticles for the delivery of drugs to avoid those limitations. NPs are now studied to deliver two or more drugs simultaneously for combination therapy, aiming to decrease frequency of dosing and number of medications a patient is receiving and thus increasing compliance. The main advantage of using NPs is that they could be modulated and specifically targeted to match the need. Therefore, the production of nanomaterials as drug delivery carriers can offer new opportunities to provide more focused and precise treatment of inflammatory diseases and improve the potential therapeutic effectiveness of available medications [17]. We covered in this chapter the advantages of nanotechnology in the medical field and the different kinds of NPs available. We also mentioned different kinds of inflammatory diseases such as arthritis, asthma, and Alzheimer's disease and how nanoparticles were able to positively contribute in their treatment. Despite the many technical, regulatory, and legal challenges, the development of these technologies on a large scale would face, there is no doubt that there is enough desire to overcome these challenges to improve the quality of life and benefit the society [2].

Abbreviations

AD	Alzheimer's disease
Aβ	amyloid β
CD	Crohn's disease
CIA	collagen-induced arthritis
C	curcumin
DMARDs	disease-modifying antirheumatic drugs
IBD	inflammatory bowel disease
5ASA	mesalamine
MTX	methotrexate
NPs	nanoparticles
NIR	near-infrared radiation
NSAIDs	nonsteroidal anti-inflammatory drugs
PLA	poly-lactic-acid
PLGA	poly-lactic-co-glycolic-acid
PEG	polyethylene glycol
RA	rheumatoid arthritis
SAR	structure activity relationship
SLN	solid lipid nanoparticles
TiO_2	titanium oxide
UC	ulcerative colitis
UV	ultraviolet
ZnO	zinc oxide

Author details

Mona A. Elsayed[1*], Ayman Norredin[2]

1 Department of Nephrology and Hypertension, University of California, Irvine, USA

2 Department of Pharmaceutical Sciences, Sharjah University, Sharjah, UAE

*Address all correspondence to: dr.mona.atta@gmail.com

References

[1] Bonifácio BV, da Silva PB, dos S Ramos MA, Negri KMS, Bauab TM, Chorilli M. Nanotechnology-based drug delivery systems and herbal medicines: A review. International Journal of Nanomedicine. 2014;**9**:1-15

[2] Murthy S, Papazoglou E, Kanagarajan NMNS. Nanotechnology: Towards the detection and treatment of inflammatory diseases. In: Stevenson CS, Marshall LA, Morgan DW, editors. In Vivo Models of Inflammation. Progress in Inflammation Research. Switzerland: Birkhäuser Basel; 2006. DOI: https://doi.org/10.1007/978-3-7643-7520-1_8. Print ISBN: 978-3-7643-7519-5. Online ISBN: 978-3-7643-7520-1

[3] Moghimi SM, Hunter AC, Murray JC. Nanomedicine: Current status and future prospects. The FASEB Journal [Internet]. 2005;**19**(3):311-330. DOI: 10.1096/fj.04-2747rev

[4] Abdulkhaleq LA, Assi MA, Abdullah R, Zamri-Saad M, Taufiq-Yap YH, Hezmee MNM. The crucial roles of inflammatory mediators in inflammation: A review. Veterinary World. 2018;**11**(5):627-635

[5] Nordqvist C. Everything You Need to Know About Inflammation. Medical News Today [Internet]. Medilexicon. 2017. Available from: https://www.medicalnewstoday.com/articles/248423.php%0A [November 15, 2018]

[6] What is an Inflammation? Informed Health Online [Internet]. Cologne, Germany: Institute for Quality and Efficiency in Health Care (IQWiG); 2006. Available from: https://www.ncbi.nlm.nih.gov/books/NBK279298 [November 23, 2010]

[7] Pahwa R, Jialal I. Chronic Inflammation. StatPearls Publishing: 2018. Available from: https://www.ncbi.nlm.nih.gov/books/NBK493173 [Updated: October 27, 2018]

[8] Sun D, Zhuang X, Xiang X, Liu Y, Zhang S, Liu C, et al. A novel nanoparticle drug delivery system: The anti-inflammatory activity of curcumin is enhanced when encapsulated in exosomes. Molecular Therapy [Internet]. The American Society of Gene & Cell Therapy. 2010;**18**(9):1606-1614. DOI: 10.1038/mt.2010.105

[9] Gendelman HE, Anantharam V, Bronich T, Ghaisas S, Jin H, Kanthasamy AG, et al. Nanoneuromedicines for degenerative, inflammatory, and infectious nervous system diseases. Nanomedicine: Nanotechnology, Biology and Medicine [Internet]. The Authors. 2015;**11**(3):751-767. DOI: 10.1016/j.nano.2014.12.014

[10] Yokota J, Kyotani S. Influence of nanoparticle size on the skin penetration, skin retention and anti-inflammatory activity of non-steroidal anti-inflammatory drugs. Journal of the Chinese Medical Association - Elsevier Ltd. 2018;**81**(6):511-519

[11] Landriscina A, Rosen J, Friedman A. Nanotechnology, inflammation and the skin barrier: Innovative approaches for skin health and cosmesis. Cosmetics [Internet]. 2015;**2**(2):177-186. Available from: http://www.mdpi.com/2079-9284/2/2/177/

[12] Hasan A, Morshed M, Memic A, Hassan S, Webster TJ, Marei HES. Nanoparticles in tissue engineering: Applications, challenges and prospects. International Journal of Nanomedicine. 2018;**13**:5637-5655

[13] Chabib L, Ikawati Z, Martien R, Ismail H, Wahyudi MDP, Arimurni DA, et al. Rheumatoid arthritis and the challenge of using nanoparticles for its treatment. MATEC Web of Conferences. 2018;**154**:1-7

[14] Blecher K, Nasir A, Friedman A. The growing role of nanotechnology in combating infectious disease. Virulence. 2011;**2**(5):395-401. DOI: 10.4161/viru.2.5.17035

[15] Wagner V, Dullaart A, Bock A-K, Zweck A. The emerging nanomedicine landscape. Nature Biotechnology. 2006;**24**:1211-1217

[16] McMillan J, Batrakova E, Gendelman HE. Cell delivery of therapeutic nanoparticles. Progress in Molecular Biology and Translational Science. 2011;**104**:563-601

[17] Oliveira IM, Gonçalves C, Reis RL, Oliveira JM. Engineering nanoparticles for targeting rheumatoid arthritis: Past, present, and future trends. Nano Research. 2018;**11**(9):4489-4506

[18] Pal SL, Jana U, Manna PK, Mohanta GP, Manavalan R. Nanoparticle: An overview of preparation and characterization. Journal of Applied Pharmaceutical Science. 2011;**1**(6):228-234

[19] Naahidi S, Jafari M, Edalat F, Raymond K, Khademhosseini A, Chen P. Biocompatibility of engineered nanoparticles for drug delivery. Journal of Controlled Release. 2013;**166**(2):182-194

[20] Yaser D, Hoda J, Jiafu C, Al-Chick Sulaiman B. Nanoparticles. In: Yaser D, editor. Nanotechnology and Functional Materials for Engineers. Philadelphia, United States: Elsevier; 2017. pp. 93-119

[21] Harish KK, Nagasamy V, Himangshu B, Anuttam K. Metallic nanoparticle: A review. Biomedical Journal of Scientific & Technical Research [Internet]. 2018;**4**(2):1-11. Available from: https://biomedres.us/pdfs/BJSTR.MS.ID.001011.pdf

[22] Franiak-Pietryga I, Ziemba B, Messmer B, Skowronska-Krawczyk D. Dendrimers as Drug Nanocarriers: The Future of Gene Therapy and Targeted Therapies in Cancer, Dendrimers - Fundamentals and Applications. In: Maria CS, editor. IntechOpen; 25 April 2018. Available from: https://www.intechopen.com/books/dendrimers-fundamentals-and-applications/dendrimers-as-drug-nanocarriers-the-future-of-gene-therapy-and-targeted-therapies-in-cancer

[23] Abbasi E, Aval SF, Akbarzadeh A, Milani M, Nasrabadi HT, Joo SW, et al. Dendrimers: Synthesis, applications, and properties. Nanoscale Research Letters. 2014;**9**(1):1-10

[24] Oliveira JM, Kotobuki N, Marques AP, Pirraco RP, Benesch J, Hirose M, et al. Surface engineered carboxymethylchitosan/poly(amidoamine) dendrimer nanoparticles for intracellular targeting. Advanced Functional Materials. 2008;**18**(12):1840-1853

[25] Lee S-M, Kim HJ, Ha Y-J, Park YN, Lee S-K, Park Y-B, et al. Targeted chemo-photothermal treatments of rheumatoid arthritis using gold half-shell multifunctional nanoparticles. ACS Nano [Internet]. 2013;**7**(1):50-57. Available from: http://www.ncbi.nlm.nih.gov/pubmed/23194301%0Ahttp://pubs.acs.org/doi/10.1021/nn301215q

[26] Ilinskaya AN, Dobrovolskaia MA. Immunosuppressive and anti-inflammatory properties of engineered nanomaterials. British Journal of Pharmacology. 2014;**171**(17):3988-4000

[27] Wiechers JW, Musee N. Engineered inorganic nanoparticles and cosmetics: Facts, issues, knowledge gaps and challenges. Journal of Biomedical Nanotechnology. Oct 2010;**6**(5):408-431

[28] Filipe P, Silva JN, Silva R, Cirne De Castro JL, Marques Gomes M, Alves LC, et al. Stratum corneum is

an effective barrier to TiO_2 and ZnO nanoparticle percutaneous absorption. Skin Pharmacology and Physiology. 2009;**22**(5):266-275

[29] Lee DW, Shirley SA, Lockey RF, Mohapatra SS. Thiolated chitosan nanoparticles enhance anti-inflammatory effects of intranasally delivered theophylline. Respiratory Research. 2006;**7**(1):-10

[30] Caramori G, Adcock I. Pharmacology of airway inflammation in asthma and COPD. Pulmonary Pharmacology & Therapeutics. 2003;**16**(5):247-277

[31] Lee DW, Powers K, Baney R. Physicochemical properties and blood compatibility of acylated chitosan nanoparticles. Carbohydrate Polymers. 2004;**58**:371-377

[32] Türker S, Onur E, Özer Y. Nasal route and drug delivery systems. Pharmacy World & Science. 2004;**26**(3):137-142

[33] Beloqui A, Coco R, Memvanga PB, Ucakar B, Des Rieux A, Préat V. PH-sensitive nanoparticles for colonic delivery of curcumin in inflammatory bowel disease. International Journal of Pharmaceutics. 2014;**473**(1-2):203-212

[34] Pertuit D, Moulari B, Betz T, Nadaradjane A, Neumann D, Ismaïli L, et al. 5-amino salicylic acid bound nanoparticles for the therapy of inflammatory bowel disease. Journal of Controlled Release. 2007;**123**(3):211-218

[35] Epstein J, Sanderson IR, MacDonald TT. Curcumin as a therapeutic agent: The evidence from in vitro, animal and human studies. The British Journal of Nutrition. 2010;**103**(11):1545-1557

[36] Jubeh TT, Barenholz Y, Rubinstein A. Differential adhesion of normal and inflamed rat colonic mucosa by charged liposomes. Pharmaceutical Research. 2004;**21**(3):447-453

[37] Ray B, Lahiri DK. Neuroinflammation in Alzheimer's disease: Different molecular targets and potential therapeutic agents including curcumin. Current Opinion in Pharmacology. 2009;**9**(4):434-444

[38] Darvesh AS, Carroll RT, Bishayee A, Novotny NA, Geldenhuys WJ, Van der Schyf CJ. Curcumin and neurodegenerative diseases: A perspective. Expert Opinion on Investigational Drugs. 2012;**21**(8):1123-1140

[39] Luppi B, Bigucci F, Corace G, Delucca A, Cerchiara T, Sorrenti M, et al. Albumin nanoparticles carrying cyclodextrins for nasal delivery of the anti-Alzheimer drug tacrine. European Journal of Pharmaceutical Sciences. 20 Nov 2011;**44**(4):559-565

[40] Nazem A, Mansoori GA. Nanotechnology for Alzheimer's disease detection and treatment. Insciences Journal. 2011;**1**(4):169-193. DOI: 10.5640/insc.0104169

[41] Mathew A, Aravind A, Fukuda T, Hasumura T, Nagaoka Y, Yoshida Y, et al. Curcumin nanoparticles—A gateway for multifaceted approach to tackle Alzheimer's disease. Proceedings of the IEEE Conference on Nanotechnology. 2011;**11**:833-836

Chapter 10

Exploring Epigenetic Drugs in the Regulation of Inflammatory Autoimmune Diseases

Cristian Doñas, Alejandra Loyola and Mario Rosemblatt

Abstract

During recent years, numerous studies have shown that epigenetics, heritable changes that do not involve alterations in the DNA sequence, play an important role in the development, function, and regulation of the immune system as well as in the onset and progress of autoimmune diseases. For that reason, in the following chapter, we will review some of the most important concepts about epigenetics and how they modulate the development and function of immune cells, specifically macrophages, dendritic cells, and T cells. Moreover, we will review the role of epigenetics on autoimmune diseases, as well as the use of pharmacological modulation of the epigenetic machinery, as an innovative way to approach a potential new treatment or improve the current treatments of autoimmune diseases.

Keywords: epigenetic, DNA methylation, histone modification, autoimmunity, therapy

1. Introduction

Conrad Waddington introduced the epigenetic term in 1942, and it was defined as the causal interactions between genes and their products that allow for phenotypic expression [1]. Currently, this term has been refined to collective heritable changes in phenotype due to processes that arise independent of DNA sequence [2]. The epigenetic information is transferred during cellular division and includes DNA methylation, post-translational modifications of histones such as acetylation and methylation, and non-coding RNA. The transcriptional effects of epigenetic regulation are multidimensional, including on/off gene regulation, maintenance of transcriptional status, and responsiveness or no-responsiveness to external stimuli.

Increasing interest in the study of epigenetic processes has emerged because changes in these mechanisms have been linked to the onset and/or development of several human diseases such as cancer, autoimmune diseases, and systemic metabolic disorders. For that reason, many epigenetic clinical trials are on the horizon. Here, we will examine some of the basic concepts about DNA methylation, post translational modifications of histones, and their effect on development, differentiation, and effector function in antigen-presenting cells (i.e., dendritic cells and macrophages) and T cells. Finally, we will summarize the epigenetic changes found in immune cell populations and how some of the epigenetic modifications affect the most prevalent autoimmune diseases such as systemic lupus erythematosus (SLE),

IntechOpen

rheumatoid arthritis (RA), multiple sclerosis (MS), and inflammatory bowel diseases (IBD). Finally, we will address how "epigenetic drugs" can be used to modulate these immunological changes.

2. A brief introduction to epigenetics

The classical concept of heritable information is that phenotypic characteristics are transmitted from parental cell to their offspring by genetic information [3]. However, several examples of heritable phenotypic variation cannot be fully explained by Mendelian genetics. In this context, epigenetic modifications such as covalent chemical modifications on the DNA, histone posttranslational modifications, and diverse no-coding RNAs can explain the inheritance of specific phenotypes that genetics cannot explain [4]. Those modifications occur in the nucleosome, the fundamental building block of eukaryotic chromatin, that consist of 147 base pairs of DNA wrapped twice around a histone octamer formed by two subunits of each of the core histones H2A, H2B, H3, and H4 [5]. A variety of modifying enzymes are responsible of the generation, maintenance, and removal of DNA methylation and histone modifications. Enzymes involved in the generation of those marks are called "writers," whereas enzymes involved in the removal of them are called "erasers"; the proteins able to bind to the marks are called "readers." Here, will provide a summary of the function and factors involved in these modifications.

2.1 DNA methylation

This modification occurs mostly in CpG dinucleotides and consists of the transfer of a methyl moiety from S-adenosylmethionine (SAM) to the 5 position of cytosines. DNA methylation in a gene regulatory region or in its coding region correlates with repression of gene expression (**Figure 1**). This reaction is catalyzed by DNA methyltransferases (DNMTs) (**Figure 2**). DNMTs comprise two families that are functionally and structurally distinct. Dnmt1 maintains DNA methylation patterns during DNA replication and repair, while Dnmt3a and Dnmt3b establish *de novo* CpG methylation patterns [6]. Methylated DNA is recognized by methyl-CpG-binding proteins (MBPs) (**Figure 2**), which bind to the methylated DNA and

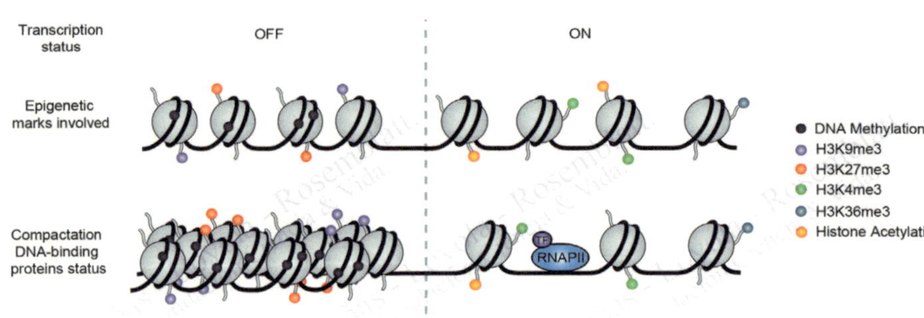

Figure 1.
Epigenetic marks associated to regulation of transcription. DNA methylation and histone modifications induce changes on chromatin structure leading to effects on transcriptional activity. On the left, DNA methylation and histone modifications such as the trimethylation of lysine 9 of H3 (H3K9me3) and the trimethylation of lysine 27 of H3 (H3K27me3) induce the chromatin compaction, making the DNA relatively inaccessible to DNA-binding proteins such as transcription factors (TFs) and RNA polymerase II (RNAPII) causing a transcriptional repression. On the right, histone modifications such as histone acetylation, H3K4me3 and H3K36me3, induce an open chromatin making the DNA to remain accessible to DNA-binding proteins such as TFs and RNAPII generating a state of active transcription.

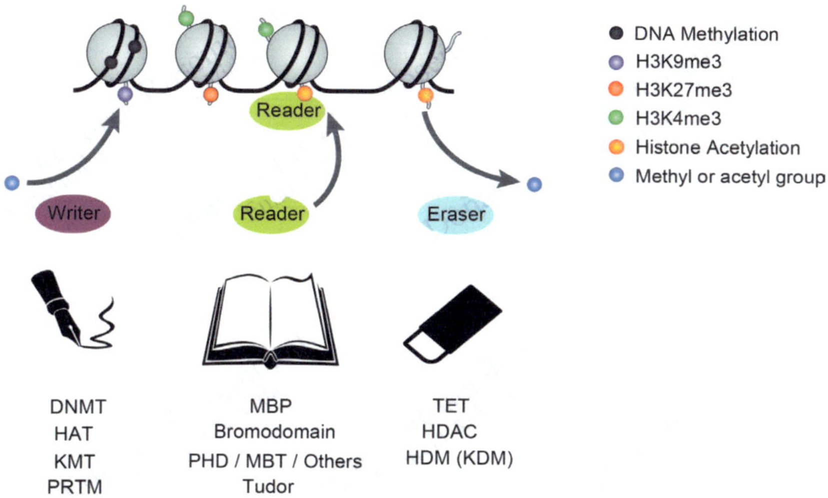

Figure 2.
Writer, readers, and erasers of epigenetic marks. A representative model of epigenetic writers, readers, and erasers and their function. Writers such as DNMT, HAT, KMT, and PRMT carry out the epigenetic modification on DNA and histone tails, while erasers such as TET, HDAC, and KDM remove those modifications. Proteins containing specific domains such as MBP, Bromodomain, PHD, MBT, and Tudor are able to "read" these epigenetic marks and promote either transcriptional activation or repression.

initiate the silencing of chromatin through the recruitment of other factors. These MBP proteins include MeCP2 and MBD1-4 [7]. On the other hand, DNA demethylation is catalyzed by ten-eleven translocation (TET) proteins (**Figure 2**) [8].

2.2 Histone modifications

Over 60 different modifications have been detected on histones. Histone amino-terminal tails are the most frequent target of modifications, including acetylation, methylation, phosphorylation, ubiquitination, sumoylation, and ADP-ribosylation. These modifications, which regulate a variety of functions, including cell cycle, DNA repair, and transcription, has led to the "histone code hypothesis" that postulates that a combination of different modifications may result in distinct and consistent cellular outcomes [9].

2.3 Acetylation

Histone acetylation consists of the transfer of an acetyl group from acetyl-CoA to the lysine 1-amino groups on the N-terminal tail of histones. Acetylation can occur on specific lysines on H3, H4, H2A, and H2B. Acetylation of histones is considered a hallmark of transcriptionally active regions (**Figure 1**) [9]. Histone acetylation is catalyzed by histone acetyltransferases (HATs) (**Figure 2**), which are also known as lysine acetyltransferases (KATs). They are divided into three families based on sequence conservation: GNAT (GNC5/PCAF), MYST (KAT6-8), and p300/CBP families [10]. In addition to neutralize the positive charge normally present on histones, hence reducing affinity between histone and DNA, lysine acetylation generates binding sites for specific protein-protein interaction domains, such as the bromodomain and tandem PHD domains that facilitate chromatin decompaction (**Figure 2**) [11, 12]. On the other hand, four distinct families of histone deacetylases (HDAC) have been described (**Figure 2**). The classes I, II, and IV are considered classical HDACs and require zinc to catalyze the reaction, whereas the class III is NAD-dependent enzymes of the Sirtuin family. HDACs are involved in multiple signaling pathways and are present in numerous repressive chromatin complexes [13, 14].

2.4 Methylation

Histone methylation occurs through the covalent addition of methyl group(s) from the donor SAM to arginine and lysine. Arginine can be mono- and dimethylated (symmetrically or asymmetrically), whereas lysine can be mono-, di- and trimethylated. Methylation mark on histones can be related to activation or repression of gene expression, depending on the residue that is modified (**Figure 1**) [9]. For example, methylation of lysine 4 of H3 (H3K4) is linked to the initiation of transcription [15], H3K36 methylation correlates to transcriptional elongation [16], whereas methylation of H3K79 is implicated both in transcriptional activation and elongation [17]. Three lysine methylation sites are correlated to transcriptional repression: H3K9, H3K27, and H4K20 [10, 18].

In the case of arginine methylation, asymmetric and symmetric dimethylations on arginine have an opposite role on gene expression. For example, asymmetric methylation on H4R3 produced by PRMT1 (protein arginine methyltransferase 1) promotes active transcription [19], whereas symmetric methylation on the same residue (H4R3) produced by the enzyme PRMT5 leads to transcriptional repression [20].

In addition, studies have shown that during early development some of the genes that are not expressed have both repressive (H3K27me3) and permissive (H3K4me3) marks on their promoters, forming the so-called bivalent domains. At the time when the differentiation process occurs, bivalent domain genes are resolved by getting rid of either the active or repressive mark. Therefore, these bivalent domains are thought to keep genes repressed at a certain developmental window but poised for activation in another developmental stage [21].

The enzymatic addition of methyl groups to histone lysine residues is mediated by lysine methyltransferases (KMT) (**Figure 2**) [22]. KMTs have a high degree of enzymatic specificity. For example, SUV39H1 and SUV39H2 convert H3K9me1 to H3K9me3, while G9a produces H3K9me2 [23]. In addition, some "writers" are able to produce all of the methylation status on a histone residue such as Ezh2 (Enhancer of zeste homolog 2) on H3K27 [24]. Methylated histone lysine residues can bind to several protein domains, including PHD, Tudor, and WD40 domains (**Figure 2**). Each domain recognizes specific methylated residues. For example, H3K4me3 is recognized by PHD domains, while WD40 domain recognizes several trimethylated lysine residues associated with repressive marks [25]. Histone lysine demethylase (KDM) removes methylation on specific histone lysine residues (**Figure 2**). These enzymes are divided into two families with distinct enzymatic mechanisms: the FAD-dependent amine oxidase family comprises two members, LSD1 and LSD2, while the iron- and α–ketoglutarate-dependent Jumonji C (JmjC) family comprises more than 30 members [26].

In the case of arginine methylation, the addition of methyl groups is mediated by arginine methyltransferases (PRMTs) (**Figure 2**). PRMTs are divided into three types: type I enzymes including PRMT1-4, 6, 8 and CARM1 generate asymmetric dimethylarginine, whereas type II enzymes such as PRMT5 generate symmetric dimethylarginine [27]. Tudor domains are one of the best-characterized domains that recognize methylated arginines (**Figure 2**) [28]. JMJD6 and JMJD1B have proved to serve as arginine demethylases [29].

Notably, DNA methylation cross-talks with histone modifications. In this context, DNA methylation correlates with the absence of activating marks, such as methylation on H3K4, and the presence of repressive marks, such as H3K9 methylation. H3K4 methylation has been suggested to protect gene promoters from *de novo* DNA methylation. On the other hand, methylated CpG can recruit HDACs to deacetylate histones around the methylated CpG [30].

3. Epigenetic regulation of immune cell development, function, and effector function

3.1 Epigenetic regulation of macrophage development

CCAAT enhancer-binding protein (C/EBP) is a key transcription factor in the development of granulocyte-monocyte progenitors that it is not expressed on hematopoietic stem cells (HSCs). However, the gene promoter that encodes this transcription factor (*Cebpa*) has a "poised" status on HSCs, thus possessing both repressive and activating marks. After the commitment to myeloid cell development, the repressive modification H3K27me3 is removed from the *Cebpa* locus, while the permissive mark H3K4me3 remains, inducing *Cebpa* gene expression [31]. Afterward during myeloid development, the dosage of the transcription factors PU.1 versus C/EBP regulates the macrophage or neutrophil lineage decision, whereas high PU.1 dosage favors macrophage development. PU.1 recruits both DNA demethylases (TET2) and methyltransferases (Dnmt3b) to modulate DNA methylation, facilitating or repressing gene expression, respectively. In contrast, DNA methylation mediated by Dnmt1 is critical for preventing premature differentiation of HSCs [32].

3.2 Epigenetic regulation of macrophage polarization and function

Stimuli and microenvironmental variables induce the polarization of macrophages into M1 or M2 phenotypes. Classical activation is mediated by proinflammatory cytokines such as TNF-α and toll-like receptor (TLR) ligands triggering differentiation to a M1 phenotype. M1 macrophages have host-defense activities that result in pathogen death and are characterized by high expression of proinflammatory cytokines (TNFα, IL-1β, IL-12), antimicrobial molecules, and oxygen reactive species [33]. Studies have shown that regulatory regions of TLR target genes are poised for induction by master transcription factors. Under steady state conditions, those promoters have permissive histone modifications such as H3K4me3 and acetylated H3, and their enhancers are enriched on H3K4me1 [33, 34]. In addition, poised promoters of genes involved in eliminating the infection are primed for a strong and rapid response by IFN-β [35]. However, macrophages under steady state also have the repressive modifications such as H3K9me3, H3K27me3, and H4K20me3 at those loci, limiting effector gene expression in the absence of TLR ligands. Upon TLR activation, repressive histone methylations are removed by inducing histone demethylases such as JMJD3 [36, 37].

The alternative activation of macrophages occurs in the presence of type 2 cytokines, such as IL-4 and IL-13, driving them towards the M2 phenotype that plays an essential role in tissue repair and the resolution of inflammation [33]. In this conversion, the IL-4/Stat6 signaling induces the expression of the histone demethylase JMJD3 that binds to genes required for M2 differentiation [38]. JMJD3 removes the repressive H3K27me3 mark from the regulatory regions of M2-activating genes such as *Irf4* [39]. In contrast, HDAC3, which is a positive regulator of M1 polarization, has been shown to repress M2 programs [40].

3.3 Epigenetic regulation of trained and tolerized macrophages

Trained and tolerized states of macrophages have been recognized as the immunological "memory" of innate immunity. During those states, macrophages have a robust and specific response upon a secondary challenge. Macrophages derived from monocytes treated with β-glucan, called trained macrophages, show an enhanced inflammatory status. β-glucan challenge showed stable changes in H3K4me3 at promoters of proinflammatory cytokines such as *Tnf*, *Il6*, and *Il18*, while no changes were observed in H3K27me3 [41]. In addition, H3K4me1 mark persists at enhancers after a pathogen challenge, contributing to the faster and stronger induction of multiple genes upon restimulation of trained macrophages [42].

In contrast, monocytes-derived macrophages pretreated with LPS produced less proinflammatory mediators such as IL-6 and TNFα upon challenge with certain toll-like receptor agonist(s). At the same time, anti-inflammatory molecules such as IL-10 and TGF-β show an increased expression following a secondary challenge compared to non-tolerized macrophages. H3K4me3 was induced in macrophages at both proinflammatory and anti-inflammatory gene promoters. However, "tolerized" macrophages treated with LPS induce a rapid and selective loss of H3K4me3 at proinflammatory gene promoters maintaining the mark on anti-inflammatory gene promoters. In this context, H4 acetylation was found on both group of genes in naïve macrophages but was reacetylated only on promoters of proinflammatory genes in tolerized macrophages [43, 44].

Additionally, the transcription factor ATF7 controls genes involved on immune response such as *Tnf*, *Ccl3*, and *Cxcl2* in unstimulated macrophages by recruiting the lysine methylase G9a and promoting H3K9me2 on these promoters. LPS treatment in trained macrophages induces phosphorylation of ATF7 via p38, leading to ATF7 release from chromatin with the concomitant removal of G9a and a decrease of the repressive H3K9me2 mark on the promoter of target genes. This partially disrupted chromatin structure leads to enhanced resistance to pathogens in trained macrophages [45].

3.4 Epigenetic regulation of DC development

The permissive mark H3K4me3 is confined to promoters of progenitor genes in multipotent progenitors (MPP) and in common dendritic cell progenitors (CDP), while H3K4me1 is found in their enhancers. H3K27me3 was observed at promoters of progenitor genes in conventional DCs (cDC) and plasmacytoid DCs (pDC). Conversely, H3K4me3 and H3K4me1 in cDCs and pDC were observed at promoter and enhancer of DC-specific genes, while H3K27me3 was seen in progenitors [46, 47].

3.5 Epigenetics and DC function

Few studies have investigated the role of epigenetic modifications on DC function. Genome-wide DNA methylation analysis showed rapid and active demethylation at thousands of loci on DCs exposed to the pathogenic bacterium *Mycobacterium tuberculosis* (MBT) [48].

Our own studies have shown that under steady state conditions *Il6* and *tgfb1* promoters have a bivalent status on splenic DCs and that treatment of DCs with LPS induces H3K4me3, decreasing H3K27me3 on the *Il6* promoter, while it decreases H3K4me3 and increases H3K27me3 on the *tgfb1* promoter. Contrary, the use of GSK-J4, a specific inhibitor of the H3K27me3 histone demethylase JMJD3, reverses this bivalent status and promotes DCs with tolerogenic functions in LPS-treated DCs [49].

Patients who survive sepsis have significant deficiencies in their immune response. One study found that these deficiencies are explained at least in part because post-septic DCs exhibit a significant and chronic suppression of IL-12. Whereas normal

DCs showed a high H3K4me3 and low H3K27me2 at both *Il12p35* and *Il12p40* promoters, suggesting a permissive chromatin structure poised for expression on exposure to stimuli, post-septic DCs showed a significant decreased H3K4me3 and increased H3K27me2 levels. In addition, post-septic DCs fail to recruit histone methyltransferases to *Il12* promoter [50].

Several studies have shown that histone deacetylase inhibitors such as valproic acid and MS-275 inhibit *Cd40, Cd80*, and *Cd86* expression as well as proinflammatory cytokines such as *Il6*, *Il12*, and *Tnf*. All these studies suggest that histone acetylation is a key player in the modulation of DC function [51, 52].

3.6 Epigenetic regulation of B cell development and immunoglobulin gene recombination

The main function of these cells is the production of antibodies. They can also act as APC for T cells. Many epigenetic changes have been described during B cell development, differentiation, and effector function. PAX5 is an essential transcription factor in B-cell differentiation and maintenance as it induces B-cell-specific genes, while repressing genes of other lineages. The permissive marks H3K9ac, H3K4me2, and H3K4me3 are important to mediate PAX5 transactivation [53]. Epigenetic marks also regulate immunoglobulin gene recombination at several levels. For example, H3K4me2 on immunoglobulin genes is correlated with V(D)J recombination, whereas methylation on H3K9 and H3K27 is inversely correlated with the efficiency of V(D)J recombination [54, 55]. DNA methylation and histone acetylation inhibits and enhances the V(D)J recombination, respectively [56, 57]. Furthermore, hypermutation required to produce antibody diversity in V(D)J recombination is mediated by activation-induced cytidine deaminase (AID). DNA methylation as well as hypoacetylation on H3 suppresses *Aicda* gene expression (encoding AID) [58]. Upon activation of B cells, *Aicda* gene is DNA demethylated and the locus becomes enriched in H3K4me3 and H3K9ac/K14ac [58].

3.7 Epigenetic regulation of plasma cell and memory B cell

B cell differentiation into antibody-secreting plasma cells (PC) is initiated by external stimuli. PCs are derived from either germinal center (naïve B cell) or memory B cells. Blimp-1, a key transcription factor required for PC differentiation, inhibits *Bcl6*, *Pax5*, and *Spib* expression by binding to the promoters of these genes and recruiting HDAC to decrease histone acetylation [59] and G9a to induce H3K9me3 [60]. On the other hand, memory B cells quickly react to a second challenge with the same antigen, thereby providing humoral immune protection. Finally, the differentiation of naïve B cells to PC or memory B cells associates with changes in DNA methylation in an DNMT3a-dependent manner [61].

3.8 Epigenetic regulation of early T cell development

Initial commitment of hematopoietic precursors to the T-cell phenotype is triggered by Notch signaling. During this process, B-cell transcription factors *Pax5* and *Ebf1* are repressed by H3K27me3 marks. The myeloid regulatory gene, *Cebpa*, is kept silent by a bivalent status (H3K27me3 and H3K4me3), while the erythroid gene, *EpoR*, is repressed via H3K27me3 [62]. Activation of T-cell-associated genes is strongly and temporally correlated with histone acetylation, although DNA methylation also regulates early T-cell development. DNA demethylation has been observed in many essential T-cell regulators, including genes that encode TCR components such as CD3 molecules and key developmental genes such as *Runx3, Rorc, Ikaros, Rag,* and *Lck* [63].

3.9 Epigenetics on the regulation of terminal differentiation and effector functions of CD4+ and CD8+ T cells

The lineage choice between CD4 and CD8 T cells is defined by the transcription factors ThPOK and Runx. ThPOK activity is necessary and sufficient for CD4 lineage commitment, and its function is abrogated in the presence of the histone deacetylase HDAC1. Runx1 and Runx3 or their common obligatory dimerization partner, Cbfβ, is necessary for the development of CD8 T cells. ThPOK and Runx factors are mutual repressors [64]. After their terminal differentiation, CD4+ T cells exert their function as either helper T cell subsets (Th1, Th2, and Th17) or Treg cells. This section describes the epigenetic regulation of naïve T (Tn) cells to a specific differentiation program upon activation. Genome wide analysis of H3K4me3 (permissive mark) and H3K27me3 (repressive mark) in Tn, Th1, Th2, Th17, and Treg cells demonstrated the enrichment of H3K4me3 in genes that encode signature transcription factors and cytokine production for the corresponding cell subsets, while these genes are enriched in the repressive mark H3K27me3 in the other subsets (**Figure 3**). For example, the permissive mark H3K4me3 is found in the *Tbx21* (encoding Tbet) and *Ifng* loci in Th1 cells, in the *Gata3* and *Il4* loci in Th2 cells, in the *Rorc* (encoding RORγt) and *Il17* loci in Th17 cells, and *Foxp3* in Treg cells. However, these same loci show the repressive mark H3K27me3 in the opposing cell subsets, for example, the *Tbx21* locus in Th2. Most interesting, the master transcription factors for each T cell subset (*Tbx21, Gata3, Rorc*, and *Foxp3*) have a bivalent status (permissive H3K4me3 and repressive H3K27me3) in the opposing cell subsets (i.e., *Tbx21* loci in Treg cells), thus suggesting functional plasticity among Th subsets and Treg cells [65] (**Figure 3**).

Suv39H1, which mediates the repressive H3K9me3 mark, is a key to keep Th1 commitment since disruption of Suv39H1 results in an aberrant induction of IFNγ in Th2 cells after re-culture under Th1 polarizing conditions. However, the absence of Suv39H1 does not disturb Th2 cell differentiation [66]. The histone demethylase JMJD3 has a controversial role in CD4+ T-cell differentiation. One study showed that JMJD3 ablation promotes Th2 and Th17 differentiation, while decreases Th1 cells [67]. However, another study shows that JMJD3 induction is crucial to induce Th17 cells. The same study described that the epigenetic drug GSK-J4, a JMJD3 inhibitor, dramatically suppressed Th17 cell differentiation *in vitro* [68]. Nevertheless, our own studies reveled that GSK-J4 promotes Treg differentiation by DCs. Also, we showed that GSK-J4 treatment decreases the plasticity of Treg to become Th1 or Th17 cells *in vivo* [49]. This is in concordance with another report where the JMJD3 deficiency also restrains plasticity in the conversion of Th2, Th17, or Treg cells into Th1 cells [67].

The vast majority of Foxp3+ Treg cells are generated during thymic development (tTreg). A small portion of Treg cells can also be converted from conventional CD4+ T cells in the periphery. They are called inducible Treg cells (iTreg). This population has specificity towards nonpathogenic foreign antigens, including commensal microbiota, food, and fetal antigens. All Treg cell types (tTreg and iTreg) rely on a proper Foxp3 expression for the acquisition of the immunosuppressive phenotype as well as for the maintenance of their phenotype and function, particularly under inflammatory conditions. Mutations within the Foxp3 gene or deletion of Foxp3 result in the development of autoimmunity [69]. H3 and H4 acetylation as well as H3K4me2 and H3K4me3 are found at the *Foxp3* promoter in Treg cells but not in other CD4+ conventional T cell phenotypes. On the contrary, H3K27me3 (repressive mark) is found in conventional CD4+ T cells, but not in Treg cells [70]. In Treg cells, the polycomb repressor complex is replaced by p300/CREB-binding protein-associated factor (PCAF), a histone acetyltransferase recruited via the zinc-finger transcription factor Krüppel-like factor 10 (KLF10) to the *Foxp3* promoter, a process that finally results in the opening of the Foxp3 promoter by permissive histone modifications [71]. In addition, our own results showed that treatment with Trichostatin A (TSA), a histone deacetylase inhibitor, increases Treg population as well as H3 acetylation [72]. The data indicate that modulating histone acetylation on Treg might also be a key to improve Treg function and stability.

Foxp3 gene has three conserved noncoding sequences (CNS) that are the primary targets of epigenetic regulation and are necessary to modulate its expression depending on the environmental cues that T cells receive. CNS1, which is a TGF-β-sensitive enhancer element and critical for the generation of Treg cells, does not contain any CpG motifs and thus is solely regulated via histone modifications [70, 73]. Indeed, H3/H4 acetylation and H3K4me2/3 are enriched in both tTreg and iTreg cells compared to other conventional CD4+ T-cell phenotypes [70]. CNS2 is a Treg cell-specific demethylated region (TSDR). Demethylation of this CpG region, mediated by TET2, is mandatory for stable Foxp3 expression. Also, CNS2 contains H3K4 methylation as well as H3/H4 acetylation in Treg cells, suggesting that DNA demethylation and permissive histone modifications generate an open chromatin status at CNS2 that promotes stabilization of *Foxp3* expression [70, 74]. Conversely, DNA methylation

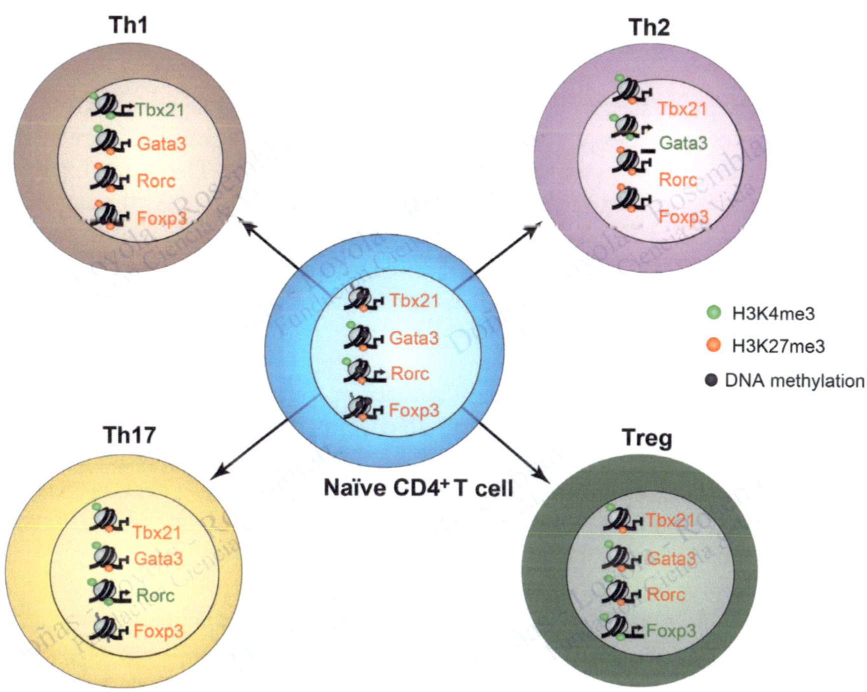

Figure 3.
Epigenetic status of "Master" transcriptional factor gene in CD4+ T cells. DNA methylation and bivalent marks (H3K27me3 repressive and H3K4me3 permissive) present on the promoter of the "master" transcription factors for Th1 (T-bet), Th2 (GATA3), Th17 (Rorγt), and Treg (Foxp3) inhibit their expression on naïve CD4+ T cells (nT cells). Upon TCR stimulation and depending on the cytokines present in the milieu, nT cells will adopt one of those phenotypes. During differentiation of nT cells to Th1, Tbx21 gene promoter (encoding T-bet) is hypomethylated, and repressive marks such as H3K27me3 removed while gaining permissive marks such as H3K4me3, thus allowing Tbx21 expression (in green) while the rest of "master" transcription factors associated to other T subsets are repressed (in red) through the acquisition of bivalent or repressive marks. The same process has been described on the promoters for the master transcription factors critical in the differentiation of the Th2, Th17, and Treg subsets, in which Gata3, Rorc, and Foxp3 are expressed, respectively. The transcription factor expressed on each phenotype is written in green, whereas transcription factors that are not expressed on that particular phenotype are written in red. It should be noted that the acquisition of bivalent marks and the absence of DNA methylation in master transcription factors associated to opposite T subsets are linked to the plasticity described on CD4+ T cells.

of CNS2 can prevent *Foxp3* expression in non-Treg cells [74]. Furthermore, Foxp3 expression cannot be maintained when Treg cells are exposed to inflammatory cytokines such as IL-4 and IL-6 upon deletion of CNS2 [75]. CNS3 has been called "pioneer element," since it plays a critical role for the initiation of Foxp3 expression in Treg cells, but is dispensable once Foxp3 is expressed. It is enriched in the permissive H3K4me1/2 marks, modifications that are increased in the Foxp3-thymocyte subsets, suggesting that CNS3 facilitates the opening of the Foxp3 locus in Treg cell precursors [70].

Epigenetic modifications also play important roles in the regulation of CD8+ T-cell effector functions. For example, H3K27me3 modification at the *Ifng* locus in naive CD8+ T cells is removed upon activation and differentiation to effector cells, whereas the permissive histone modifications H3K9ac and H3K4me3 are deposited in this locus. The *Ifng* locus has reduced levels of total histone H3 in activated CD8+ T cells, suggesting that the depletion of nucleosomes from the locus allows the transcriptional machinery to access the promoter [76]. The *Gzmb* locus, which encodes another CD8+ T-cell effector molecule, granzyme B, also shows similar epigenetic regulation during differentiation from naive to effector cells [77].

4. Epigenetic regulation of autoimmune diseases and the prospect of epigenetic drug as therapeutic agents

Autoimmune diseases are a complex group of diseases in which each one present with a unique epidemiology, pathology, symptoms, and origin. There are intrinsic and extrinsic components that predispose to autoimmunity. The following section describes some important epigenetic changes in systemic lupus erythematosus (SLE), rheumatoid arthritis (RA), multiple sclerosis (MS), and inflammatory bowel diseases (IBD), and how epigenetic drugs can modulate these changes.

4.1 Systemic lupus erythematosus (SLE)

It is a chronic inflammatory disease with a significant long-term morbidity that affects principally women, with an estimated population frequency in the United States of about 150 for white women to about 400 for African-American women per 100,000. SLE is a systemic multiorgan autoimmune disease characterized by an autoantibody response to nuclear and/or cytoplasmic antigens. Autoreactive T and B cells lead to a gradual loss of self-tolerance leading over time to high levels of autoantibodies.

A global DNA hypomethylation occurs on several promoter regions in CD4+ T cells derived from SLE patients, including genes related to immune response such as *Itgal*, *Cd40l*, *Cd70*, *Ifgnr2*, *Il-4*, and *Il-13*. These hypomethylated regions are correlated with an upregulation in the expression of those genes causing cell hyperactivity and, consequently, perpetuation of inflammatory responses. DNA is hypomethylated on interferon genes in B cells, monocytes, and neutrophils, leading to the upregulation of these genes and a predisposition to produce an increased interferon response, a factor that plays a key role in SLE pathogenesis [78]. Consistently, DNA methyltransferase inhibitors, such as procainamide and hydralazine, induce lupus-like disease in mice [79]. So far, the accumulative evidence show that changes on DNA methylation in immune cells are key during SLE development.

Modified histones, such as H3K4me3, H3K27me3, H4K8ac, H4K16ac, and H2BK12ac, are known to be relevant autoantigens in SLE. These autoantigens trigger NETosis, a phenomenon whereby neutrophils extrude their nuclear material (Neutrophils Extracellular Traps) to kill pathogens [80]. However, very little attention has been paid to histone modifications in SLE and in the induction or repression of gene expression. In SLE monocytes, H3K4me3 is enriched on type I interferon response genes, which is consistent with the type I interferon effect in lupus [81]. Nevertheless, the histone methyltransferase Ezh2 seems to be important in autoimmune responses of CD4+ T cells. Ezh2 is highly enriched on genes such as *Il-4, Il-10, Il-13, Cd70*, and *Tnf* [82]. Since Ezh2 mRNA levels are decreased in human lupus CD4+ T cells, this leads to an elevated expression of these genes [98]. Gene expression profile of CD4+ T cells generated from Ezh2-deficient mice shows a similar behavior to lupus CD4+ T cells [82]. These results suggest that Ezh2 and histone modifications have a relevant role in SLE.

4.2 Rheumatoid arthritis (RA)

RA is a disease characterized by the progressive destruction of joints by invasive synovial fibroblasts. RA synovial fibroblasts (RASFs) play a major role in this pathology. This disease is characterized by painful joint swelling, cartilage damage, bone erosion, severe joint deformation, disability, and premature mortality.

Global DNA hypomethylation is observed in RASF, T cells, B cells, and monocytes. In RA, Cxcl12 gene is hypomethylated in RASF cells, which allows for overexpression of Cxcl12 and thus promoting infiltration of inflammatory cells in the synovium [83]. The promoter of the transcription factor Tbx5 is also DNA hypomethylated, and its overexpression induces pro-inflammatory cytokines production [84]. In monocytes, DNA methyltransferase expression is reduced leading to a reduction of DNA methylation in inflammatory response promoter genes. For example, hypomethylation in the *Il6* promoter gene causes an overexpression of IL-6, furthering B cell response [85]. In CD4+ T cells, *Cd40l* promoter is DNA demethylated in female patients, leading to the overexpression of this gene and an increased immune response. On the other hand, Tregs responses fail to control the activity of T helper cells in RA. Foxp3 is the master transcription factor for the differentiation of Tregs, and DNA methylation controls its expression (see T cell section above). Methotrexate, a drug that inhibits S-adenosylmethionine (SAM) synthesis (the donor methyl group during methylation reaction), restores the suppressive function of Tregs by demethylating the Foxp3 promoter [86].

Destruction of cartilage on RA synovial tissue is characterized by an imbalance between HAT and HDAC activities (acetylation vs. deacetylation). For example, hyperacetylation on p16 and p21 gene promoters induce their expression with a subsequent decrease in TNFα synthesis leading to an improvement of RA symptoms in a murine RA model [87]. Many studies have described the beneficial effects of HDAC inhibitors *in vitro* and in an *in vivo* mouse model of arthritis. HDAC inhibitors such as Givinostat [NCT00570661] have already started to be used in clinical trials, revealing benefits in patients with systemic-onset juvenile idiopathic arthritis after 12 weeks of treatment. On the other hand, HDAC class III enzymes showed a contradictory function in RA. For example, the levels of the NAD-dependent protein deacetylase SIRT6 are increased in the joint tissues of collagen-induced arthritis (CIA) in mice, and further studies revealed that SIRT6 overexpression attenuates the severity of arthritis by reducing both the inflammatory response and tissue destruction, whereas SIRT1 levels were increased and its overexpression contributed inflammatory cytokine production [88, 89]. Finally, Pan-inhibitors against the BET protein family (acetylation readers) have anti-inflammatory and anti-destructive properties *in vitro* [90] and in CIA mice [91, 92]. The effects of BET inhibitors in CIA are attributed to the suppression of Th17 cell differentiation and function, suggesting that BET inhibitors are potential targets for RA treatment [91].

4.3 Multiple sclerosis (MS)

MS is an autoimmune disease of the central nervous system (CNS) characterized by the abnormal entry of inflammatory cells into the CNS followed by chronic inflammation, myelin destruction, and axonal loss. MS affects more than 2 million people worldwide and has an incidence rate of approximately 5–6 per 100,000 population per year in the United States and 83 per 100,000 in Europe. MS is caused by an autoimmune response against myelin proteins in neurons.

CD44 is an interesting protein in the MS pathophysiology because the signaling induced by its activation modifies DNA methylation patterns in key immune response genes that have been associated to MS in T cells. CD44-ligand interaction leads to hypomethylation of the IFNγ and Il-17 genes and promotes differentiation towards Th1 and Th17 cells [93]. CD44 deficiency decreases Th1 and Th17 differentiation and promotes Th2 differentiation via hypomethylation of the Il-4 promoter. This may explain why CD44-deficient mice are protected against experimental autoimmune encephalomyelitis (EAE) (a mouse model of MS) [94]. Similar effect has been showed in CD4+ T cells from MS patients, where Th17 differentiation and IL-17 expression are increased following DNA hypomethylation of Il-17α gene promoter [95]. On the other hand, the Foxp3 promoter is DNA hypermethylated in CD4+ T cells of relapsing-remitting MS patients leading to a reduction of the Treg population and their control of immune response [96]. Decitabine (5-aza-2′-deoxicytidine), which is a DNMT inhibitor, induces Foxp3 expression in mice exposed to experimental autoimmune encephalomyelitis (EAE, a MS murine model) by demethylating CpG islands in the gene encoding Foxp3. As a result, this drug decreases spinal infiltration and ameliorates disease progression [97]. A cross-talk has been described between DNA methylation and histone acetylation. For example, MeCP2, a reader of methylated DNA, suppresses the brain neurotrophic factor expression, which is necessary for myelin repair, whereas histone acetyltransferase expression and HDAC inhibitors reduce MeCP2 expression and thus favor remyelination [97].

The oligodendrocytes are a key to maintain the central nervous system by providing support and insulation to axons. Stem cell commitment to oligodendrocyte is modulated by histone acetylation levels since deacetylation promotes oligodendrocyte differentiation, while acetylation is associated with inhibition of differentiation. For example, HDAC1 and HDAC2 are needed for oligodendrocyte differentiation, while an increase in H3 acetylation is associated with high levels of oligodendrocyte-differentiation inhibitors such as TCF7 and SOX2 [98]. In PBMCs, high H3K9ac levels correlate with a decrease in the expression of SIRT1, a class III deacetylase (HDAC) during MS relapse when compared to stable MS patients and controls [99]. Therefore, SIRT1 expression has been proposed as an activity marker as well as therapeutic target in MS. Resveratrol, a SIRT1 activator, has shown promising results when tested in EAE mice, preventing neuronal loss during optic neuritis, providing neuroprotection, and a demonstrated secondary benefit in clinical dysfunction [100]. These results have also been shown using other SIRT1 activators. However, these treatments did not prevent inflammatory cell infiltration in these tissues.

Histone acetylation also plays a direct role on immune response. For example, IL-17 expression is regulated by the T cell transcription factor TCF1 through the acetylation of histones. Hyperacetylation on IL-17 promoter was found in TCF1 knockout mice and correlated with more susceptibility to EAE induction [101]. Modification of histone acetylation has emerged as therapeutic treatment for MS. In this context, HDAC inhibitors have potential therapeutic value in MS because of their anti-inflammatory and neuroprotective effects both *in vitro* and *in vivo*. For example, sodium phenylacetate (SPA) suppresses neurological damage in mice pretreated with myelin basic protein (MBP)–primed T-cells [102]. Valproic acid reduces the duration and severity of EAE by regulating inflammation through a decrease of macrophage and lymphocyte infiltration into the spinal cord and of proinflammatory cytokines such as IFNγ, TNFα, and IL-17 [103]. Several a histone deacetylase inhibitors have been used in the EAE mouse model as potential drugs for human treatment. Trichostatin A (TSA) treatment after myelin oligodendrocyte glycoprotein (MOG) immunization reduces inflammation, cell infiltration, demyelination, and neuronal loss in the spinal cord and ameliorates the disability of EAE relapse [104]. Likewise, Largazole, another powerful class I histone deacetylase (HDAC) inhibitor, decreases IL-17 and IFNγ production, reduces CNS inflammatory infiltrates, and produces a clinical effect on the incidence, severity, and disability scores in MS murine model [105]. Vorinostat prevents human CD14 monocyte-derived dendritic cell differentiation and reduces Th1 and Th17-mediated inflammation and demyelination in the CNS of EAE mice [106]. Curcumin reduces cytokine synthesis such as IL-17, TGFβ, IL-6, and IL-21 and transcription factors STAT3 and RORγt as well as reduces inflammatory cell infiltration into the spinal cord, thus leading to reduction in clinical severity in EAE mice and MBP-reactive lymphocyte proliferation in a dose-dependent manner [107, 108]. Studies using inhibitors of histone demethylase in EAE model are less extended. However, GSK-J4, a JMJD3 inhibitor, improves EAE disease by the generation of tolerogenic DCs and enhancing Treg function leading to a decrease in CNS inflammatory infiltrates [49]. Histone modifying drugs are promising MS therapies based on their properties to modulate overactive immune system and neuroprotective pathways to prevent CNS damage.

4.4 Inflammatory bowel diseases (IBD)

IBD is the term used to describe disorders that involve chronic inflammation of the digestive tract. Crohn's disease and ulcerative colitis are the main subtypes of IBD. Crohn's disease represents a discontinuous, transmural inflammation that can occur anywhere in the gastrointestinal tract, whereas ulcerative colitis is a continuous inflammation of the mucosal layer of the colon. In addition to the gastrointestinal tract inflammation, so-called extraintestinal symptoms are common, affecting the joints, eyes, skin, and liver.

Active inflamed tissue from ulcerative colitis patients is characterized by global DNA hypomethylation compared to patients with inactive ulcerative colitis or to healthy individuals [109]. The higher turnover of colonic epithelial cells leads to an increase in DNA methylation in tumor-suppressor genes and a decrease on pro-tumorigenic elements which could lead to genome instability and cancer development [110]. A comparison between colonic mucosa from ulcerative colitis patients with dysplasia and/or carcinoma and quiescent mucosa from the same patients showed differential DNA methylation on several genes. For example, the gene encoding cell adhesion molecule E-cadherin (CDH1) is hypermethylated in dysplasia and/or carcinoma samples, a modification that leads to the downregulation of CDH1 expression [111]. In addition, the protein levels of DNA methyltransferases DNMT1 and DNMT3b are increased in inflamed mucosa from ulcerative colitis patients compared with noninflamed paired samples [112].

There are fewer studies regarding histone methylation and acetylation in IBD. Histone acetylations such as H4K8ac and H4K12ac were found in inflamed mucosa compared with non-inflamed mucosa from mice treated with sodium dextran sulfate (DSS) and 2,4-trinitrobenzene sulfonic acid (TNBS). Identical acetylation pattern is observed in biopsies from patients with Crohn's disease [113]. The administration of HDAC inhibitors in DSS and TNBS-induced experimental colitis reduces the expression of proinflammatory cytokines and, consequently, disease severity [114]. Furthermore, HDAC9 inhibition prevents colitis in mice as a consequence of an increase in both, Treg frequency and its suppressive function [115]. An interesting perspective when talking about IBD is the effect of the gut microbiota. Bacterial metabolites, such as short-chain fatty acids (SCFAs), possess HDAC inhibitory activity [116]. Many bacteria from the Firmicutes and Bacteroides produce SCFAs, such as acetate, propionate, and butyrate, at high concentration, and IBD patients have reported to have a reduced number of those SCFA-producing bacteria [117]. In the same line, ulcerative colitis patients treated with microbiota therapy with *Roseburia*, a bacterium known to produce butyrate, an HDAC inhibitor, showed a positive effect in patient recovery by reducing inflammatory cytokines production [118]. The potential mechanism is through the generation of Tregs from naïve CD4+ T cells. Butyrate increases H3 acetylation on *Foxp3* loci, the master transcription factor required for Treg cell differentiation [116]. In addition, butyrate might modulate the function of intestinal macrophages since macrophages treated with butyrate downregulated LPS induced IL-12 and IL-6 cytokine expressions [119]. Thus, the commensal microbiota may play a beneficial role in IBD treatment via epigenetic regulation of gene expression.

5. Conclusions

During the recent years, several studies have focused on a better understanding of epigenetic processes as well as its connection with biological processes such as immune response and inflammation (**Figure 4**). Currently, many epigenetic studies are being carried out in cells of the immune system related to the inflammasome such as DCs, macrophages, and lymphocytes. Most of those studies are related to the epigenetic mechanisms associated to the development, differentiation, and function of these cells, leading to a better knowledge about how epigenetics of the immune system relates to its function in pathogenesis. However, further studies on the epigenetics of immune cells and/or the associated biological processes are much needed as a means for improving our understanding of the role of epigenetics in inflammation.

The interactions between genetic and epigenetic factors significantly contribute to inflammation and autoimmune diseases. Epigenetic research has grown and is providing new insights into inflammatory autoimmune diseases, insight that will allow us to explain the etiology of these diseases. Furthermore, studies on epigenetic changes could lead us to understand disease progression and to identify future markers for therapy. Although further studies are needed to address the potential of epigenetic factors to act as biomarkers and drug targets, epigenetic enzymes are the current target of drug development and new therapeutic trials.

Epigenetic analyses, including DNA methylation and histone modifications, require a large number of cells making these studies difficult. Recent advances in technologies such as in single-cell analysis provide a new solution to this problem. Nevertheless, an important issue to be addressed is the limited information obtained so far for several cell subsets, specifically those with small representation within the immune system. As conclusion, although some important advances have been achieved in our understanding on the epigenetics of immune cells, inflammation, and autoimmune diseases, new technologies are required to improve our knowledge on these processes.

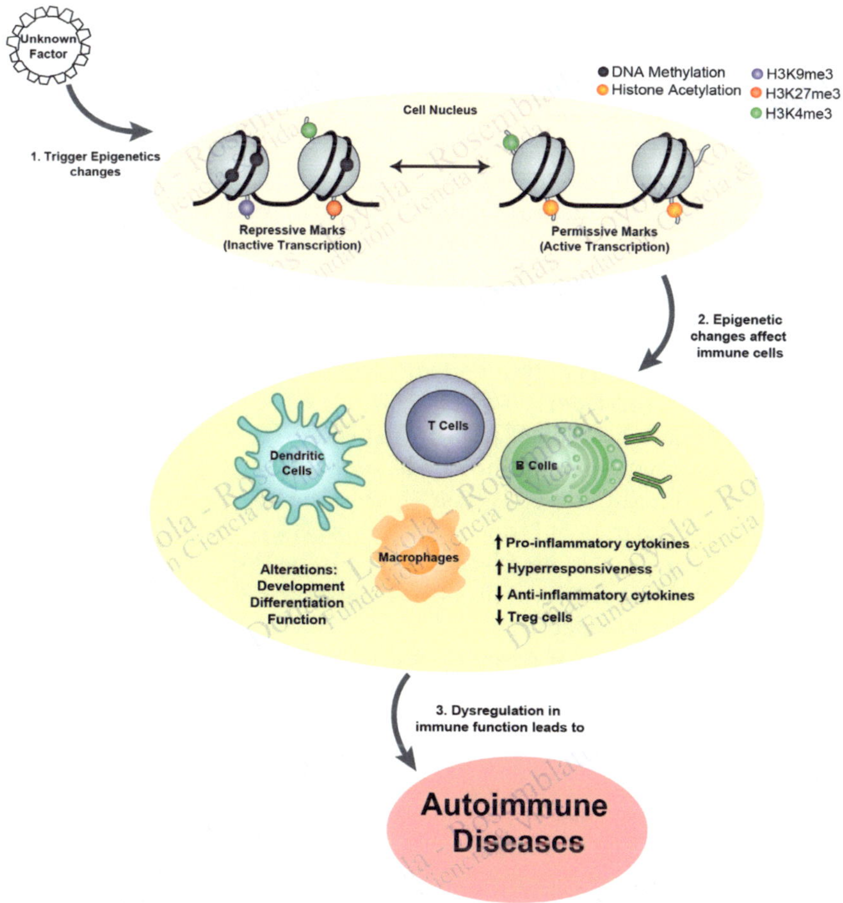

Figure 4.
Epigenetics influences on the development of autoimmune diseases. Epigenetic changes on the promoter of several genes are triggered by yet unknown factors, inducing transcriptional activation or repression. These changes bring up alterations in development, differentiation, and effector function of immune cells. All these changes result in aberrant immune responses, including increased production of proinflammatory cells and cytokines or the reduction of anti-inflammatory cells and cytokines that lead to increased inflammation and autoimmune diseases.

Acknowledgements

Financed by Programa de Apoyo a Centros con Financiamiento Basal AFB 170004, Fundación Ciencia para la Vida and Fondecyt 1160480.

Glossary

AID	activation-induced cytidine deaminase
APC	antigen-presenting cells
ATF	activating transcription factor
BET	bromodomain and extra-terminal motif proteins
Bcl6	B-cell lymphoma 6 protein
Blimp1	B lymphocyte-induced maturation protein-1
cDC	conventional DCs
CDP	common dendritic cell progenitors
CIA	collagen-induced-arthritis

CNS	conserved non-coding sequences
Cxcl12	C-X-C motif chemokine 12
C/EBP	CCAAT enhancer-binding protein
DCs	dendritic cells
DNTMs	DNA methyltransferases
DSS	dextran sulfate sodium
EAE	experimental autoimmune encephalomyelitis
Ezh2	enhancer of zeste homolog 2
Foxp3	forkhead box P3
GATA3	GATA-binding protein 3
Gzmb	granzyme B
H2BK12ac	acetylation of lysine 12 on histone H2B
H3ac	H3 acetylated
H3K4me3	trimethylation of lysine 4 on histone H3
H3K9ac	acetylation of lysine 9 on histone H3
H3K9me3	trimethylation of lysine 9 on histone H3
H3K14ac	acetylation of lysine 14 on histone H3
H3K27me3	trimethylation of lysine 27 on histone H3
H3K36me3	trimethylation of lysine 36 on histone H3
H4ac	H4 acetylated
H4K8ac	acetylation of lysine 18 on histone H4
H4K16ac	acetylation of lysine 16 on histone H4
H4R3	arginine 3 of histone H4
HAT	histone acetyltransferases
HDAC	histone deacetylases
HSCs	hematopoietic stem cells
IBD	inflammatory bowel diseases
Ifgnr	interferon receptor
IRF	interferon regulatory factor
iTreg	inducible Treg cells
JmjC	Jumonji C
KAT	lysine acetyltransferases
KDM	histone lysine demethylase
KLF10	Krüppel-like factor 10
KMT	lysine methyltransferases
MBP	myelin basic protein
MBPs	methyl-CpG-binding proteins
MBT	*Mycobacterium tuberculosis*
MPP	multipotent progenitors
MS	multiple sclerosis
Pax5	paired box gene 5
PC	plasma cells
PCAF	p300/CREB-binding protein-associated factor
pDC	plasmacytoid DCs
PHD	plant homeodomain
PRTM	protein arginine methyltransferase
RA	rheumatoid arthritis
RAG	recombination-activating gene
RASFs	RA synovial fibroblasts
RNAPII	RNA polymerase II
Rorγt	RAR-related orphan receptor gamma t
Runx1	runt-related transcription factor 1
Runx3	runt-related transcription factor 3

SAM	S-adenosylmethionine
SCFAs	short-chain fatty acids
SIRT	sirtuin
SLE	systemic lupus erythematosus
SPA	sodium phenylacetate
Sox	Sry-related HMG box
Tbet	T-box transcription factor
TCF7	transcription factor tau 7
TET	ten-eleven translocation
TGF-β	transforming growth factor beta
Th	T helper
ThPOK	Th-inducing POZ-Kruppel factor
TNBS	2,4-trinitrobenzene sulfonic acid
TSA	trichostatin A
TSDR	Treg cell-specific demethylated region
Treg	regulatory T cell
tTreg	thymic development

Author details

Cristian Doñas[1,2], Alejandra Loyola[2] and Mario Rosemblatt[2,3,4*]

1 Department of Medicine, Karolinska Institute, Sweden

2 Fundacion Ciencia and Vida, Santiago, Chile

3 Faculty of Life Sciences, Andres Bello University, Santiago, Chile

4 Faculty of Sciences, Department of Biology, University of Chile, Santiago, Chile

*Address all correspondence to: mrosemblatt@cienciavida.org

References

[1] Waddington CH. The epigenotype. Endeavour. 1942;**1**:18-20

[2] Liu L, Li Y, Tollefsbol TO. Gene-environment interactions and epigenetic basis of human diseases. Current Issues in Molecular Biology. 2008;**10**:25-36

[3] Skvortsova K, Iovino N, Bogdanović O. Functions and mechanisms of epigenetic inheritance in animals. Nature Reviews. Molecular Cell Biology. 2018;**19**:774-790

[4] Greally JM. A user's guide to the ambiguous word 'epigenetics'. Nature Reviews. Molecular Cell Biology. 2018;**19**:207-208

[5] Luger K, Mader AW, Richmond RK, Sargent DF, Richmond TJ. Crystal structure of the nucleosome core particle at 2.8 A resolution. Nature. 1997;**389**:251-260

[6] Chen T, Li E. Establishment and maintenance of DNA methylation patterns in mammals. Current Topics in Microbiology and Immunology. 2006;**301**:179-201

[7] Moore LD, Le T, Fan G. DNA methylation and its basic function. Neuropsychopharmacology. 2012;**38**:23

[8] Ito S, Shen L, Dai Q, Wu SC, Collins LB, Swenberg JA, et al. Tet proteins can convert 5-methylcytosine to 5-formylcytosine and 5-carboxylcytosine. Science. 2011;**333**:1300-1303

[9] Kouzarides T. Chromatin modifications and their function. Cell. 2007;**128**:693-705

[10] Shahbazian MD, Grunstein M. Functions of site-specific histone acetylation and deacetylation. Annual Review of Biochemistry. 2007;**76**:75-100

[11] Dhalluin C, Carlson JE, Zeng L, He C, Aggarwal AK, Zhou MM. Structure and ligand of a histone acetyl-transferase bromodomain. Nature. 1999;**399**(6735):491-496

[12] Zeng L, Zhang Q, Li S, Plotnikov AN, Walsh MJ, Zhou MM. Mechanism and regulation of acetylated histone binding by the tandem PHD finger of DPF3b. Nature. 2010;**466**(7303):258-262

[13] Wang Z, Zang C, Cui K, Schones DE, Barski A, Peng W, et al. Genome-wide mapping of HATs and HDACs reveals distinct functions in active and inactive genes. Cell. 2009;**138**(5):1019-1031

[14] Sauve AA, Youn DY. Sirtuins: NAD(+)-dependent deacetylase mechanism and regulation. Current Opinion in Chemical Biology. 2012;**16**(5-6):535-543

[15] Santos-Rosa H, Schneider R, Bannister AJ, Sherriff J, Bernstein BE, Emre NC, et al. Active genes are tri-methylated at K4 of histone H3. Nature. 2002;**419**:407-411

[16] Kizer KO, Phatnani HP, Shibata Y, Hall H, Greenleaf AL, Strahl BD. A novel domain in Set2 mediates RNA polymerase II interaction and couples histone H3 K36 methylation with transcript elongation. Molecular and Cellular Biology. 2005;**25**:3305-3316

[17] Schubeler D, MacAlpine DM, Scalzo D, Wirbelauer C, Kooperberg C, van Leeuwen F, et al. The histone modification pattern of active genes revealed through genome-wide chromatin analysis of a higher eukaryote. Genes & Development. 2004;**18**:1263-1271

[18] Vermeulen M, Eberl HC, Matarese F, Marks H, Denissov S, Butter F, et al. Quantitative interaction proteomics and genome-wide profiling of epigenetic histone marks and their readers. Cell. 2010;**142**:967-980

[19] Huang S, Litt M, Felsenfeld G. Methylation of histone H4 by arginine methyltransferase PRMT1 is essential *in vivo* for many subsequent histone modifications. Genes & Development. 2005;**19**(16):1885-1893

[20] Zhao Q, Rank G, Tan YT, Li H, Moritz RL, Simpson RJ, et al. PRMT5-mediated methylation of histone H4R3 recruits DNMT3A, coupling histone and DNA methylation in gene silencing. Nature Structural & Molecular Biology. 2009;**16**(3):304-311

[21] Zhao XD, Han X, Chew JL, Liu J, Chiu KP, Choo A, et al. Whole-genome mapping of histone H3 Lys4 and 27 trimethylations reveals distinct genomic compartments in human embryonic stem cells. Cell Stem Cell. 2007;**1**:286-298

[22] Allis CD, Berger SL, Cote J, Dent S, Jenuwien T, Kouzarides T, et al. New nomenclature for chromatin-modifying enzymes. Cell. 2007;**131**(4):633-636

[23] Shinkai Y, Tachibana M. H3K9 methyltransferase G9a and the related molecule GLP. Genes & Development. 2011;**25**(8):781-788

[24] Kuzmichev A, Jenuwein T, Tempst P, Reinberg D. Different EZH2-containing complexes target methylation of histone h1 or nucleosomal histone H3. Molecular Cell. 2004;**14**(2):183-193

[25] Musselman CA, Lalonde M-E, Cote J, Kutateladze TG. Perceiving the epigenetic landscape through histone readers. Nature Structural & Molecular Biology. 2012;**19**(12):1218-1227

[26] Black JC, Van Rechem C, Whetstine JR. Histone lysine methylation dynamics: establishment, regulation, and biological impact. Molecular Cell. 2012;**48**(4):491-507

[27] Molina-Serrano D, Schiza V, Kirmizis A. Cross-talk among epigenetic modifications: lessons from histone arginine methylation. Biochemical Society Transactions. 2013;**41**(3):751-759

[28] Yang Y, Lu Y, Espejo A, Wu J, Xu W, Liang S, et al. TDRD3 is an effector molecule for arginine-methylated histone marks. Molecular Cell. 2010;**40**(6):1016-1023

[29] Li S, Ali S, Duan X, Liu S, Du J, Liu C, et al. JMJD1B demethylates H4R3me2s and H3K9me2 to facilitate gene expression for development of hematopoietic stem and progenitor cells. Cell Reports. 2018;**23**:389-403

[30] Ooi SK, Qiu C, Bernstein E, Li K, Jia D, Yang Z, et al. DNMT3L connects unmethylated lysine 4 of histone H3 to de novo methylation of DNA. Nature. 2007;**448**(7154):714-717

[31] Sun D, Luo M, Jeong M, Rodriguez B, Xia Z, Hannah R, et al. Epigenomic profiling of young and aged HSCs reveals concerted changes during aging that reinforce self-renewal. Cell Stem Cell. 2014;**14**(5):673-688

[32] de la Rica L, Rodriguez-Ubreva J, Garcia M, Islam AB, Urquiza JM, Hernando H, et al. PU.1 target genes undergo Tet2-coupled demethylation and DNMT3b-mediated methylation in monocyte-to-osteoclast differentiation. Genome Biology. 2013;**14**(9):R99

[33] Biswas SK, Mantovani A. Macrophage plasticity and interaction with lymphocyte subsets: cancer as a paradigm. Nature Immunology. 2010;**11**(10):889-896

[34] Escoubet-Lozach L, Benner C, Kaikkonen MU, Lozach J, Heinz S, Spann NJ, et al. Mechanisms establishing TLR4-responsive activation states of inflammatory response genes. PLoS Genetics. 2011;7(12):e1002401

[35] Gough DJ, Messina NL, Clarke CJ, Johnstone RW, Levy DE. Constitutive

type I interferon modulates homeostatic balance through tonic signaling. Immunity. 2012;**36**(2):166-174

[36] De Santa F, Narang V, Yap ZH, Tusi BK, Burgold T, Austenaa L, et al. Jmjd3 contributes to the control of gene expression in LPS-activated macrophages. The EMBO Journal. 2009;**28**(21):3341-3352

[37] Stender JD, Pascual G, Liu W, Kaikkonen MU, Do K, Spann NJ, et al. Control of proinflammatory gene programs by regulated trimethylation and demethylation of histone H4K20. Molecular Cell. 2012;**48**(1):28-38

[38] Satoh T, Takeuchi O, Vandenbon A, Yasuda K, Tanaka Y, Kumagai Y, et al. The Jmjd3-Irf4 axis regulates M2 macrophage polarization and host responses against helminth infection. Nature Immunology. 2010;**11**(10):936-944

[39] Ishii M, Wen H, Corsa CA, Liu T, Coelho AL, Allen RM, et al. Epigenetic regulation of the alternatively activated macrophage phenotype. Blood. 2009;**114**(15):3244-3254

[40] Mullican SE, Gaddis CA, Alenghat T, Nair MG, Giacomin PR, Everett LJ, et al. Histone deacetylase 3 is an epigenomic brake in macrophage alternative activation. Genes & Development. 2011;**25**(23):2480-2488

[41] Quintin J, Saeed S, Martens JH, Giamarellos-Bourboulis EJ, Ifrim DC, Logie C, et al. Candida albicansinfection affords protection against reinfection via functional reprogramming of monocytes. Cell Host & Microbe. 2012;**12**(2):223-232

[42] Ostuni R, Piccolo V, Barozzi I, Polletti S, Termanini A, Bonifacio S, et al. Latent enhancers activated by stimulation in differentiated cells. Cell. 2013;**152**(1-2):157-171

[43] Foster SL, Hargreaves DC, Medzhitov R. Gene-specific control of inflammation by TLR-induced chromatin modifica-tions. Nature. 2007;**447**(7147):972-978

[44] Mages J, Dietrich H, Lang R. A genome-wide analysis of LPS tolerance in macrophages. Immunobiology. 2007;**212**(9-10):723-737

[45] Yoshida K, Maekawa T, Zhu Y, Renard-Guillet C, Chatton B, Inoue K, et al. The transcription factor ATF7 mediates lipopolysaccharide-induced epigenetic changes in macrophages involved in innate immunological memory. Nature Immunology. 2015;**16**(10):1034-1043

[46] Paul F, Arkin Y, Giladi A, et al. Transcriptional heterogeneity and lineage commitment in myeloid progenitors. Cell. 2015;**163**:1663-1677

[47] Lin Q, Chauvistré H, Costa IG, et al. Epigenetic programand transcription factor circuitry of dendritic cell development. Nucleic Acids Research. 2015;**43**:9680-9693

[48] Pacis A, Tailleux L, Morin AM, Lambourne J, MacIsaac JL, Yotova V, et al. Bacterial infection remodels the DNA methylation landscape of human dendritic cells. Genome Research. 2015;**25**:1801-1811. DOI: 10.1101/gr.192005.115

[49] Donas C, Carrasco M, Fritz M, Prado C, Tejon G, Osorio-Barrios F, et al. The histone demethylase inhibitor GSK-J4 limits inflammation through the induction of a tolerogenic phenotype on DCs. Journal of Autoimmunity. 2016;**75**:105-117. DOI: 10.1016/j.jaut.2016.07.011

[50] Wen H, Dou Y, Hogaboam CM, Kunkel SL. Epigenetic regulation of dendritic cell-derived interleukin-12 facilitates immunosuppression after a

severe innate immune response. Blood. 2008;**111**(4):1797-1804

[51] Misaki K, Morinobu A, Saegusa J, Kasagi S, Fujita M, Miyamoto Y, et al. Histone deacetylase inhibition alters dendritic cells to assume a tolerogenic phenotype and ameliorates arthritis in SKG mice. Arthritis Research & Therapy. 2011;**13**:R77

[52] Frikeche J, Simon T, Brissot E, Grégoire M, Gaugler B, Mohty M. Impact of valproic acid on dendritic cells function. Immunobiology. 2012b;**217**:704-710. DOI: 10.1016/j.imbio.2011.11.010

[53] McManus S, Ebert A, Salvagiotto G, Medvedovic J, Sun Q, Tamir I, et al. The transcription factor Pax5 regulates its target genes by recruiting chromatin-modifying proteins in committed B cells. The EMBO Journal. 2011;**30**(12):2388-2404

[54] Morshead KB, Ciccone DN, Taverna SD, Allis CD, Oettinger MA. Antigen receptor loci poised for V(D)J rearrangement are broadly associated with BRG1 and flanked by peaks of histone H3 dimethylated at lysine 4. Proceedings of the National Academy of Sciences of the United States of America. 2003;**100**:11577-11582

[55] Johnson K, Pflugh DL, Yu D, Hesslein DG, Lin KI, Bothwell AL, et al. B cell-specific loss of histone 3 lysine 9 methylation in the V(H) locus depends on Pax5. Nature Immunology. 2004;**5**:853-861

[56] Selimyan R, Gerstein RM, Ivanova I, Precht P, Subrahmanyam R, Perlot T, et al. Localized DNA demethylation at recombination intermediates during immunoglobulin heavy chain gene assembly. PLoS Biology. 2013;**11**(1):e1001475

[57] McBlane F, Boyes J. Stimulation of V(D)J recombination by histone acetylation. Current Biology. 2000;**10**:483-486

[58] Crouch EE, Li Z, Takizawa M, Fichtner-Feigl S, Gourzi P, Montano C, et al. Regulation of AID expression in the immune response. The Journal of Experimental Medicine. 2007;**204**:1145-1156

[59] Yu J, Angelin-Duclos C, Greenwood J, Liao J, Calame K. Transcriptional repression by blimp-1 (PRDI-BF1) involves recruitment of histone deacetylase. Molecular and Cellular Biology. 2000;**20**:2592-2603

[60] Gyory I, Wu J, Fejer G, Seto E, Wright KL. PRDI-BF1 recruits the histone H3 methyltransferase G9a in transcriptional silencing. Nature Immunology. 2004;**5**:299-308

[61] Luckey CJ, Bhattacharya D, Goldrath AW, Weissman IL, Benoist C, Mathis D. Memory T and memory B cells share a transcriptional program of self renewal with long-term hematopoietic stem cells. Proceedings of the National Academy of Sciences of the United States of America. 2006;**103**:3304-3309

[62] Zhang JA, Mortazavi A, Williams BA, Wold BJ, Rothenberg EV. Dynamic transformations of genome-wide epigenetic marking and transcriptional control establish T cell identity. Cell. 2012;**149**(2):467-482

[63] Rodriguez RM, Lopez-Larrea C, Suarez-Alvarez B. Epigenetic dynamics during CD4(+) T cells lineage commitment. The International Journal of Biochemistry & Cell Biology. 2015;**67**:75-85

[64] He X, He X, Dave VP, Zhang Y, Hua X, Nicolas E, et al. The zinc finger transcription factor Th-POK regulates CD4 versus CD8 T-cell lineage commitment. Nature. 2005;**433**(7028):826-833

[65] Wei G, Wei L, Zhu J, Zang C, Hu-Li J, Yao Z, et al. Global mapping of H3K4me3 and H3K27me3 reveals specificity and plasticity in lineage fate determination of differentiating CD4+ T cells. Immunity. 2009;**30**(1):155-167

[66] Allan RS, Zueva E, Cammas F, Schreiber HA, Masson V, Belz GT, et al. An epigenetic silencing pathway controlling T helper 2 cell lineage commitment. Nature. 2012;**487**(7406):249-253

[67] Li Q, Zou J, Wang M, Ding X, Chepelev I, Zhou X, et al. Critical role of histone demethylase Jmjd3 in the regulation of CD4+ T-cell differentiation. Nature Communications. 2014;**5**:5780. DOI: 10.1038/ncomms6780

[68] Liu Z, Cao W, Xu L, Chen X, Zhan Y, Yang Q, et al. The histone H3 lysine-27 demethylase Jmjd3 plays a critical role in specific regulation of Th17 cell differentiation. Journal of Molecular Cell Biology. 2015;7:505-516. DOI: 10.1093/jmcb/mjv022

[69] Hori S, Nomura T, Sakaguchi S. Control of regulatory T cell development by the transcription factor Foxp3. Science. 2003;**299**:1057-1061

[70] Floess S, Freyer J, Siewert C, Baron U, Olek S, Polansky J, et al. Epigenetic control of the foxp3 locus in regulatory T cells. PLoS Biology. 2007;**5**:e38

[71] Xiong Y, Khanna S, Grzenda AL, Sarmento OF, Svingen PA, Lomberk GA, et al. Polycomb antagonizes p300/CREB-binding protein-associated factor to silence FOXP3 in a Kruppel-like factor-dependent manner. The Journal of Biological Chemistry. 2012;**287**:34372-34385

[72] Donas C, Fritz M, Manriquez V, Tejon G, Bono MR, Loyola A, et al. Trichostatin A promotes the generation and suppressive functions of regulatory T cells. Clinical & Developmental Immunology. 2013;**2013**:679804. DOI: 10.1155/2013/679804

[73] Zheng Y, Josefowicz S, Chaudhry A, Peng XP, Forbush K, Rudensky AY. Role of conserved non-coding DNA elements in the Foxp3 gene in regulatory T-cell fate. Nature. 2010;**463**:808-812

[74] Feng Y, Arvey A, Chinen T, van der Veeken J, Gasteiger G, Rudensky AY. Control of the inheritance of regulatory T cell identity by a cis element in the Foxp3 locus. Cell. 2014;**158**:749-763

[75] Li X, Liang Y, LeBlanc M, Benner C, Zheng Y. Function of a Foxp3 cis-element in protecting regulatory T cell identity. Cell. 2014;**158**:734-748

[76] Denton AE, Russ BE, Doherty PC, Rao S, Turner SJ. Differentiation-dependent functional and epigenetic landscapes for cytokine genes in virus-specific CD8+ T cells. Proceedings of the National Academy of Sciences of the United States of America. 2011;**108**(37):15306-15311

[77] Juelich T, Sutcliffe EL, Denton A, He Y, Doherty PC, Parish CR, et al. Interplay between chromatin remodeling and epigenetic changes during lineage-specific commitment to granzyme B expression. Journal of Immunology. 2009;**183**(11):7063-7072

[78] Javierre BM, Fernandez AF, Richter J, et al. Changes in the pattern of DNA methylation associate with twin discordance in systemic lupus erythematosus. Genome Research. 2010;**20**(2):170-179

[79] Hong KM, Kim HK, Park SY, et al. CD3z hypermethylation is associated with severe clinical manifestations in systemic lupus erythematosus and reduces CD3ζ-chain ex-pression in T cells. Rheumatology (Oxford). 2017;**56**:467-476

[80] Saha S, Tieng A, Pepeljugoski KP, Zandamn-Goddard G, Peeva E. Prolactin, systemic lupus erythematosus, and auto-reactive B cells: lessons learnt from murine

models. Clinical Reviews in Allergy and Immunology. 2011;**40**(1):8-15. DOI: 10.1007/s12016-009-8182-6

[81] Shi L, Zhang Z, Song L, Leung YT, Petri MA, Sullivan KE. Monocyte enhancers are highly altered in systemic lupus erythematosus. Epigenomics. 2015;7(6):921-935. DOI: 10.2217/epi.15.47

[82] Coit P et al. Epigenetic reprogramming in naive CD4+ T cells favoring T cell activation and non-Th1 effector T cell immune response as an early event in lupus flares. Arthritis & Rhematology. 2016;**68**(9):2200-2209

[83] Karouzakis E, Rengel Y, Jungel A, Kolling C, Gay RE, Michel BA, et al. DNA methylation regulates the expression of CXCL12 in rheumatoid arthritis synovial fibroblasts. Genes and Immunity. 2011;**12**(8):643-652

[84] Karouzakis E, Trenkmann M, Gay RE, Michel BA, Gay S, Neidhart M. Epigenome analysis reveals TBX5 as a novel transcription factor involved in the activation of rheumatoid arthritis synovial fibroblasts. Journal of Immunology. 2014;**193**(10):4945-4951

[85] Kuchen S, Seemayer CA, Rethage J, et al. The L1 retroelement-related p40 protein induces p38δMAP kinase. Autoimmunity. 2004;**37**(1):57-65

[86] Cribbs AP, Kennedy A, Penn H, Amjadi P, Green P, Read JE, et al. Methotrexate restores regulatory t cell function through demethylation of the FOXP3 upstream enhancer in patients with rheumatoid arthritis. Arthritis & Rhematology. 2015;**67**(5):1182-1192

[87] Nishida K, Komiyama T, Miyazawa SI, et al. Histone deacetylase inhibitor suppression of autoantibody-mediated arthritis in mice via regulation of p16INK4a and p21WAF1/Cip1 expression. Arthritis and Rheumatism. 2004;**50**(10):3365-3376

[88] Lee HS, Ka SO, Lee SM, Lee SI, Park JW, Park BH. Overexpression of sirtuin 6 suppresses inflammatory responses and bone destruction in mice with collagen-induced arthritis. Arthritis and Rheumatism. 2013;**65**(7):1776-1785

[89] Engler A, Tange C, Frank-Bertoncelj M, Gay RE, Gay S, Ospelt C. Regulation and function of SIRT1 in rheumatoid arthritis synovial fibroblasts. Journal of Molecular Medicine. 2016;**94**(2):173-182

[90] Klein K, Kabala PA, Grabiec AM, Gay RE, Kolling C, Lin LL, et al. The bromodomain protein inhibitor I-BET151 suppresses expression of inflammatory genes and matrix degrading enzymes in rheumatoid arthritis synovial fibroblasts. Annals of the Rheumatic Diseases. 2016;**75**(2):422-429

[91] Mele DA, Salmeron A, Ghosh S, Huang HR, Bryant BM, Lora JM. BET bromodomain inhibition suppresses TH17-mediated pathology. The Journal of Experimental Medicine. 2013;**210**(11):2181-2190

[92] Xiao Y, Liang L, Huang M, Qiu Q, Zeng S, Shi M, et al. Bromodomain and extra-terminal domain bromodomain in-hibition prevents synovial inflammation via blocking ikappab kinase-dependent nf-kappab activation in rheumatoid fibroblast-like synoviocytes. Rheumatology. 2016;**55**(1):173-184

[93] Naor D, Sopmpv RV, Ish-Shalom D. CD44: structure, function and association with the malignant process. Advances in Cancer Research. 1997;**71**:241-319

[94] Guan H, Nagarkatti PS, Nagarkatti M. CD44 reciprocally regulates the differentiation of encephalitogenic Th1/Th17 and Th2/Treg cells through epigenetic modulation involving DNA methylation of cytokine gene promoters thereby controlling the development of experimental autoimmune

encephalomyelitis. Journal of Immunology. 2011;**186**(12):6955-6964

[95] Janson PC, Linton LB, Bergman EA, Maritis P, et al. Profiling CD4+ T cells with epigenetic immune lineage analysis. Journal of Immunology. 2011;**186**(1):92-102

[96] Koch MW, Metz LM, Kovalchuk O. Epigenetics changes in patients with multiple sclerosis. Nature Reviews. Neurology. 2012;**9**:35-43

[97] Mangano K, Fagone P, Bendtzen K, Meroni PL, Quattrocchi C, Mammana S, et al. Hypomethylating agent 5-aza-2′-deoxycytidine (DAC) ameliorates multiple sclerosis in mouse models. Journal of Cellular Physiology. 2014;**229**(12):1918-1925

[98] Pedre X, Mastronardi F, Bruck W, Lopez-Rodas G, Kuhlmann T, Casaccia P. Changed histone acetylation patterns in normal-appearing white matter and early multiple sclerosis lesions. The Journal of Neuroscience. 2011;**31**:3435-3445

[99] Tegla CA, Azimzadeh P, Andrian-Albescu M, Martin A, Cudrici CD, Trippe R, et al. SIRT1 is decreased during re-lapses in patients with multiple sclerosis. Experimental and Molecular Pathology. 2014;**96**:139-148

[100] Shindler KS, Ventura E, Dutt M, Elliott P, Fitzgerald DC, Rostami A. Oral reservatrol reduces neuronal damage in a model of multiple sclerosis. Journal of Neuro-Ophthalmology. 2010;**30**(4):328-339

[101] Ma J, Wang R, Fang X, Ding Y, Sun Z. Critical role of TCF-1 in repression of the IL-17 gene. PLoS One. 2011;**6**(9):e24768

[102] Faraco G, Cavone L, Chiarugi A. The therapeutic potential of HDAC inhibitors in the treatment of multiple sclerosis. Molecular Medicine. 2011;**17**(5-6):442-447

[103] Zhang Z, Zhang ZY, Wu Y, Schluesener H. Valproic acid ameliorates inflammation in experimental autoimmune encephalomyelitis rats. Neuroscience. 2012;**221**:140-150

[104] Camelo S, Iglesias AH, Hwang D, Due B, Ryu H, Smith K, et al. Transcriptional therapy with the histone deacetylase inhibitor trichostatin A ameliorates experimental autoimmune encephalomyelitis. Journal of Neuroimmunology. 2005;**164**(1-2):10-21

[105] Chen F, Chai H, Su MB, Zhang YM, Li J, Xie X, et al. Potent and orally efficacious bisthiazole-based histone deacety-lase inhibitors. ACS Medicinal Chemistry Letters. 2014;**5**(6):628-633

[106] Ge Z, Da Y, Xue Z, Zhang K, Zhuang H, Peng M, et al. Vorinostat, a histone deacetylase inhibitor, suppresses dendritic cell function and ameliorates experimental autoimmune encephalomyelitis. Experimental Neurology. 2013;**241**:56-66

[107] Xie L, Li XK, et al. Amelioration of experimental autoimmune encephalomyelitis by curcumin treatment through inhibition of IL-17 production. International Immunopharmacology. 2009;**9**(5):575-581

[108] Feng J, Tao T, Yan W, Chen CS, Qin X. Curcumin inhibits mitochondrial injury and apoptosis from the early stage in EAE mice. Oxidative Medicine and Cellular Longevity. 2014;**2014**:728751

[109] Glória L, Cravo M, Pinto A, de Sousa LS, Chaves P, Leitão CN, et al. DNA hypomethylation and proliferative activity are increased in the rec-tal mucosa of patients with long-standing ulcerative colitis. Cancer. 1996;**78**(11):2300-2306

[110] Issa JP, Ahuja N, Toyota M, Bronner MP, Brentnall TA. Accelerated age-related CpG island methylation in ulcerative colitis. Cancer Research. 2001;**61**(9):3573-3577

[111] Azarschab P, Porschen R, Gregor M, Blin N, Holzmann K. Epigenetic control of the E-cadherin gene (CDH1) by CpG methylation in colecto-my samples of patients with ulcerative colitis. Genes, Chromosomes & Cancer. 2002;**35**(2):121-126

[112] Saito S, Kato J, Hiraoka S, Horii J, Suzuki H, Higashi R, et al. DNA methylation of colon mucosa in ulcerative colitis patients: Correlation with inflammatory status. Inflammatory Bowel Diseases. 2011;**17**(9):1955-1965

[113] Tsaprouni LG, Ito K, Powell JJ, Adcock IM, Punchard N. Differential patterns of histone acetylation in inflammatory bowel diseases. Journal of Inflammation. 2011;**8**(1):1

[114] Glauben R, Batra A, Fedke I, Zeitz M, Lehr HA, Leoni F, et al. Histone hyperacetylation is associated with amelioration of experimental colitis in mice. Journal of Immunology. 2006;**176**(8):5015-5022

[115] de Zoeten EF, Wang L, Sai H, Dillmann WH, Hancock WW. Inhibition of HDAC9 increases T regulatory cell function and prevents colitis in mice. Gastroenterology. 2010;**138**(2):583-594

[116] Arpaia N, Campbell C, Fan X, Dikiy S, van der Veeken J, de Roos P, et al. Metabolites produced by commensal bacteria promote peripheral regulatory T-cell generation. Nature. 2013;**504**(7480):451-455. Published on-line November 13, 2013

[117] Louis P, Flint HJ. Diversity, metabolism and microbial ecology of butyrate-producing bacteria from the human large intestine. FEMS Microbiology Letters. 2009;**294**(1):1-8

[118] Fofanova TY, Petrosino JF, Kellermayer R. Microbiome-epigenome interactions and the environmental origins of inflammatory bowel diseases. Journal of Pediatric Gastroenterology and Nutrition. 2016;**62**(2):208-219

[119] Chang PV, Hao L, Offermanns S, Medzhitov R. The microbial metabolite butyrate regulates intestinal macrophage function via histone deacetylase inhibition. Proceedings of the National Academy of Sciences of the United States of America. 2014;**111**(6):2247-2252

Chapter 11

The Experimental Bioengineering of Complete Spinal Cord Injury in Adult Rats

I.N. Bolshakov, A.V. Svetlakov, A.V. Eremeev and Yu.I. Sheina

Abstract

The chapter is devoted to the research of experimental complete mechanical spinal injury in adult rats and attempts at bioengineering restoration of the structure and function of the spinal cord using a protein-polysaccharide construct that includes bovine collagen, highly purified crab chitosan ascorbate, nanostructuring additives in the form of sodium chondroitin sulfate, sodium hyaluronate, heparin sulfate in the presence of complete nutrient medium DMEM, neural supplement N2, conditioned nutrient medium, obtained about brain cell mouse embryos and mouse embryonic stem cells, retinoic acid, and mouse neural progenitor cells derived from embryonic stem cells. After a complete intersection of the spinal cord at the level of the ninth tho racic vertebra, the authors directly implanted a collagen-chitosan construct into the gap between the ends of the spinal cord. Analysis of the recovery of motor and sensory and vegetative functions of the spinal cord for 20 weeks after surgery using the cytological immune-fluorescent method showed a high viability of the transplanted neural cell precursors during the entire observation period and the early emergence of activity of mediators of nerve signal transmission in the implantation zone of the structure with accompaniment active dynamics of reducing neurodeficiency.

Keywords: collagen-chitosan scaffold, complete intersection of the spinal cord, mouse neuronal progenitor cells, adult rats, neurological deficiency, neurotransmitters, immunofluorescence analysis

1. Introduction

Solid biodegradable constructs as an implant in the spinal cord based on proteins and polysaccharides are able to create favorable conditions for the adaptation, proliferation, differentiation, and sprouting of the precursors of neural cells placed in the implant. At the same time, direct transplantation of the structure together with the precursors of neural cells substantially eliminates weight loss during cell transfer and the apoptosis reaction and increases the survival time of cells in new conditions, and the polysaccharide components of the matrix not only play the role of shielding the protein base from the immune system, and also provide a high function cell transfer system to the central and peripheral ends of the central nervous system. The problem of spinal injury remains acute without addressing the issues of effectively eliminating neuro-inflammation in the area of injury and creating conditions for the formation of pathways and sprouting axons under the conditions of glial scar formation.

1.1 Embryonic stem cells in the correction of spinal cord injury

A significant improvement of the neurological deficit was achieved by Bottai et al. by intravenous administration of undifferentiated ESCs at a dose of 1 million cells 2 hours after injury [1]. The protective role of multipotent cells was demonstrated during the development of an inflammatory reaction, accompanied by a decrease in the intensity of infiltration of the affected area with elements of microglia. The presence of hESCs in the spinal cord injury zone in adult rats or mini-pigs for 4.5 months induces the formation of embryoid bodies with expression of specific (hNUMA, HO14, hNSE, and hSYN) and nonspecific (DCX, MAP2, CHAT, GFAP, and ACP) antigens. Research results of Yang et al., in a rat spinal cord contusion injury model using green fluorescent protein-labeled pig embryonic stem cells (pES/GFP (+)), indicate a decrease in expression of green fluorescent protein within 3 months, and positively stained cells for neural are detected in the transplant area of specific antigens: anti-NFL, anti-/MBP, anti-SYP, and anti-Tuj 1 [2]. The use of undifferentiated cells significantly reduces the efficiency of functional restoration of the hind limbs in rats, compared to the use of neural progenitors derived from ESCs. The value of indicators of the neurological status on the BBB scale was 15.20 ± 1.43 points on the 24th week of the posttransplant period.

1.2 Neural stem cells and their precursors

Under certain conditions, these cells are able to differentiate into neurons, astrocytes, and oligodendrocytes. Neuronal progenitors and precursors of oligodendrocytes showed positive dynamics in reducing neuro-deficiency in spinal cord injury models. The use of two cell populations with neurogenic and gliogenic activity leads to the restoration of locomotor functions and stimulates angiogenesis, the growth of axons, and their re-myelination [3–11]. A monolayer of neural precursors (NPs) from ESCs is obtained by a combination of diffusion of nutrients and growth factors; it includes extracellular matrices such as laminin, poly-d-lysine, and matrigel [12]. A three-dimensional matrix with the precursors of neuronal cells or oligodendrocytes creates the conditions for the formation of intercellular contacts, ensures survival, differentiation, and proliferation [13, 14]. Cultivation of neural precursors on a three-dimensional substrate forms oligodendrocyte precursors with the expression of Nestin and PAX6 [15, 16]. At the same time, NP cultivation conditions and their micro-environment are of key importance [17].

1.3 Neurotrophic support in the area of spinal cord injury

Re-myelination of damaged axons and improvement of their conductivity are possible with transplantations of neural progenitors in the experiment [18, 19]. The effect of transplantation is enhanced by trophic support of neurons and immune modulation [20–23]. Transplantation of spinal cord precursors of neuronal cells to the zone of spinal cord injury is accompanied by activation of axon growth, their locomotion, and registration of G-CSF, BDNF, CNTF, FGF, EGF, and NT-3 growth factors in cells [24–27]. Consequently, neurotrophic support is a prerequisite for the regeneration of specialized nervous tissue when it is lost. The presence of neurospheres of exogenous growth factors such as EGF, bFGF, and CNTF in the environment creates conditions for the long-term cultivation of viable precursors of neurons, differentiation into mature neurons, and successful transfer to the area of spinal injury [28]. Spinal cord regeneration with the help of neural cell progenitors indicates the important role of stem cells under conditions of intensive neurotrophic support by NGF, BDNF, CNTF, GDNF, and IGF-1 molecules [24, 29].

1.4 Use of degradable biopolymer substrates as implants in the damaged spinal cord

Modern technologies for obtaining biomaterials with unique consumer properties make them the most important link in the task of reconstruction of spinal cord injury. Neuroprotection from re-inflammatory response is possible, provided that the growth of neurites is artificially oriented with the inclusion of neurotrophic support in this system. Studies confirm that the creation of such conditions leads to the restoration of lost tissue, enhancement of axonal growth and active sprinting to the head and caudal segments of the damaged area, suppression of astrocytosis, and the appearance of inter-synaptic connections.

The strategy of reconstruction of the damaged spinal cord includes the use of prepared cell mass in solid or liquid, biodegradable, highly compatible 3D matrices with favorable conditions for its cultivation, proliferation, and differentiation. Such constructions allow direct transfer of cellular material to the area of spinal cord injury.

Matrigel, laminin, type-1-collagen, fibronectin, chitosan, glycosaminoglycans, poly-d-lysine, and fibrin are used in experimental practice. The final results of the studies do not allow asserting one of the mentioned polymers as the best sample, despite the use of combined materials with a neurotrophic microenvironment [30].

The differentiation of hESC in contact with neuronal progenitors occurred more actively when laminin was used [31]. In other conditions of cultivation of neuronal precursors, the efficiency of using Matrigel is confirmed [32, 33]. A number of authors obtained satisfactory results when using a combination of collagen IV, laminin, and poly-L-lysine [12, 16, 34]. Such nonstandardized approaches to the creation of culture conditions do not exclude the risk of immune reactions.

1.5 Materials based on chitosan to obtain neural substrates

Chitosan, a linear copolymer consisting of N-acetylglucosamine and N-glucosamine, when in contact with the wound surface biodegrades without causing toxic reactions from surrounding somatic cells and is capable of screening protein molecules from the immune system during biodegradation. The number of scientific publications on the use of chitosan polymers as the basis of the matrix for implantation in the spinal cord in trauma is immeasurably small compared to the use of other biopolymers in spinal injury models. The strategy for using chitosan polymers for spinal cord reconstruction is developed by Freier et al. [35] and Nomura et al. [36]. The advantages of liquid and solid substrates are known for cell mass transplantation and neurotrophic support in the spinal cord in trauma. However, sponge structures are capable of covering extensive defects in the damage zone. An important aspect of the technology is the formation of oriented microchannels in the matrix for the directed growth of axons and, thus, enhanced sprouting of cells in the graft area and beyond. The polycationic properties of chitosan ensure constant contact of cells with a biopolymer, which enhances cell migration and axon regeneration [37] and lengthens and thickens neurites [35], and in low concentrations, the biopolymer is able to shield stem and progenitor cells [38].

In 2008, experimental transplantation of neural cell precursors as part of a chitosan microchannel biomaterial was performed first after complete transection of the spinal cord. The use of NSPS in the spinal cord of Sprague-Dawley rats as a base of a highly de-acetylated chitosan hydrochloride micro-channel substrate confirmed that massive cellular transitional bridges containing a high number of differentiated cells are formed in the spinal cord within 100 days after the surgical intervention. Cell-free channel matrices also formed transition zones, but the thickness of the transitions was significantly less [39]. If precultured neural progenitor cells (NSPCs) are placed in the micro-channels of the chitosan substrate, in the damaged rat spinal cord, one can demonstrate very high cell survival for 5 weeks and their differentiation not only into neurons but also astrocytes and oligodendrocytes [40]. High cell survival and differentiation of not only neurons but also glial cells in chitosan extramedullary channels and in the spinal cord after transplantation and active sprouting from the central to the caudal segment of the spinal cord with the formation of active transitional brain tissue are accompanied by significant restoration of the motor and sensory functions of the hind limbs [41]. The inflammatory process in the area of spinal cord injury stimulates the synthesis of type IV collagen in endothelial cells, fibroblasts, and Schwann cells, which leads to the formation of a massive glial scar. Productive inflammation in the connective tissue inhibits the growth of axons [42–44]. Exogenous suppression of the synthesis of collagen type IV prolongs axonal growth. The introduction of type I collagen into the system enhances the growth of axons and neural connections between the central and peripheral zone of injury [45, 46]. It is convincingly shown that the presence of stem cells in the composition of the polymer chitosan in the area of spinal cord injury improves cell viability and stimulates their differentiation and the expression of neurotrophic factors. As a result, functional neurodeficiency is reduced. Prolonged presence of chitosan in the brain tissue and its biodegradation do not stimulate the immune response [47, 48].

Preliminary studies have resulted in 4 variants of the neural matrix that can support long-term human ESC and animals (rats) in complete medium and translate them into a state of differentiation with reception on the 5th day of cells with neuronal markers exposed on its membrane (neuro-filament, MBP, and GFAP) [49]. The approaches proposed in this work to the reconstruction of the spinal cord in experimental complicated spinal injury (total mechanical spinal cord transection) are based on modern biodegradable polysaccharide matrices containing the necessary microenvironment, including the products of growth and differentiation of stem cells and neuronal cells and neuronal precursor cells for the reconstruction of spinal cord to restore its motor and sensory functions. Consumer properties of the proposed cellular matrix showed competitive advantages due to the lack of matrices satisfying the task. They are as follows: high biocompatibility, biodegradability, nontoxicity, the system of information transfer, the creation of a strict orientation of the tissues in tissue engineering implant thanks to a rigid linear structure of chitosan, the regulation of collagen synthesis, stimulation of breeding passaged cell precursor neuronal tissue, vascular endothelial cell proliferation, and tumor micro-vessel recovery of the intracellular substrate. Implantation of such a matrix can be done in an open manner of the operative spinal cord diastasis.

2. Materials and methods

2.1 Neuronal matrix getting

To create a neural matrix base poly-ion complex consisting of nano-micro-structured ascorbate chitosan with a molecular weight of 695 kDa and a degree of deacetylation of 98%, when the content of 1 g dry chitosan 1.8 g of ascorbic acid, comprising anionic salt forms chondroitin acid (Sigma) (20 mg\d), hyaluronic acid (Sigma) (10 mg\d) and heparin (5 mg\d) (Russia), serum growth factors in cattle "adgelon" (110 mcg\d) were used.

To obtain the basic collagen-chitosan complex, we used a triply purified chitosan obtained in Vostok-Bor-1, Dal'negorsk, Russia with a molecular weight of 695 kDa and a deacetylation degree above 95%, protonated with an ascorbic acid solution (dissolution of the polymer in ascorbic solution acid in a ratio of 1: 1.5). Introduction of a heparin solution, serum low-molecular growth factor "adgelon" (SLL "Endo-Pharm-A," Moscow region, Shchyolkovo, Russia), neural supplement N2 (Sigma), and retinoic acid (Sigma) stimulated embryonic stem cells (ESCs) in the chitosan gel to neuronal differentiation. A conditioned nutrient medium obtained after culturing embryonic neuronal cells of brain tissue of mice or conditioned nutrient medium obtained after culturing embryonic allogeneic stem cells of mice was added to the base poly-ionic complex (Krasnoyarsk Center for Reproductive Medicine, Russia). Embryonic stem cells (ESCs) were obtained from mouse blastocysts by eluting the uterus with DMEM medium of the anesthetized animal on the 4th–5th day after copulation. Getting the inner cell mass (ICM) and the further expansion of ESC colonies was performed according to the protocol [50, 51]. Overage human blastocysts were taken from patients undergoing IVF. Full consultation was done and informed consent was received before embryo processing. This research followed the directives of the Russian Association of Human Reproduction. Embryos were obtained for research use only, without other restrictions and compensation.

Cultivation of cells was performed in DMEM supplemented with 10% fetal calf serum (FCS F0926, Sigma), 100 mg/ml kanamycin sulfate (Sigma), 1 mM L-glutamine (G7513, Sigma) in bottles Corning, gelatin-coated (Sigma).

In the experiments to obtain the conditioned medium from neural stem embryonic mouse cells (cells from the brains of 17–20 day fetus outbred mice (Institute of biophyisic SD RAS, Russia) after the dispersion and processing of 0.5% collagenase solution (Sigma) for 30 minutes in medium DMEM (Sigma) at 37°C for increasing cell biomass used DMEM under light microscopy with 10% fetal calf serum (FCS), 100 mg/ml canamycin sulfate, 1 mM L-glutamine, which is added 4 ng\ml basic fibroblast growth factor (bFGF, Sigma), 1 mM solution of essential amino acids (Sigma-Aldrich). The cell biomass was grown at 37°C in vials coated with 0.1% gelatin solution. The environment was collected daily. The condition of cells was estimated by light microscope. After subculturing with 0.5% collagenase solution, the matrix cells were cultured in medium supplemented with neuronal differentiation agent—N2 component, according to the manufacturer's instructions. The medium was collected, filtered through a 0.22 mcm cellulose acetate filter, and used hereinafter as a conditioned medium.

Next performed covalent compounds derived polysaccharide gel structure (The Developer is SBEU HPT Krasnoyarsk State Medical University, Russia) with bovine collagen gel (SLL Belkosin, Russia) in a ratio of 1: 3, a freeze-drying deep frozen samples to install FC500 (Germany). This mixture was poured on pallets of duralumin, a layer thickness of 2 mm, frozen at −20°C, and then freeze-dried at 10^{-5} Pa for 8 hours; the product is packaged and sterilized by the electron beam method (neuronal dry matrix courtesy SLL "Medical Company Collachit," Krasnoyarsk Region, Russia).

The manipulation above yielded a neuronal matrix of the size 50 × 50 × 2 mm, suitable for not only the culture and in vitro differentiation of embryonic stem cells into neurons and oligodendrocyte progenitor of mice, but also for direct transplantation into the spinal cord gap in experimental injury in adult rats.

When using a sponge matrix, they need to be previously soaked in sterile bicarbonate buffer (Sigma) to reduce their acid properties. After neutralization phase of collagen-chitosan substrate was washed three times with sterile phosphate-buffered Dulbecco's modified eagle's medium (Biolot), placed in a vial, and carefully layered on top of them the cell suspension in a medium with all the components, depending on the cell type.

The cultivation of pluripotent cell experiments on collagen-chitosan substrates initially used for biomass growth basal medium DMEM (Sigma) supplemented with 10% SR (serum substitute), 100 μg/ml kanamycin sulfate, 1 mM L-glutamine, 4 ng/ml primary engine of growth fibroblast (bFGF), 1 mM solution of amino acids, and the inhibitor Rock 5 ng/ml kinase (Sigma). Capacity cell biomass was performed in flasks coated with 0.1% gelatin. The environment was changed daily. The colonial state was assessed visually using a microscope AxioVert-200. To assess the state of maintenance of pluripotency, limmune-cytochemical analysis of the expression of markers—oct4, TRA-1-60, SSEA4, and cd30 (Sigma)—was performed.

To differentiate embryonic cells in the neuronal direction, they were seeded into vials in a medium with all additives except bFGF, with the addition of retinoic acid and N2 component.

Every three days, formaldehyde fixation was performed followed by immune-cytochemistry of the cells with antibodies (Abcam, USA) against GFAP glial fibrillar acid protein, neuro-filament, and nestin. Detection of markers was carried out by the method according to the instructions of the antibody manufacturer. The cell nuclei were stained with DAPI (Sigma) (0.1 μg/ml) for 10 minutes. The Olympus BX-51 fluorescence microscope (Japan) and the software products "Applied Spectral Imaging" (USA) were used to obtain images and analysis. For the analysis of each marker, the experiment was repeated three times, increasing three vials, each of which was randomly assigned into 6 zones for carrying out immunocytochemistry. Microscopy was carried out for each zone in 30 fields of vision.

2.2 The experimental complete transection of the spinal cord in rats

The conditions of biological test systems in the CDI CI correspond to Guide for the Care and Use of Laboratory Animals, 8th edition, 2011, NRC, USA (Manual on the content and use of laboratory animals, 8th edition, 2011, national research Committee, USA). The content of animals in individually ventilated cells from polysulfone seal-safe, 461 × 274 × 228 mm (production TECHNIPLAST.P. A.)

The rooms contain biological test systems, controlled temperature (18–24°C), humidity (30–70%), illumination (12/12 hours), and the multiplicity of air (X11 without recirculation). Control of climatic parameters is carried out in accordance with the SOP "control of climatic parameters in the premises of the vivarium."

Distribution of feed and water is carried out at a fixed time; the change of litter is made once a week in accordance with the SOP "preparation of cells for biological test systems. Marking. Change of bedding, feed, water."

Biological test systems receive food " CHARA" for the maintenance of laboratory animals of the SPF-category, production of LLC "Assortment agro" and "VAKA," and production of LLC "BIOSPHERE," auto-clavable, with confirmation of the absence of microbial contamination. The feed is balanced in amino acid composition, minerals, and vitamins, made of high quality components. Laboratory tests for toxicity have been carried out. The food is not toxic, but a environmentally friendly product. Certificates of feed quality are present. Sterilization of feed is carried out in the steam sterilizer TOUCHCLAVE LAB K14 369 manufactured by LTE Scientific LTD, with confirmation of sterilization (multi-parameter chemical indicators of sterilization 3 M Comply Steri Gage manufactured by 3 M). After sterilization, the feed is stored in closed containers for no more than 7 days (SOP "operation of steam sterilizer with automatic control Touchclave-LAB model TC/R300E/PL/PASS").

For watering of biological test systems, we used water that had been trained in the reverse osmosis production unit JSC "Scientific-production company

Mediana-Filter," confirming the absence of microbial contamination, and bottled in pro-anti-cianidinas bottle. Access to food and water is unrestricted throughout the study.

The cells consist of a mixture of litter "Golden cat," produced by "the zone" "the Gold Ear," Russia and "Lignosol," produced by J. Rettenmaier and Sohne Gmbh, Germany, in the ratio of 1:4 subjected to autoclaving, control of microbiological purity in accordance with SOP "Operation of a steam sterilizer with automatic control Touchclave-LAB model TC/R300E/PL/PASS."

Veterinary protocol was considered and approved at the meeting of the Commission on Bioethics, minutes of the meeting No 57 dated 01.10.2016.

The research methods used in the planned experiment, capable of causing pain and stress to animals, cannot be replaced by more humane ones. The possible negative effects on animals are minimized and the principles of their humane use are observed.

Premedication: 30 minutes prior to surgery—Sol. Tramadoli 2.5 mg/m; Sol. Atropini sulfatis 0.1%–0.1 ml/m; Sol. Dimedroli 0.1%–0.1 ml/m Anesthesia: anesthesia (diethyl ether). About 12 white female rats, Wistar line, weighing 250 g with Carl Zeiss optics, individually reproduced model of spinal cord injury at the IX-X thoracic vertebrae with a complete transverse intersection of the spinal cord after first performing a laminectomy.

2.3 Operation course

After preliminary treatment of the operating field with a 70% solution of ethyl alcohol under anesthesia, an incision was made along the midline of the animal's back at a level of Th7 to L4 4–5 cm in length. Hemostasis was performed during the operation. After dissection of the skin, subcutaneous fat layer, the wound edges were mobilized and diluted with Edson's retractors. The acristoid-trapezius and the broadest muscle were cut off from the places of their attachment to the spinous processes of Th9-L3. The muscles of the deep layer were separated from the spine and diluted with a microsurgical retractor, and the Th9-Th12 vertebrae were bared. The Th10 arch resection was performed, and the dura mater was dissected and diluted to the sides in the horizontal plane.

A complete transverse intersection of the spinal cord was performed using a microscalpel and micro-scissors and individual optics of Carl Zeiss. A neuronal cell matrix with a size of about 2 mm^3 containing about 100 thousand precursors of neuronal cell implant was placed immediately in the formed neural tissue defect. The bony wound was closed as a film with polysaccharide hydrogel mass "bolchit" [52], which does not contain animal collagen. The wound was closed layer by layer using suture material Vicril 4–0 (muscle) and Polyester 3–0 (skin). The stitches were treated with an alcohol solution of iodine (**Figures 1–6**).

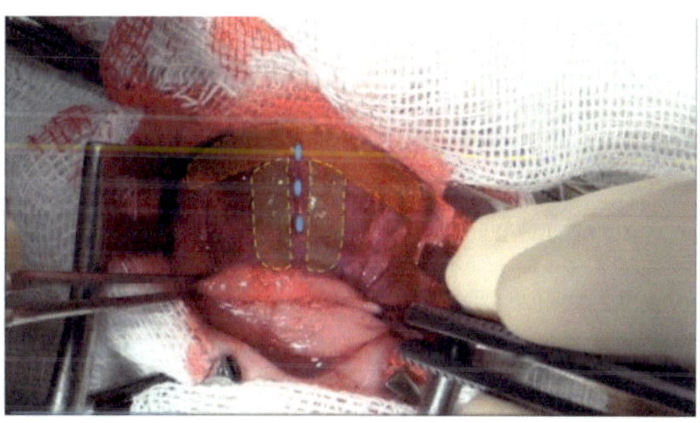

Figure 1.
Quick access to back extensor and awned appendages of vertebras Th VIII-X.

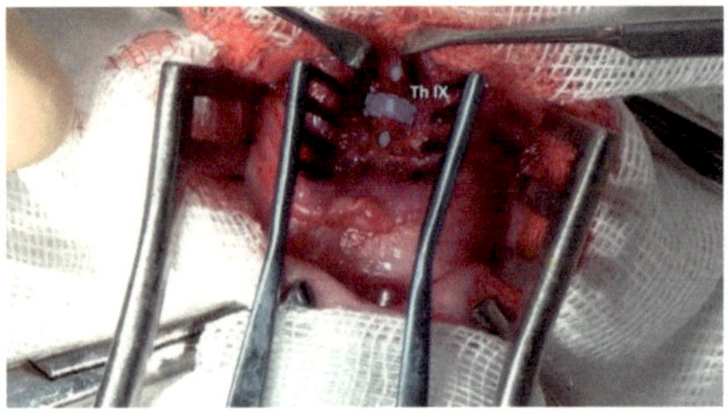

Figure 2.
Skeletization of the ninth chest vertebra handle.

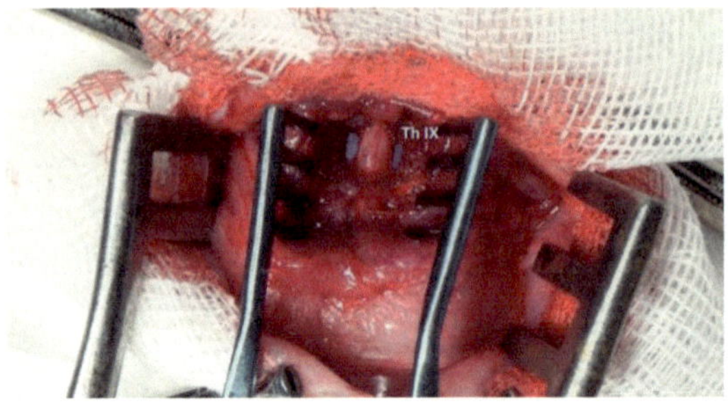

Figure 3.
Resection of the ninth chest vertebra handle with removal of a firm brain cover, and spinal cord exposure.

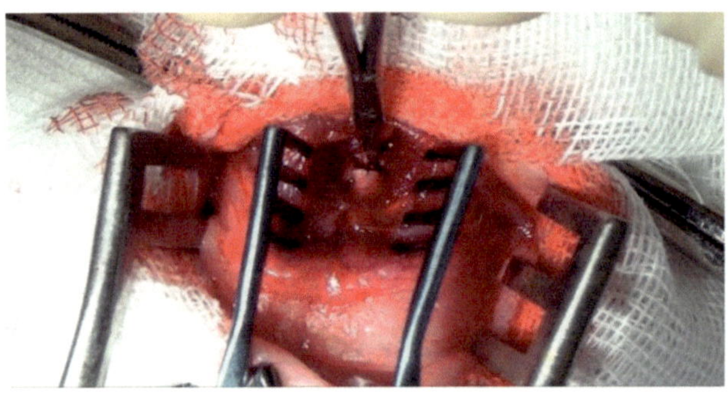

Figure 4.
Full spinal cord transection.

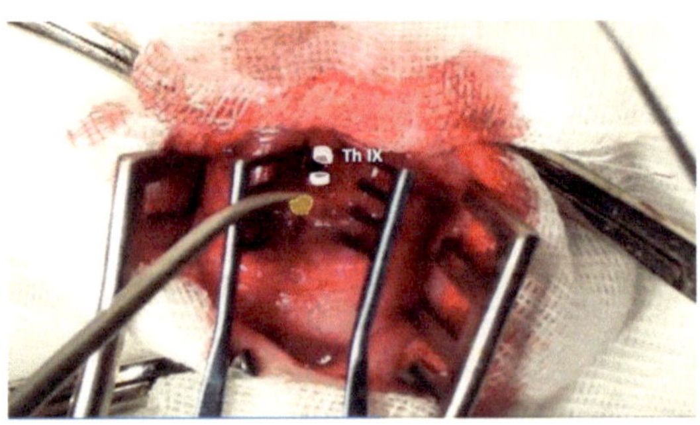

Figure 5.
Cellular neuromatrix implantation of spinal cord diastases.

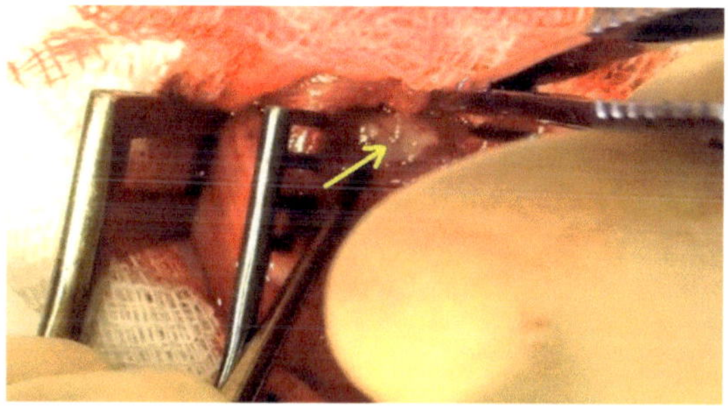

Figure 6.
Restoration of vertebral channel integrity by means of a chitosan film (it is pointed by an arrow).

2.3.1 The composition of transplantable matrices

On the basis of collagen-chitosan structures, two different implants were prepared containing the following components:

1. A lyophilic collagen-chitosan matrix obtained as described above, which does not contain cells, including in its composition the complete DMEM nutrient medium, conditioned medium from neuronal cells and neural supplement N2, and retinoic acid (6 rats of the control group);

2. A lyophilic collagen-chitosan matrix, obtained as indicated above in the control group, containing about 100,000 neuronal precursor cells obtained by culturing and differentiating mouse embryonic stem cells (ESCm) (6 rats in the test group).

Variants of porous matrix substrates were cut into 1 or 2 mm^3 before embryonic stem cells were placed on them and, in sterile conditions, were unfolded in the wells of a 96-well plate without coating with 0.1% gelatin solution. The cells from the culture flasks were removed with a 0.5% collagenase solution, then washed three times with DMEM medium from the enzyme and transferred to wells with a cut matrix in the ESC medium. Cells were cultured for at least 3 days prior to the appearance of neuronal markers under humid conditions at 37°C and 6% CO_2. The number of attached cells was evaluated by dispersing 5–6 pieces of the matrix in the enzyme solution, followed by counting the cells in the Goryaev chamber. Each future neuron implant during cultivation contained about 100 thousand of neuronal precursor cells. Before the implantation in the spinal cord, the pieces with a micro pincer were carefully transferred to microtubes with DMEM/F12 culture medium (Nutrient mixture F-12 HAM, Sigma) and transported to the operating room.

2.4 Postoperative care

Within 3–5 days after the operation, the animals received Sol as an analgesic; Tramadoli 2.5 mg 3 times daily IM. Sutures were removed after 10 days. During the first 24 hours, animals were admitted to the water. Feeding was performed 48 hours after the operation solely with a mixture of "Polyproten-nephro" (SLL "Protenpharma," Russia) for 1–4 weeks. The rats were kept in separate boxes with a double bottom. Drug support was provided with a broad-spectrum antibiotic, antispasmodics, and vessel-dilator drugs.

2.5 Dynamic neurological control

To assess the neurological disturbances and recovery dynamics, a scale was used to assess the severity of the neurological deficit for complete transection (BBB scale) [53] within 20 weeks after implantation.

2.6 The immunofluorescence analysis of sections of the spinal cord after direct implantation of cellular neuronal matrices in the dislocation of a spinal trauma

Histological sections were subjected to immunofluorescence treatment for the search for transplanted cells expressing the green fluorescent protein GFP and the presence of neurotransmitters in the upper and lower areas of the spinal cord adjacent to the graft, as well as in the collagen chitosan transplant itself: acetylcholine, serotonin, and GABA (Abcam, USA). The Olympus BX-51 fluorescence microscope and the software products "Applied Spectral Imaging" (USA) were used to obtain images and analysis.

Spinal cord preparations obtained by careful and judicious selection of tissue from the spinal canal through the 20 weeks after surgery.

3. Results and discussion

Analysis of neurological deficits in rats after complete spinal cord transection indicates that transplantation of the cell-free collagen-chitosan matrix into spinal cord diastase at the level of thoracic vertebra IX leads to a marked reduction in the volume of violations by restoring the function of the pelvic organs in full, and provides 5–6 level recovery of motor and sensory functions of the spinal cord within 20 weeks of follow-up (**Table 1**). Implantation into the spinal cord diastasis collagen-chitosan substrate of about 100,000 mouse neuronal precursor cells leads to virtually eliminate neuronal lack, reaching over 20 weeks 19.5 replacement level (**Table 1**, **Figure 7**). The serial photo shows the animals in the control and experiment at different times of the postoperative period with different levels of reduction of neurological deficit (**Figures 8–14**).

3.1 Immunofluorescent analysis of neurotransmitters in the spinal cord sections at its complete transection

Immunofluorescence neurotransmitter control of serial sections of the cerebral spinal cord rats 20 weeks after its full transection (the zone above the transplant area) shows that the interstitial tissue filled with nuclear cell mass actively express GABA, acetylcholine, and serotonin. The number of these cells is the uniformity of the distribution center to the area of the graft (**Figure 15**).

Serial immunofluorescence zone collagen-chitosan graft shows that 20 weeks after the operation area is filled with interstitial brain tissue with a large number of viable neuronal cells, maternal spinal cord actively expresses markers GABA, acetylcholine, and serotonin. Furthermore, zone graft contains many newly formed micro-capillaries containing the body of erythrocytes with auto-fluorescence effect. The number of nucleated cells in maternal spinal cord transplant decreases toward the tail region (**Figure 16**). In the rear area of the spinal cord (below the graft), the number of nucleated cells is substantially less than in the head area and in the control graft. However, viable cells express neurotransmitters GABA, acetylcholine, and serotonin (**Figure 17**).

Lower limb\week			1	2	3	4	5	6	7	8	9	10	11	12	13	14	15	16	17	18	19	20
Neuronal lack's level	Experimental group (with predecessors NC)	left paw	0	1	2.5	5	7	7	7.5	9	10	11.5	12.5	13	14.5	16	19	19.5	19.5	19.5	19.5	19.5
		right paw	0	1	1	4	4.5	5.5	7	8.5	10.5	11.5	12.5	13	14.5	16	19	19.5	19.5	19.5	19.5	19.5
Neuronal lack's level	The control group (without predecessor NC	left paw	0	0	0.5	1.2	1.8	3.4	4.8	5	5.4	5.4	5.4	5.4	5.4	5.4	5.4	5.4	5.4	5.4	5.4	5.4
		right paw	0	0.4	0.8	0.8	2.2	4.4	4.8	4.8	4.8	4.8	4.8	4.8	4.8	4.8	4.8	4.8	4.8	4.8	4.8	4.8

Table 1.
Analysis results with complete neurological spinal cord transection and transplantation of collagen-chitosan matrix predecessor mouse neuronal cells (PNCm).

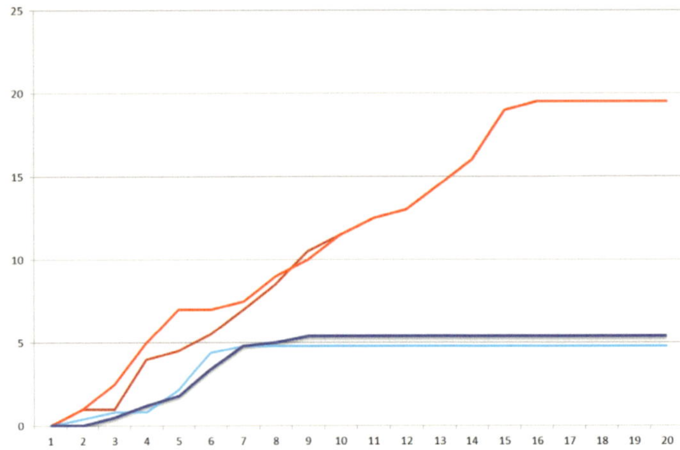

Figure 7.
The neurological analysis results of a full transection of a spinal cord. Red (left) and burgundy (right) color (experience) back extremities, blue (right) and navy blue (left) color (control) back extremities. Down – levels of reduction of neuronal deficiency, across – weeks of supervision.

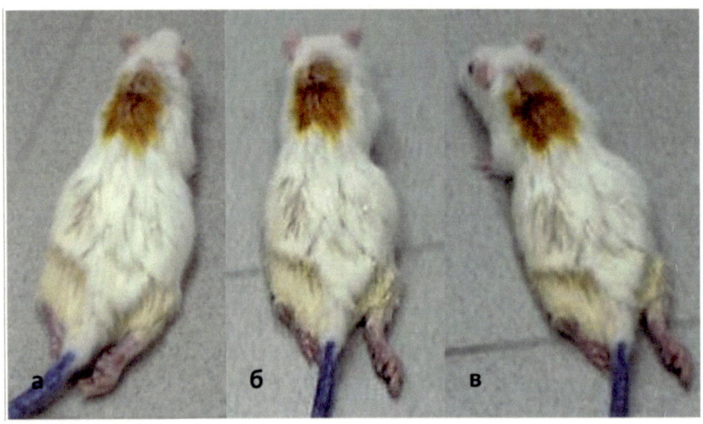

Figure 8.
The first week after transplantation, level of reduction of neurological deficiency 0 (control).

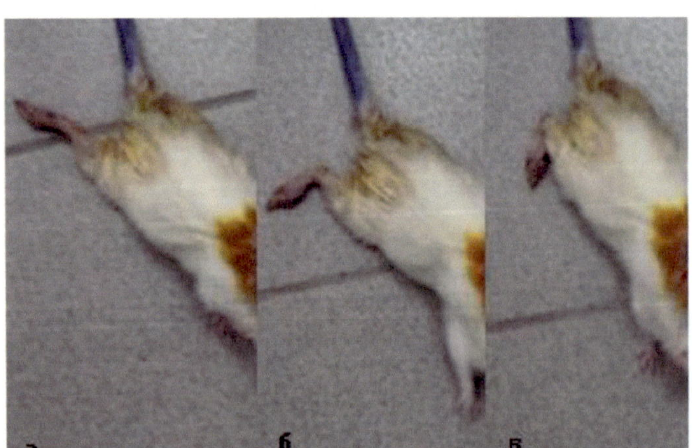

Figure 9.
The fourth week after transplantation, level of reduction of neurological deficiency 1 (control).

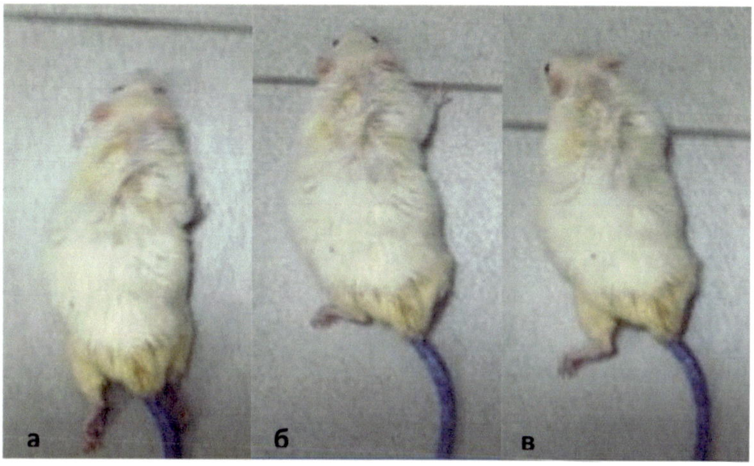

Figure 10.
The sixth week after transplantation, level of reduction of neurological deficiency 3.9 (control).

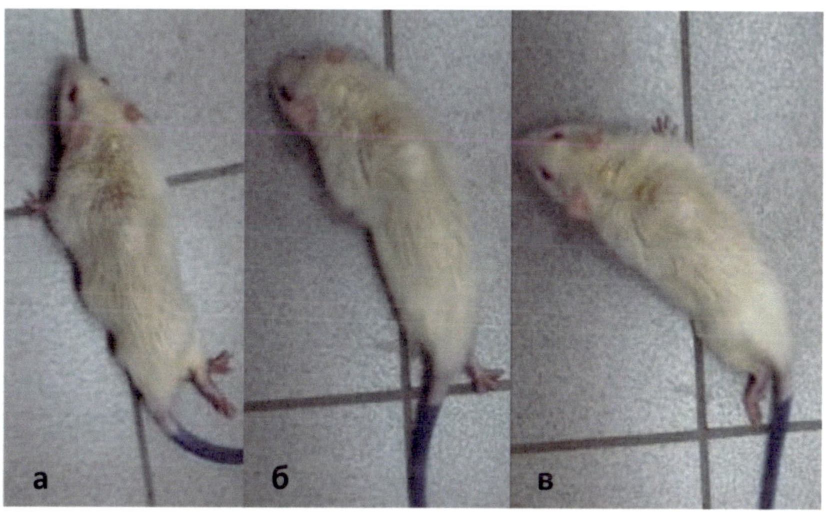

Figure 11.
The eighth week after transplantation, level of reduction of neurological deficiency 4.9 (control).

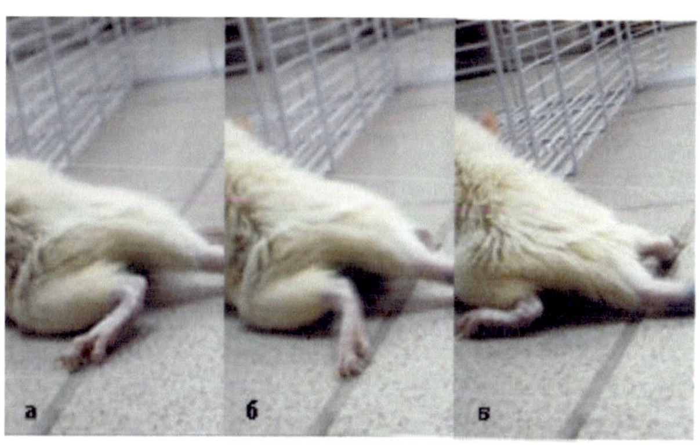

Figure 12.
The twentieth week after transplantation, level of reduction of neurological deficiency 5.1 (control).

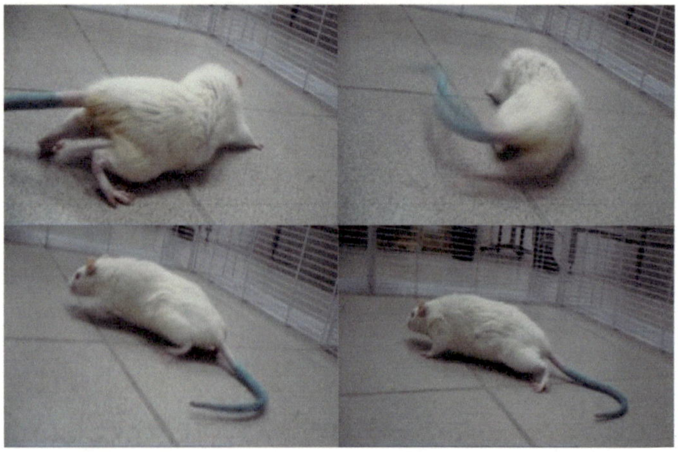

Figure 13.
The eighteenth week after transplantation, level of reduction of neurological deficiency 19.5 (experience).

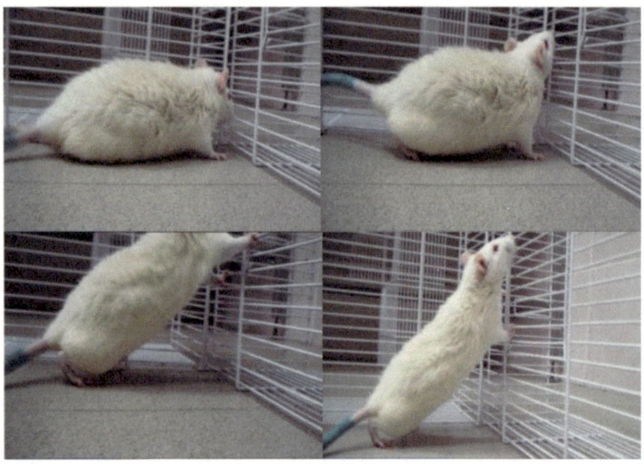

Figure 14.
The eighteenth week after transplantation, level of reduction of neurological deficiency 19.5 (experience).

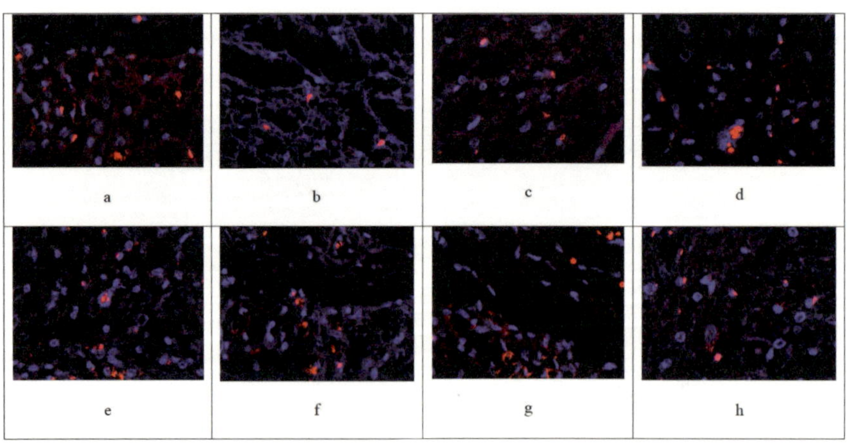

Figure 15.
The immune fluorescent analysis of serial cut neurotransmitters (from top to down, control): head department of a spinal cord in 20 weeks after its full transection (above-transplant zone): GABA (a and b), acetylcholine (c–e), and serotonin (f–h).

DOI: http://dx.doi.org/10.5772/intechopen.85353

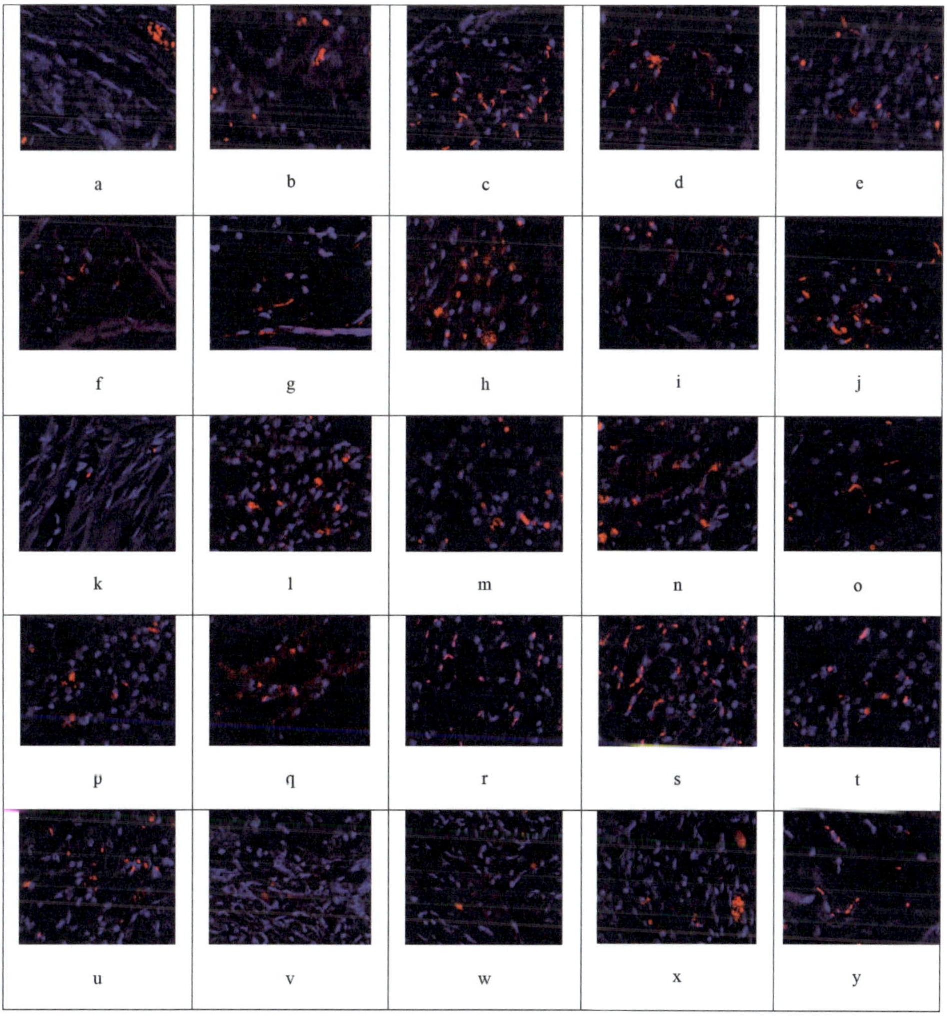

Figure 16.
The immune fluorescent analysis of serial cut neurotransmitters (from top to down, control): zones of a spinal cord transplant in 20 weeks after its full transection: GABA (a–g), acetylcholine (h–o), and serotonin (p–y).

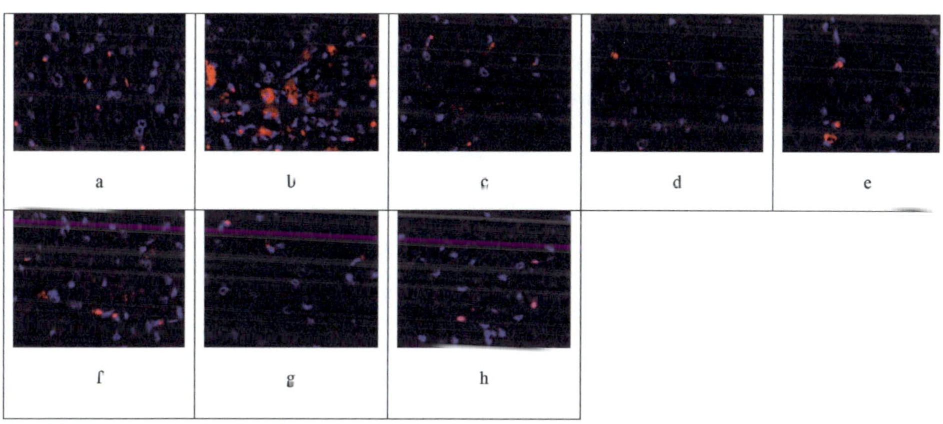

Figure 17.
The immune fluorescent analysis of serial cut neurotransmitters (from top to down, control): a tail zone of a spinal cord in 20 weeks after its full transection: GABA (a and b), acetylcholine (c–e), and serotonin (f–h).

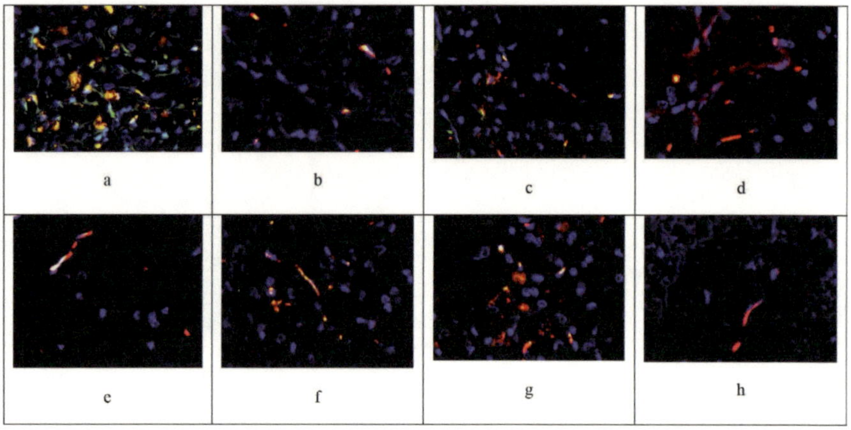

Figure 18.
The immune fluorescent analysis of serial cut neurotransmitters (from top to down, experience): head department of a spinal cord in 20 weeks after its full transection (above-transplant zone): GABA (a and b), acetylcholine (c–e), and serotonin (f–h).

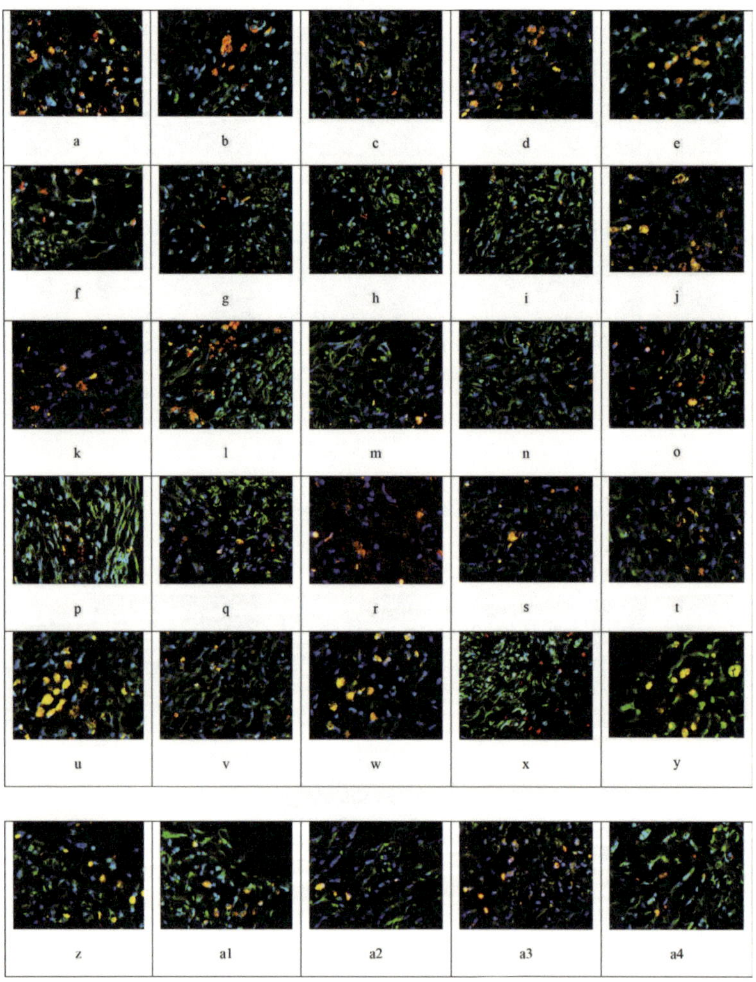

Figure 19.
The immune fluorescent analysis of serial cut neurotransmitters (from top to down, experience) zones collagen-chitosan of a transplant of a spinal cord in 20 weeks after its full transection: GABA (a–i), acetylcholine (j–r), and serotonin (s-a4).

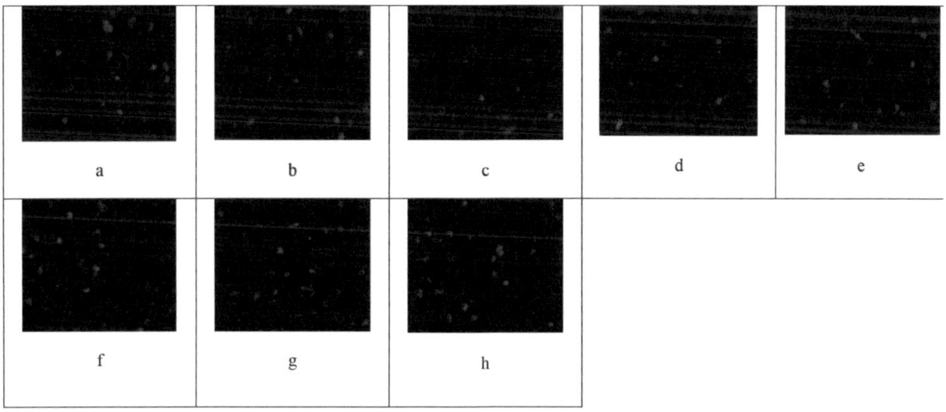

Figure 20.
The immune fluorescent analysis of serial cut neurotransmitters (from top to down, experience): a tail zone of a spinal cord in 20 weeks after its full transection: GABA (a and b), acetylcholine (c–e), and serotonin (f–h).

Research prototypes spinal cord, containing besides the neuronal microenvironment of growth factors 100,000 neuronal progenitor cells of mice, showed that by the transplant register sprouting cells producing GFP, in the area of the central end of the parent spinal cord. Broadcast nucleated cells are accompanied by the expression of neurotransmitter GABA, acetylcholine, and serotonin (**Figure 18**). A detailed analysis of the serial sections of the actual donor cells in the spinal cord indicates a rich content of viable neurons, producing GFP while expressing neurotransmitters. Transplanted cell mass in addition to the parent who came to neuronal cell occupies the entire volume of collagen-chitosan scaffold (**Figure 19**). In the tail of the spinal cord of the experimental group, the number of registered nucleated cells with expression and without expression of neurotransmitters reduced. The study of serial sections below collagen-chitosan cell transplant (tail of the spinal cord) did not reveal the GFP-cell sprouting phenomenon (**Figure 20**).

4. Conclusion

Thus, the results obtained in the course of the studies suggest that the collagen-chitosan matrix containing the neural progenitor cells is suitable for the repair of the damaged cells in the artificial three-dimensional environment. Transplantation of acellular collagen-chitosan substrate at full experimental spinal cord transection is accompanied by active sprouting maternal cell mass neuronal origin, actively expressing markers of neurotransmitters. This change is accompanied by a partial recovery of motor, sensory, and autonomic functions of the spinal cord, reaching the level of reduction, which is 5.6 point neuronal lack in BBB scale. Transplantation of collagen-chitosan matrix containing 100,000 progenitor neuronal cells followed for 20 weeks of the maintenance of their viability, in addition to expressing neuronal marker mediators of transmission of nerve signals. Transplanted cell mass broadcast their axons in the maternal side of the central segment of spinal cord beyond the graft. The tail part of the spinal cord after its complete intersection demonstrates a reduced number of viable neurons. However, the transplantation of a matrix containing precursors of neurons, resulting in significant recovery of lost motor and sensory functions of the spinal cord, reaching the level of reduction neuronal lack is equal to 19.5 on a BBB scale. Recent studies show that the inclusion of implantable structures and aminated polysaccharide polymer in a state of compaction to nanoscale alert direct contact of immune cells with allogeneic or xenogeneic cells of nervous tissue that is included in the implant, which substantially reduces the immunological conflict in this area of privilege [54–56].

It is known that primary objectives of SCI therapy are processes of neuron re-myelination, reduction in apoptosis, damaged neuron and oligodendrocyte regeneration, neural cell sprouting, formation of new synaptic connections, reduction in astrogliosis intensity, neurotrophic support, reduction in leucocytes, and macrophage reactions. [57]. Combined therapy of SCI is dictated by complicated mechanisms of pathophysiological changes in critical and chronic periods after trauma [36, 58–61]. Based on the multifactorial mechanism of spinal trauma the main directions of the problem solution of spinal cord bioengineering after its damage are formed. The authors of the paper confirm that the cell therapy is an attractive therapeutic way of spinal cord function regeneration. The main idea formulates the necessary regeneration of deficiency in specialized cells, remaining after the injury, which leads to auto-allo-transplantation of exogenic neural stem cells (NSCs) and neural precursor cells (NPCs), and stimulation of endogenic potential of neural cells. Using optimal neurotrophic support for spinal cord cells such as exogenic injections including cocktails from conditioned environments and endogenic stimulation is an indispensable component of an integral strategy for repairing spinal cord injury. The use of cells as part of biodegrading and highly compatible 3D matrix, constituting carcass and benevolent conditions for cultivation, proliferation, and differentiation of cell material and the possibility of direct translation into problematic areas in spinal cord constitute an important part of the algorithm in the treatment of spinal cord injury. Biopolymer substrates should play the role of protection against permeabilization and progressing destruction of neural tissue, and also should regenerate barrier function of damaged membranes.

Acknowledgements

This work was supported by grants from State Educational Institution, Krasnoyarsk State Medical University, prof. V.F.Voyno Yasenetsky MH-SD RF (2009), and grants the State Fund for Assistance to Small Innovative Enterprises in Science and technology (contract number 6746r/9167 from 10.04.2009, contract No 8775 dated 11.01.2011 r/13993 city, contract number 10494 r/16892 from 06.08.2012).

Conflict of interest

The authors declare that there is no conflict of interest regarding the publication of this paper.

Author details

I.N. Bolshakov[1], A.V. Svetlakov[2]*, A.V. Eremeev[3] and Yu.I. Sheina[2]

1 State Federal Educational Institution of Higher Education Krasnoyarsk State Medical University named after Prof. V. F. Voino-Yasenetsky, Krasnoyarsk, Russia

2 Krasnoyarsk Center of Reproductive Medicine, Laboratory of Cellular Technologies, Krasnoyarsk, Russia

3 Federal State Budgetary Institution, Federal Scientific and Clinical Center of Physical and Chemical Medicine of Federal Medical and Biological Agency, Moscow, Russia

*Address all correspondence to: krasivf@mail.ru

References

[1] Bottai D, Cigognini D, Madaschi L, Adami R, Nicora E, Menarini M, et al. Embryonic stem cells promote motor recovery and affect inflammatory cell infiltration in spinal cord injured mice. Experimental Neurology. 2010;**223**(2):452-463. DOI: 10.1016/j.expneurol.2010.01.010

[2] Yang JR, Liao CH, Pang CY, Huang LLH, Chen YL, Shiue YL, et al. Transplantation of porcine embryonic stem cells and their derived neuronal progenitors in a spinal cord injury rat model. Cytotherapy. 2013;**15**(2):201-208. DOI: 10.1016/j.jcyt.2012.09.001

[3] Sharp J, Frame J, Siegenthaler M, Nistor G, Keirstead HS. Human embryonic stem cell-derived oligodendrocyte progenitor cell transplants improve recovery after cervical spinal cord injury. Stem Cells. 2010;**28**. DOI: 1:152-163. DOI:10.1002/stem.245

[4] Cui YF, Xu JC, Hargus G, Jakovcevski I, Schachner M, Bernreuther C. Embryonic stem cell-derived L1 overexpressing neural aggregates enhance recovery after spinal cord injury in mice. PLoS One. 2011;**6**(3):e17126. DOI: 10.1371/journal.pone.0017126

[5] Cloutier F, Siegenthaler MM, Nistor G, Keirstead HS. Transplantation of human embryonic stem cell-derived oligodendrocyte progenitors into rat spinal cord injuries does not cause harm. Regenerative Medicine. 2006;**1**(4):469-479. DOI: 10.2217/17460751.1.4.469

[6] Perrotta S, Cucciolla V, Ferraro M, Ronzoni L, Tramontano A, Rossi F, et al. EPO receptor gain-of-function causes hereditary polycythemia, alters CD34 cell differentiation and increases circulating endothelial precursors. PLoS One. 2010;**5**(8):e12015. DOI: 10.1371/journal.pone.0012015

[7] McDonald JW, Liu XZ, Qu Y, Liu S, Mickey SK, Turetsky D, et al. Transplanted embryonic stem cells survive, differentiate and promote recovery in injured rat spinal cord. Nature Medicine. 1999;**5**(12):1410-1412. DOI: 10.1038/70986

[8] Kerr DA, Lladó J, Shamblott MJ, Maragakis NJ, Irani DN, Crawford TO, et al. Human embryonic germ cell derivatives facilitate motor recovery of rats with diffuse motor neuron injury. The Journal of Neuroscience. 2003;**23**(12):5131-5140

[9] Roy NS, Nakano T, Keyoung HM, Windrem M, Rashbaum WK, Alonso ML, et al. Telomerase immortalization of neuronally restricted progenitor cells derived from the human fetal spinal cord. Nature Biotechnology. 2004;**22**(3):297-305. DOI: 10.1038/nbt944

[10] Hori J, Ng TF, Shatos M, Klassen H, Streilein JW, Young MJ. Neural progenitor cells lack immunogenicity and resist destruction as allografts. Ocular Immunology and Inflammation. 2007;**15**(3):261-273. DOI: 10.1080/09273940701382242

[11] Harper JM, Krishnan C, Darman JS, Deshpande DM, Peck S, Shats I, et al. Axonal growth of embryonic stem cell-derived motoneurons in vitro and in motoneuron-injured adult rats. Proceedings of the National Academy of Sciences of the United States of America. 2004;**101**(18):7123-7128. DOI: 10.1073/pnas.0401103101

[12] Hu Z, Li T, Zhang X, Chen Y. Hepatocyte growth factor enhances the generation of high-purity oligodendrocytes from human embryonic stem cells. Differentiation. 2009;**78**(2-3):177-184. DOI: 10.1016/j.diff.2009.05.008

[13] Hong S, Kang UJ, Isacson O, Kim KS. Neural precursors derived from human embryonic stem cells maintain long-term proliferation without losing the potential to differentiate into all three neural lineages, including dopaminergic neurons. Journal of Neurochemistry. 2008;**104**(2):316-324. DOI: 10.1111/j.1471-4159.2007.04952.x

[14] Campos LS. Neurospheres: Insights into neural stem cell biology. Journal of Neuroscience Research. 2004;**78**(6):761-769. DOI: 10.1002/jnr.20333

[15] Nistor GI, Totoiu MO, Haque N, Carpenter MK, Keirstead HS. Human embryonic stem cells differentiate into oligodendrocytes in high purity and myelinate after spinal cord transplantation. Glia. 2005;**49**(3):385-3960. DOI: 10.1002/glia.20127.

[16] Sundberg M, Skottman H, Suuronen R, Narkılahti S. Production and isolation of NG2+ oligodendrocyte precursors from human embryonic stem cells in defined serum-free medium. Stem Cell Research. 2010;**5**(2):91-103. DOI: 10.1016/j.scr.2010.04.005

[17] Itsykson P, Ilouz N, Turetsky T, Goldstein RS, Pera MF, Fishbein I, et al. Derivation of neural precursors from human embryonic stem cells in the presence of noggin. Molecular and Cellular Neurosciences. 2005;**30**(1):24-36. DOI: 10.1016/j.mcn.2005.05.004

[18] Eftekharpour E, Karimi-Abdolrezaee S, Wang J, El Beheiry H, Morshead C, Fehlings MG. Myelination of congenitally dysmyelinated spinal cord axons by adult neural precursor cells results in formation of nodes of Ranvier and improved axonal conduction. The Journal of Neuroscience. 2007;**27**(13):3416-3428. DOI: 10.1523/JNEUROSCI.0273-07.2007

[19] Mothe AJ, Tator CH. Transplanted neural stem/progenitor cells generate myelinating oligodendrocytes and Schwann cells in spinal cord demyelination and dysmyelination. Experimental Neurology. 2008;**213**(1):176-190. DOI: 10.1016/j.expneurol.2008.05.024

[20] Karimi-Abdolrezaee S, Eftekharpour E, Wang J, Morshead CM, Fehlings MG. Delayed transplantation of adult neural precursor cells promotes remyelination and functional neurological recovery after spinal cord injury. The Journal of Neuroscience. 2006;**26**(13):3377-3389. DOI: 10.1523/JNEUROSCI.4184-05.2006

[21] Karimi-Abdolrezaee S, Eftekharpour E, Wang J, Schut D, Fehlings MG. Synergistic effects of transplanted adult neural stem/progenitor cells, chondroitinase, and growth factors promote functional repair and plasticity of the chronically injured spinal cord. The Journal of Neuroscience. 2010;**30**:1657-1676. DOI: 10.1523/JNEUROSCI.3111-09.2010

[22] Emgård M, Holmberg L, Samuelsson E-B, Bahr BA, Falci S, Seiger A, et al. Human neural precursor cells continue to proliferate and exhibit low cell death after transplantation to the injured rat spinal cord. Brain Research. 2009;**1278**:15-26. DOI: 10.1016/j.brainres.2009.04.012

[23] Hawryluk GWJ, Spano S, Chew D, Wang S, Erwin M, Chamankhah M, et al. An examination of the mechanisms by which neural precursors augment recovery following spinal cord injury: A key role for remyelination. Cell Transplantation. 2014;**23**:365-380. DOI: 10.3727/096368912X662408

[24] Lu P, Jones LL, Snyder EY, Tuszynski MH. Neural stem cells constitutively secrete neurotrophic factors and promote extensive host axonal growth after spinal cord injury. Experimental Neurology. 2003;**181**(2):115-129

[25] Guo J-S, Zeng Y-S, Li H-B, Huang W-L, Liu R-Y, Li X-B, et al. Cotransplant of neural stem cells and NT-3 gene modified Schwann cells promote the recovery of transected spinal cord injury. Spinal Cord. 2007;**45**(1):15-24. DOI: 10.1038/sj.sc.3101943

[26] Pan HC, Cheng FC, Lai SZ, Yang DY, Wang YC, Lee MS. Enhanced regeneration in spinal cord injury by concomitant treatment with granulocyte colonystimulating factor and neuronal stem cells. Journal of Clinical Neuroscience. 2008;**15**(6):656-664. DOI: 10.1016/j.jocn.2007.03.02

[27] Cao Q, He Q, Wang Y, Cheng X, Howard RM, Zhang Y, et al. Transplantation of ciliary neurotrophic factor-expressing adult oligodendrocyte precursor cells promotes remyelination and functional recovery after spinal cord injury. The Journal of Neuroscience. 2010;**30**(8):2989-3001. DOI: 10.1523/JNEUROSCI.3174-09.2010

[28] Åkesson E, Piao JH, Samuelsson EB, Holmberg L, Kjældgaard A, Falci S, et al. Long-term culture and neuronal survival after intraspinal transplantation of human spinal cord-derived neurospheres. Physiology & Behavior. 2007;**92**(1-2):60-66. DOI: 10.1016/j.physbeh.2007.05.056

[29] Hawryluk GW, Mothe A, Wang J, Wang S, Tator C, Fehlings MG. An in vivo characterization of trophic factor production following neural precursor cell or bone marrow stromal cell transplantation for spinal cord injury. Stem Cells and Development. 2012;**21**(12):2222-2238. DOI: 10.1089/scd.2011.0596

[30] Pashuck ET, Stevens MM. Designing regenerative biomaterial therapies for the clinic. Biomaterials. 2012;**4**(160):160sr4. DOI: 10.1126/scitranslmed.3002717

[31] Ma W, Tavakoli T, Derby E, Serebryakova Y, Rao MS, Mattson MP. Cell-extracellular matrix interactions regulate neural differentiation not human embryonic stem cells. BMC Developmental Biology. 2008;**8**:90. DOI: 10.1186/1471-213X-8-90

[32] Kang SM, Cho MS, Seo H, Yoon CJ, Oh SK, Choi YM, et al. Efficient induction of oligodendrocytes from human embryonic stem cells. Stem Cells. 2007;**25**(2):419-424. DOI: 10.1634/stemcells.2005-0482

[33] Kerr CL, Letzen BS, Hill CM, Agrawal G, Thakor NV, Sterneckert JL, et al. Efficient differentiation of human embryonic stem cells into oligodendrocyte progenitors for application in a rat contusion model of spinal cord injury. The International Journal of Neuroscience. 2010;**120**(4):305-313. DOI: 10.3109/00207450903585290

[34] Hu Z, Li T, Zhang X, Chen Y. Hepatocyte growth factor enhances the generation of high-purity oligodendrocytes from human embryonic stem cells. Differentiation. 2009;**78**(2-3):177-184. DOI: 10.1016/j.diff.2009.05.008

[35] Sundberg M, Skottman H, Suuronen R, Narkilahti S. Production and isolation of NG2+ oligodendrocyte precursors from human embryonic stem cells in defined serum-free medium. Stem Cell Research. 2010;**5**(2):91-103. DOI: 10.1016/j.scr.2010.04.005

[36] Sundberg M, Hyysalo A, Skottman H, Shin S, Vemuri M, Suuronen R, et al. A xeno-free culturing protocol for pluripotent stem cell-derived oligodendrocyte precursor cell production. Regenerative Medicine. 2011;**6**(4):449-460. DOI: 10.2217/rme.11.36

[37] Freier T, Montenegro R, Shan Koh H, Shoichet MS. Chitin-based tubes for tissue engineering in the nervous system. Biomaterials. 2005;**26**(22):4624-4632. DOI: 10.1016/j.biomaterials.2004.11.040

[38] Nomura H, Tator CH, Shoichet MS. Bioengineered strategies for spinal cord repair. Journal of Neurotrauma. 2006;**23**(3-4):496-507. DOI: 10.1089/neu.2006.23.496

[39] Yuan Y, Zhang P, Yang Y, Wang X, Gu X. The interaction of Schwann cells with chitosan membranes and fibers in vitro. Biomaterials. 2004;**25**(18):4273-4278. DOI: 10.1016/j.biomaterials.2003.11.029

[40] Cho Y, Shi RY, Borgens RB. Chitosan produces potent neuroprotection and physiological recovery following traumatic spinal cord injury. The Journal of Experimental Biology. 2010;**213**(9):1513-1520. DOI: 10.1242/jeb.035162

[41] Nomura H, Zahir T, Kim H, Katayama Y, Kulbatski I, Morshead CM, et al. Extramedullary chitosan channels promote survival of transplanted neural stem and progenitor cells and create a tissue bridge after complete spinal cord transection. Tissue Engineering Part A. 2008;**14**(5). DOI: 10.1089/tea.2007.0180

[42] Zahir T, Nomura H, Guo XD, Kim H, Tator C, Morshead C, et al. Bioengineering neural stem/progenitor cell-coated tubes for spinal cord injury repair. Cell Transplantation. 2008;**17**(3):245-254. DOI: 10.3727/096368908784153887

[43] Hofstetter CP, Holmstrom NA, Lilja JA, Schweinhardt P, Hao J, Spenger C, et al. Allodynia limits the usefulness of intraspinal neural stem cell grafts; directed differentiation improves outcome. Nature Neuroscience. 2005;**8**(3):346-353. DOI: 10.1038/nn1405

[44] Klapka N, Muller HW. Collagen matrix in spinal cord injury. Journal of Neurotrauma. 2006;**23**(3-4):422. DOI: 10.1089/neu.2006.23.422

[45] Iseda T, Nishio T, Kawaguchi S, Kawasaki T, Wakisaka S. Spontaneous regeneration of the corticospinal tract after transection in young rats: Collagen type IV deposition and astrocytic scar in the lesion site are not the cause but the effect of failure of regeneration. The Journal of Comparative Neurology. 2003;**464**(3):343-355. DOI: 10.1002/cne.10786

[46] Liesi P, Kauppila T. Induction of type IV collagen and other basement-membrane-associated proteins after spinal cord injury of the adult rat may participate in formation of the glial scar. Experimental Neurology. 2002;**173**(1):31-45. DOI: 10.1006/exnr.2001.7800

[47] Yoshii S, Oka M, Shima M, Taniguchi A, Taki Y, Akagi M. Restoration of function after spinal cord transection using a collagen bridge. Journal of Biomedical Materials Research. 2004;**70**(4):569-575. DOI: 10.1002/jbm.a.30120

[48] Yoshii S, Oka M, Shima M, Taniguchi A, Akagi M. Bridging a 30-mm nerve defect using collagen filaments. Journal of Biomedical Materials Research. 2003;**67**:467-474

[49] Kim YC, Kim YH, Kim JW, Ha KY. Transplantation of mesenchymal stem cells for acute spinal cord injury in rats: Comparative study between intralesional injection and scaffold based transplantation. Journal of Korean Medical Science. 2016;**31**(9):1373-1382. DOI: 10.3346/jkms.2016.31.9.1373

[50] Kim H, Tator CH, Shoichet MS. Chitosan implants in the rat spinal cord: Biocompatibility and biodegradation. Journal of Biomedial Materials Research Part A. 2011;**97A**(4):395-404. DOI: 10.1002/jbm.a.33070

[51] Eremeev AV, Svetlakov AA, Bolshakov IN, Sheina Yu I, Polstyanoy AM. Method for Producing a Neural Matrix. PCT/RU000213; No WO/2011/142691. 2011

[52] Thomson JA, Itskovitz-Eldor J, Shapiro SS, Waknitz MA, Swiergiel JJ, Marshall VS, et al. Embryonic stem cell lines derived from human blastocysts. Science. 1998;**282**(5391):1145-1147

[53] Kima HS, Oha SK, Parkb YB, Ahnb HJ, Ki CS, Kanga MJ, et al. Methods for derivation of human embryonic. Stem Cells. 2005;**23**(9):1228-1233

[54] Patent RU 2301675. 2007

[55] Basso DM, Beattie MS, Bresnahan JC. A sensitive and reliable locomotor rating scale for open field testing in rats. Journal of Neurotrauma. 1995;**12**:1-21

[56] Bolshakov IN, Eremeev AV, Sheina YI, Polstyanoy AM, Karapetyan AM, Ignatov AV, et al. The collagen-chitosan matrix for cultivation and differentation of embryonic stem cells in the neuronal nature cells. Markers investigation. Fundamental Research. 2012;**1**:18-23

[57] Bolshakov IN, Krivopalov VA, Kaptyuk GI, Karapetyan AM, Ignatov AV. The transplantation of cellular polyssacharide scaffold by incomplete spinal cord injury of rats. Dinamic neurological control. Fundamental Research. 2012;**2**:31-34

[58] Bolshakov IN, Eremeev AV, Svetlakov AV, YuI S, Rendashkin IV, Polstyanoy AM, et al. Using neuronal polyssacharide matrix in the treatment of experimental spinal cord injury. Questions of Reconstructive and Plastic Surgery. 2012;**15**(1):34-42

[59] Ronsyn MW, Berneman ZN, VanTendeloo VF, Jorens PG, Ponsaerts P. Cancell therapy heal a spinal cord injury? Spinal Cord. 2008;**46**(8):532-539. DOI: 10.1038/sc.2008.13

[60] McCreedy DA, Sakiyama-Elbert SE. Combination therapies in the CNS: Engineering the environment. Neuroscience Letters. 2012;**519**(2):115-121. DOI: 10.1016/j.neulet.2012.02.025

[61] Pego AP, Kubinova S, Cizkova D, Vanicky I, Mar FM, Sousa MM, et al. Regenerative medicine for the treatment of spinal cord injury: More than just promises? Journal of Cellular and Molecular Medicine. 2012;**16**(11):2564-2582. DOI: 10.1111/j.1582-4934.2012.01603.x